T0256012

Clinics in Developmental Medicine No. 170
THE MANAGEMENT OF DISORDERS OF
BLADDER AND BOWEL CONTROL IN
CHILDHOOD

© 2006 Mac Keith Press
30 Furnival Street, London EC4A 1JQ

Editor: Hilary M. Hart
Managing Editor: Michael Pountney
Project Manager: Sarah Pearsall

First published in this edition 2006

British Library Cataloguing-in-Publication data
A catalogue record for this book is available from the British Library

ISSN: 0069 4835
ISBN: 1 898683 45 X

Typeset by Keystroke, Jacaranda Lodge, Wolverhampton
Printed by The Lavenham Press Ltd, Water Street, Lavenham, Suffolk
Mac Keith Press is supported by Scope

Clinics in Developmental Medicine No. 170

The Management of Disorders of Bladder and Bowel Control in Childhood

ALEXANDER VON GONTARD
Saarland University Hospital, Homburg, Germany

TRYGGVE NEVÉUS
Uppsala University Children's Hospital, Uppsala, Sweden

2006
Mac Keith Press

Distributed by 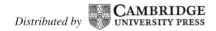 **CAMBRIDGE** UNIVERSITY PRESS

CONTENTS

AUTHORS' APPOINTMENTS

Alexander von Gontard   Professor, Chair for Child and Adolescent
Psychiatry, Saarland University Hospital,
Homburg, Germany

Tryggve Nevéus   Associate Professor, Consultant in Paediatric
Nephrology, Uppsala University Children's
Hospital, Uppsala, Sweden

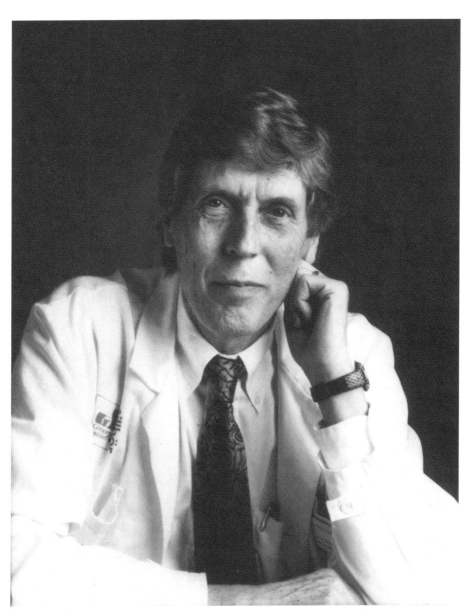

Kelm Hjälmås

PREFACE

Voiding disorders are common disturbances in childhood, affecting bladder and bowel control both during the day and at night-time. These disorders are based on multiple, interacting aetiologies: both genetic and environmental factors are involved, affecting somatic as well as behavioural domains. Voiding disorders are often highly distressing for children and parents. Although many can be treated effectively, many myths and preconceptions prevail.

The groundbreaking work in the field, which endeavours to put approaches to enuresis on an 'evidence-based' foundation, dates back to 1973. *Bladder Control and Enuresis*, edited by Kolvin, Mac Keith and Meadow, is an excellent compilation of basic scientific texts – some in review format, others in the form of original research articles. This volume in the Mac Keith Press series has inspired a generation of practitioners and researchers and has, over time, become a classic text which is still being quoted today.

Thirty years later, the body of scientific findings has increased dramatically. Most research has centred on nocturnal enuresis, followed by functional faecal incontinence (encopresis) and finally daytime wetting, which has received the least attention. Unfortunately, in many countries most of this research has not trickled down to primary care practitioners. Therefore, when we were approached by Dr Martin Bax to take on the job of writing a new book in the Mac Keith Press series, we gladly accepted. In no way do we want to attempt to replicate or update the classic enuresis book of 1973. Our aim is both more modest and broader. As some children have more than one voiding disorder and these are interconnected, we have included functional faecal incontinence (encopresis). Our basic idea was to produce a book that would be useful to researchers in the field, by reviewing the current state of the art, and to provide a clinical handbook that could be used in primary practice. Therefore, case reports, illustrations, summaries of chapters, clinical guidelines and an appendix with charts and instruments have been included.

Different medical disciplines deal with voiding disorders: paediatric urology, paediatrics with the subspecialties of paediatric nephrology and paediatric gastroenterology, as well as child psychiatry (and child psychology, which, of course, is not a medical specialty). In order to reflect the approaches of these different disciplines, three authors decided to put their know-how together and collaborate on this project: Kelm Hjälmås, a paediatric urologist, Tryggve Nevéus, a paediatric nephrologist, and Alexander von Gontard, a paediatrician and child psychiatrist. All three can be considered experts in the field. The first productive meeting of the three authors took place in February 2004 in Göteborg, Sweden. It was a promising first step in a creative, multidisciplinary endeavour. Unfortunately, it was not meant to be. Shortly after that, Kelm Hjälmås died suddenly and unexpectedly.

Kelm Hjälmås trained as a paediatric surgeon and urologist and can be considered to be the 'founding father' of enuresis and bladder research. Starting in the 1960s he devoted a large part of his research career to this topic. In contrast to many of his colleagues, he was not just interested in structure but in function, showing again and again that a primary physiological dysfunction (such as of the bladder) can induce a cascade of secondary, even structural, effects. Only a functional understanding will enable treatment of the primary aetiological cause, thus avoiding or mitigating many of the consequences. A true humanist, Kelm's focus was much broader than pure surgery and included both the child as an individual and the family as a whole. He was truly interested in the subjective, emotional world of the child – the child's feelings and perceptions, as well as his or her social environment. He showed the same personal attention not only towards his patients, but also towards his colleagues – young trainees and researchers as well as his peers. He was a friend, a mentor and a father figure to many of us – and we miss him dearly.

After Kelm's death, we – the two remaining co-authors – decided to carry on the task we had taken on. We did not change the structure of the book but divided up Kelm's chapters as best we could. It is not, of course, the book we originally planned in February 2004. Kelm's experience and profound knowledge in paediatric urology cannot be replaced easily. To ensure that the content reflects current paediatric urological practice and thinking, we asked a renowned expert in the field to check and correct the text. Fortunately, Professor Göran Läckgren of Uppsala, Sweden generously agreed to read the text and to suggest corrections and additions where they were needed. In Kelm's name, we would like to thank Göran very much and acknowledge his invaluable contribution.

Dr Nevéus is also grateful for the help of Lars-Göran Andersson, Marie Raiend, Birgitta Karanikas and Anna Sandin of Uppsala University Hospital. We would also like to thank Dr Hilary Hart and Michael Pountney of Mac Keith Press for their kind support and helpful editorial guidance throughout the writing process.

Now that the project has been completed, we would like to dedicate this book entirely to Kelm Hjälmås with feelings of thankfulness for his great inspiration and dear friendship.

May 2006
Alexander von Gontard, Homburg, Germany,
Tryggve Nevéus, Uppsala, Sweden

ABBREVIATIONS

ABU	Asymptomatic bacteriuria
ADHD	Attention deficit hyperactivity disorder
ATP	Adenosine triphosphate
CBCL	Child Behavior Checklist
CIC	Clean intermittent catheterization
CNS	Central nervous system
CPAP	Continuous positive airway pressure
CT	Computed tomography
DMSA	Dimercapto-succinylic acid
DW	Daytime wetting
ECG	Electrocardiography
EEG	Electroencephalography
EMG	Electromyography
ICCS	International Children's Continence Society
LC	Locus coeruleus
MAG3	dimercaptoacetyltriglycine
MCU	Micturating cystourethrography
MMC	Myelomeningocele
MRI	Magnetic resonance imaging
NW	Night-time wetting
OAB	Overactive bladder
ODD	Oppositional defiant disorder
PEG	Polyethylene glycol
PMC	Pontine micturition centre
PUV	Posterior urethral valve
RAS	Reticular activation system
REM	Rapid eye movement
TRS	Toilet refusal syndrome
UTI	Urinary tract infection
VUR	Vesico-ureteric reflux

1
INTRODUCTION

Disorders of bladder and bowel control are very common disorders of childhood. Of 7-year-olds, 10 per cent wet at night, 2 to 3 per cent wet during the daytime, and 1 to 3 per cent soil. Often, these disorders coexist. Despite a high remission rate, 1 to 2 per cent of all adolescents are still affected by nocturnal enuresis and less than 1 per cent by either daytime wetting or functional faecal incontinence (encopresis). The vast majority of voiding disorders are functional, i.e. not due to neurological, structural or medical causes.

In all cultures, there has always been a minority of children who have shown problems with gaining bladder and bowel control at the age that their caregivers expect them to do so. This has elicited a wide range of responses in the past – some supportive and understanding, others punitive (Glicklich 1951). Even though some misconceptions of the past prevail, the latter part of the twentieth century finally brought about a scientific approach. Voiding disorders are viewed as medical conditions, which can be assessed and treated quite effectively.

According to current classification schemes such as ICD-10 (WHO 1993), enuresis is defined as wetting from the age of 5 years onwards (encopresis, from the age of 4 years) – after organic causes have been ruled out. In the past two decades, several distinct subtypes of voiding disorders have been identified, which differ regarding aetiology, clinical symptoms and treatment. While some disorders (such as nocturnal enuresis) are primarily genetically determined, in others (such as voiding postponement) environmental factors predominate. Also, the rate of comorbid behavioural disturbances differs greatly from one syndrome to another: in some (such as encopresis) the rate of concomitant behavioural disorders is high, while in others (such as primary monosymptomatic nocturnal enuresis) the rate is no different from that among controls. Because of this variety and heterogeneity, each voiding disorder requires a specific approach in assessment and treatment. Unfortunately, the traditional classification schemes (such as ICD-10) lag behind these new developments. Therefore, this book will closely follow more recent attempts at classification and terminology as laid down by the International Children's Continence Society (Nevéus et al 2006).

The aim of this book is to provide an evidence-based state-of-the-art overview of the different voiding disorders. Approaches and perspectives of the three main medical disciplines dealing with children with voiding disorders – i.e. paediatric urology, paediatric nephrology and child psychiatry – are integrated. As approaches and practices can differ from one country to another, we present different options as long as they are equally effective.

In addition to providing a theoretical overview, the book is intended as a practical handbook, useful to all those involved in primary care. Therefore, short case vignettes are provided. Each chapter is followed by a short summary, and guidelines are provided in the form of easy-to-follow charts and diagrams. Important points are illustrated by relevant photos and line drawings. The appendices include questionnaires, calendars and charts which can be copied and used directly in clinical practice.

Specifically, the book deals first with general principles and basic approaches applicable to voiding disorders in general. Individual syndromes and disorders are discussed in the second part of the book.

Chapter 2 deals with issues of classification and definition and provides an up-to-date summary regarding terminology. Basic information regarding embryology, anatomy and physiology follows in Chapter 3. An understanding of 'normal' development will provide a sound basis for comprehending and integrating pathological processes. Chapters 4 and 5 give an overview of general principles in assessment and treatment, which will, again, provide a basis for understanding the individual syndromes and disorders.

As the most common voiding disorder, nocturnal enuresis is dealt with first in the second part of the book. This is followed by an overview of daytime wetting, which encompasses different syndromes of functional urinary incontinence. Each of the daytime wetting syndromes is dealt with separately, including urge incontinence, voiding postponement, dysfunctional voiding, stress and giggle incontinence, detrusor decompensation and other forms of urinary incontinence. Finally, a short – and in no way comprehensive – overview of organic causes of urinary incontinence is provided. For more detailed information, readers are referred to textbooks of paediatric urology.

The final chapters concentrate on syndromes of functional faecal incontinence (encopresis). The two main subtypes are faecal incontinence with and without constipation. Rarer disorders include toilet refusal syndrome and toilet phobia. Finally, a short, non-comprehensive overview of organic faecal incontinence points to signs and symptoms in those rare cases in which organic non-functional causes predominate.

We hope that this book will be of interest to all professionals working in the field, including paediatric surgeons, urologists, general paediatricians, paediatric nephrologists, general practitioners, child psychiatrists, psychologists, psychotherapists, nurses and social workers, as well as interested parents.

2
CLASSIFICATION AND DEFINITIONS

Classification according to ICD-10 and DSM-IV

Enuresis is defined by both the ICD-10 and DSM-IV classification schemes as involuntary wetting of children 5 years of age or older after organic causes have been ruled out. The ICD-10 criteria (WHO 1993) are compiled and shown in Table 2.1, the DSM-IV criteria (APA 1994) in Table 2.2.

In keeping with ICD-10 and DSM-IV, the wetting must have occurred for three months or longer to be considered a disorder. According to ICD-10, the frequency required for diagnosis is twice a month in children under 7 years of age and once a month in children 7 years and older. The criteria according to DSM-IV are less precise: the voiding must occur at least twice a week for at least three months or else must cause clinically significant distress or impairment in social, academic (occupational) or other important areas of functioning. This loose definition is not helpful in clinical practice. Also, different definitions of the frequency of wetting have been used in studies, so that a careful comparison of definitions is required (Butler 1991).

These standardized criteria are no longer up to date as new concepts and findings have evolved in the past decades. Thus, voluntary voiding should not be termed enuresis. Enuretic

---

TABLE 2.1
Diagnostic criteria for non-organic enuresis (F98.0)
according to ICD-10 (research criteria) (WHO 1993)

A. The child's chronological and mental age is at least 5 years.

B. Involuntary or intentional voiding of urine into bed or clothes occurs at least twice a month aged under 7 years, and at least once a month in children aged 7 years or more.

C. The enuresis is not a consequence of epileptic attacks or of neurological incontinence, and not a direct consequence of structural abnormalities of the urinary tract or any other non-psychiatric medical condition.

D. There is no evidence of any other psychiatric disorder that meets the criteria for other ICD-10 categories.

E. Duration of the disorder is at least three months.

A fifth character may be used, if desired, for further specification:

F98.00 Nocturnal enuresis only
F98.01 Diurnal enuresis only
F98.02 Nocturnal and diurnal enuresis

TABLE 2.2
Diagnostic criteria for enuresis (307.6) according to DSM-IV (APA 1994)

A. Repeated voiding of urine into bed or clothes (whether involuntary or intentional).

B. The behaviour is clinically significant as manifested by either a frequency of twice a week for at least three consecutive months or the presence of clinically significant distress or impairment in social, academic (occupational), or other important areas of functioning.

C. Chronological age is at least 5 years (or equivalent developmental level).

D. The behaviour is not due exclusively to the direct physiological effect of a substance (e.g. a diuretic) or a general medical condition (e.g. diabetes, spina bifida, a seizure disorder).

Specify type:

Nocturnal only
Diurnal only
Nocturnal and diurnal

voidings are always involuntary during the night. In those rare cases of voluntary wetting during the daytime, this can usually be understood as a sub-symptom of a child psychiatric disorder.

Also, the restrictions laid down by ICD-10 in case of comorbid disorders are not really useful in practical terms. Instead, enuresis, as well as any other comorbid disorder, should be diagnosed in a descriptive manner. In practical terms, this approach is highly relevant, as each disorder might require a separate individual type of treatment, e.g. a child might have nocturnal enuresis, encopresis and ADHD. Though occurring together, each separate problem should be addressed.

Also, ICD-10 does not differentiate between enuresis and urinary incontinence. In the terminology used by most modern researchers (Nørgaard et al 1998), enuresis denotes involuntary wetting with completely normal bladder function. Most cases of nocturnal wetting probably represent enuresis in a strict sense. In contrast, nearly all children with daytime wetting problems have additional signs of bladder dysfunction. For all practical reasons, enuresis is extremely rare in daytime wetting and hardly ever occurs. Therefore, the term diurnal enuresis should be abandoned and urinary incontinence – in most cases functional – should be adopted.

ICCS classification

Recently, a new system of terminology and classification was suggested by the International Children's Continence Society (Nevéus et al 2006), and this system will be followed in this book. The ICCS suggestions are, where applicable, congruent with the terminology of lower urinary tract function put forward by the International Continence Society (Abrams et al 2002) and represent an updated version of the paediatric terminology previously put forward by the International Children's Continence Society (ICCS) (Nørgaard et al 1998). The full, updated ICCS document can be found in Nevéus et al (2006).

4

ENURESIS

Enuresis means wetting in discrete amounts while asleep in a child who has passed his or her fifth birthday. The word nocturnal may be added for extra clarity, but it has to be underlined that the previous definition of enuresis denoting 'a urodynamically normal, complete emptying of the bladder' (Nørgaard et al 1998) is no longer valid, since this would require ambulatory cystometric investigations before being able to use the correct terminology. Thus, bedwetting is properly called enuresis regardless of whether it occurs in a child with concomitant daytime incontinence or not, regardless of the suspected underlying pathogenetic mechanisms, and regardless of the results of cystometric evaluation of the same child. Enuresis just means wetting while asleep.

A child exhibiting incontinence during both day and night has two diagnoses: enuresis (or nocturnal enuresis) and daytime incontinence. The confusing term 'diurnal enuresis' is obsolete, and the term 'nocturnal incontinence' – previously denoting bedwetting episodes that were presumed not to be due to normal complete emptying of the bladder – should now either be avoided or taken as being completely synonymous with enuresis.

Two subdivisions of enuresis are deemed important enough to warrant specifically defined terminology by the ICCS: primary/secondary enuresis and monosymptomatic/non-monosymptomatic enuresis (Table 2.3). *Primary enuresis* is when the child has previously been spontaneously dry for less than six months (or not at all), whereas *secondary enuresis* means that a relapse after a dry period of at least six months has occurred. The dry interval can occur in any age group, i.e. even in infancy. Also, it is not relevant if a child became dry spontaneously or if dryness was achieved by treatment. In the past, some authors have used a different definition for the length of the dry interval. Thus, definitions of one, three, six and twelve months have been in use. Experience shows that the six months definition is of practical relevance, as it does differentiate well between children with a low rate of comorbid behavioural symptoms and disorders (primary nocturnal enuresis), and children with a higher risk for comorbid disorders (secondary nocturnal enuresis) (von Gontard et al 1997, von Gontard 2002).

Children with enuresis who do not have daytime symptoms suggesting disturbances of bladder function are suffering from *monosymptomatic* enuresis, whereas children who do have such symptoms have *non-monosymptomatic* enuresis. The symptoms deemed relevant in this respect are the following (defined below): daytime incontinence, increased/decreased daytime voiding frequency, urgency, voiding postponement, holding manoeuvres and intermittent urine stream. The terms monosymptomatic and non-monosymptomatic are based entirely on history and verified by voiding diaries. Note that in previous terminology the word monosymptomatic was used in a wider sense, denoting just enuretic children without concomitant daytime incontinence. The greater precision of the current definition reflects the fact that several daytime bladder symptoms – not just incontinence – give crucial clues as to the pathogenesis of enuresis in the individual case. Also, this differentiation is of great practical relevance. In non-monosymptomatic nocturnal enuresis, daytime symptoms have to be treated first before addressing the night-time wetting. In contrast, in monosymptomatic cases, the nocturnal wetting can be approached without further preliminary procedures.

5

TABLE 2.3
Basic subdivisions of nocturnal enuresis according to ICCS terminology

		Maximal dry interval <6 months	Maximal dry interval >6 months
No signs of bladder dysfunction* during daytime	Mono-symptomatic nocturnal enuresis (MNE)	Primary nocturnal enuresis (PNE) Primary monosymptomatic nocturnal enuresis (PMNE)	Secondary nocturnal enuresis (SNE) Secondary monosymptomatic nocturnal enuresis (SMNE)
Signs of bladder dysfunction* during daytime present	Non-monosymptomatic nocturnal enuresis (NMNE)	Primary non-monosymptomatic nocturnal enuresis (PNMNE)	Secondary non-monosymptomatic nocturnal enuresis (SNMNE)

* Daytime incontinence, urgency, holding manoeuvres, interrupted flow, etc.

URINARY INCONTINENCE

Incontinence means any involuntary loss of urine at a socially unacceptable place and time by a child aged 5 years or more whose general cognitive and neurological development indicates that bladder control should have been achieved. We often talk about *daytime incontinence* to distinguish it from nocturnal enuresis. In this book it should be clear from the context that the word incontinence is usually used to denote daytime incontinence. Most cases of daytime incontinence can be considered to be functional forms of urinary incontinence. Organic urinary incontinence is extremely rare and can be due to structural, iatrogenic, neurogenic or other paediatric causes.

The main syndromes of functional urinary incontinence that will be dealt with in this book are: urge incontinence, voiding postponement, dysfunctional voiding, stress incontinence, giggle incontinence, detrusor underactivity and other subtypes (see Table 2.4). These can develop as separate entities in some children. In others, a natural development from one type to another can be observed. Voiding postponement can develop from urge incontinence as a result of habitually increasing the micturition intervals, and dysfunctional voiding can develop as a result of unphysiological use of pelvic floor muscles. The end stage of this process can be an underactive bladder with detrusor decompensation. This progression can be prevented by appropriate management (Hoebeke et al 2001).

URINE PRODUCTION

Polyuria means a urine output of >2 litres per square metre of body surface area or >40 ml per kg body weight during 24 hours. Nocturnal urine production is calculated as the proportion of the 24-hour urine output that is produced at night when the patient is in bed, including the first morning micturition. *Nocturnal polyuria* is present in a child when nocturnal urine production is more than 130 per cent of his/her expected bladder capacity (defined below). The reason for bothering with these definitions is that nocturnal polyuria is believed to be a central pathogenetic mechanism in nocturnal enuresis.

TABLE 2.4
Classification of functional urinary incontinence with main distinguishing symptoms

Type of daytime wetting	Main symptoms and features
Urge incontinence	Urge symptoms. Often increased daytime voiding frequency and small voided volumes
Voiding postponement	Infrequent micturitions <5 times per day; postponement
Dysfunctional voiding*	Straining to initiate and during micturition; interrupted stream of urine
Stress incontinence	Wetting during coughing, sneezing; small volumes
Giggle incontinence	Wetting during laughing; large volumes with apparently complete emptying
Detrusor underactivity	Interrupted stream; emptying of bladder possible only by straining

* Although the child with dysfunctional voiding is not by definition incontinent this is often the case, and the condition is therefore included in the table.

BLADDER VOLUME

Since the bladder is a distensible organ which is under more or less complete cortical control, and it has been shown that children usually void when they want to, not necessarily because the bladder is 'full' (Mattsson et al 2003), measurements of bladder volume – especially in children – are difficult and have engendered a confusing array of different strategies and definitions. We will therefore avoid the earlier notion of 'bladder capacity' and instead use the more vague but also more accurate term, *voided volume*, when talking about the perceived size of the bladder (outside of the cystometric setting). The *maximum voided volume* is the largest voided volume as detected from a voiding diary that has been kept for a couple of days. This is the term used in preference to the previous notion of 'functional bladder capacity'. However, when a comparison is needed, we express the maximum voided volume as a percentage of the *expected bladder capacity* which is derived from the standard formula [30 + (age in years x 30) ml] (Koff 1983). This does not mean that we regard the expected bladder capacity as necessarily 'normal' for the child's age, but just that we need a universal value of comparison. For measurements of cystometric bladder capacity, see below.

MICTURITION FREQUENCY

Increased daytime frequency is the spontaneous voiding (incontinence episodes excluded) eight or more times per day in a child who drinks and voids *ad libitum*. *Decreased daytime frequency* is when the child voids four times or less per day in the same circumstances. These data are obviously acquired via the voiding chart.

SYMPTOMS AND SYNDROMES OF URINARY TRACT MALFUNCTION

Urgency denotes the sudden experience of an imminent need to micturate. *Urge incontinence* means involuntary leakage of urine concomitant with urgency. The child with urgency symptoms suffers from an *overactive bladder* regardless of whether he or she is incontinent or not. In the absence of urge incontinence, the term *urgency–frequency syndrome* can be used. Urgency is the subjective symptom of detrusor overactivity (see under cystometric findings below).

Voiding postponement is the term used for children who can be observed to habitually delay micturition in typical situations by various *holding manoeuvres*, such as squatting with the heel pressed to the perineum, standing on toes or keeping the legs crossed. This is usually combined with urgency of increasing intensity and wetting when the child has postponed micturition too long. Traditionally, this syndrome has been considered to be an acquired disorder caused by voluntary 'abuse' of the urethral sphincter and pelvic floor muscles until the bladder becomes overfilled. Recent research, however, has indicated that voiding postponement can occur as an entity in itself, without a preceding phase of bladder over-activity (von Gontard et al 1998a, Hoebeke et al 2001, Lettgen et al 2002). These children, for obvious reasons, are usually infrequent voiders, and they often have some degree of psychiatric comorbidity.

Dysfunctional voiding is defined as an intermittent and/or fluctuating flow rate due to intermittent contractions of the external sphincter and/or pelvic floor during voiding, in neurologically normal individuals. It is thus synonymous with older entities such as 'non-neurogenic neurogenic bladder', 'occult neuropathic bladder' and 'detrusor–sphincter dyscoordination'. Note that dysfunctional voiding always denotes a disturbance during the emptying phase and says nothing about the storage phase. A child may thus, very possibly, have both bladder overactivity and voiding dysfunction.

The term 'dysfunctional voiding' as an umbrella term to include all forms of lower urinary tract malfunction is not used in this book. When we say dysfunctional voiding we are talking about the voiding only, and define it as stated above.

Hesitancy denotes observable difficulties in initiating voiding. *Straining* means that the child has to contract the abdominal muscles to initiate and maintain micturition. *Intermittency* or *intermittent/interrupted stream* are the terms used when urine is not voided in a continuous stream but in several discrete portions. These pathological phenomena may be due to urethral obstruction, but are also typical of the child with detrusor underactivity. *Detrusor underactivity* is the term used when the child needs to use abdominal muscle contractions to void. The previous term 'lazy bladder' for the same condition is now obsolete. These children are usually infrequent voiders (i.e. fewer than four voidings per day), they void increased volumes and have residual urine detectable by ultrasound.

Stress incontinence occurs on exertion and is caused by an underactive or damaged sphincter. It is very rare in neurologically normal children. The same can be said about *mixed incontinence*, i.e. the combination of stress and urge incontinence. Both these conditions can, however, frequently be present in children with neurogenic bladder disturbance.

Giggle incontinence is a rare form of incontinence occurring specifically during laughter (rather than during giggling, but the term 'laughter incontinence' has never gained acceptance). These children are usually otherwise fully continent and the urine that escapes during laughter seems to represent a complete and presumably urodynamically normal emptying of the bladder.

CYSTOMETRIC FINDINGS

Detrusor overactivity is the term used for cystometrically observed involuntary detrusor contractions, previously known as detrusor instability. It is the consistent objective urodynamic finding in patients with bladder overactivity. *Neurogenic detrusor overactivity* replaces the older term detrusor hyperreflexia used in children with neurogenic bladder disturbance, and *idiopathic detrusor overactivity* is the word used in neurologically normal children with involuntary detrusor contractions found on cystometry.

Cystometric bladder capacity is the bladder volume reached during cystometry when bladder filling is stopped due to strong urgency, pain, significant leakage, spontaneous micturition or elevated basal detrusor pressure. For more detailed cystometric definitions and terminology the reader is referred to the ICCS document (Nevéus et al 2006) and to the ICS document (Abrams et al 2002).

FUNCTIONAL FAECAL INCONTINENCE (ENCOPRESIS)

Functional faecal incontinence is defined as voluntary and involuntary passage of faeces in inappropriate places from the age of 4 years onwards – after organic causes have been ruled out. Synonymously, the term encopresis can be used, and the terms will be used interchangeably in this book. The two main subtypes are those with and without accompanying constipation. Detailed aspects of classification are covered in Chapter 9.

TREATMENT TERMINOLOGY

The definition of treatment success, in the clinical setting, is, obviously, made by the child and family. In the research setting, and when comparing studies and reports of various therapies, we do, however, need more rigid and objective criteria.

When evaluating *initial treatment success* we are comparing the number of days or nights with wetting or soiling episodes during two weeks before treatment and two weeks during treatment. The definitions are given in Table 2.5.

TABLE 2.5
ICCS recommendations (Nevéus et al 2006) for treatment outcome

Initial success
Non-response: 0 to 49% reduction
Partial response: 50 to 89% reduction
Response: >90% reduction
Full response: 100% or less than one accident per month

Long-term success
Relapse: more than one accident per month
Continued success: no relapse in six months after treatment
Complete success: no relapse in two years after treatment

3
NORMAL BLADDER AND BOWEL DEVELOPMENT

Bladder and urinary tract

EMBRYOLOGY AND ANATOMY

The major part of the urogenital system derives from the intermediate part of the intraembryonic mesoderm. The pronephros, the first renal precursor, appears at the end of the fourth week of gestation. Although it rapidly disappears, the second precursor, the mesonephros, develops and gives rise to tubular structures that are destined to become parts of the gonads. Lateral to the mesonephros, the mesonephric ducts gradually advance caudally to fuse with the terminal portion of the hindgut. During the fifth week of gestation the future ureters appear as outgrowths or buds on the mesonephric ducts.

The metanephros develops at the same time caudally to the mesonephros and is the final and definitive progenitor of the kidneys. The fusion of the ureteric bud with this structure at approximately day 32 triggers the start of *nephron-forming*, or nephrogenesis, a process that is not finished until approximately week 36, when the final number of nephrons – $0.5–1.0 \times 10^6$ (Hinchliffe et al 1991) – is reached. The ureteric buds give rise to the renal pelvis and calyces as well as the collecting ducts, whereas the rest of the nephron is derived from the metanephros. It is important to understand that the development of the ureteric buds and the development of the metanephros are interdependent, so that a primary defect in either component will affect the development of the other and give rise to combined malformations (Schwartz et al 1981).

The cloaca, or the terminal portion of the primitive hindgut, gives rise to the lower urinary tract, and is partitioned some time between the fourth and sixth week of gestation by the urogenital septum into the urogenital and the anorectal canals. The bladder evolves from the upper portion of the urogenital canal at the same time as the ureters separate from the mesonephric ducts (which will become the vas deferens in the male and more or less disappear in the female). The genital tubercle, situated anterior to the orifice of the urogenital canal, will evolve into the phallus in the presence of testosterone, or the clitoris without such stimulation. The female urethra is derived entirely from the urogenital canal, whereas the distal part of the male urethra is formed, from the seventh week onwards, by the ingrowth of superficial mesenchyme into the evolving phallus. For a more comprehensive review of the embryology and developmental pathogenesis of the urinary tract, see Woolf and Winyard (2002).

All three major neural systems – somatic, sympathetic and parasympathetic – converge to the lower urinary tract. The largest neural input to the bladder is cholinergic, via the pelvic nerves (El-Badawi and Schenk 1966). The thoracolumbar sympathetic branch of the autonomic nervous system reaches the bladder via the hypogastric and pelvic plexa (Nergårdh and Boréus 1972). Somatic efferents and afferents of the urethra and bladder travel through the pudendal nerve (Kuru 1965, de Groat and Booth 1980). The motor neurons of the striated muscles of the sphincter and pelvic floor are located in the conus medullaris of the spinal medulla.

NORMAL BLADDER FUNCTION

The role of the bladder (including the urethra) is, of course, to store and release urine in a physiologically and socially acceptable way. Ideally, the detrusor should be completely relaxed during storage, bladder size should allow for several hours' interval between micturitions, and voiding should be characterized by coordinated detrusor contraction and sphincter relaxation resulting in a complete emptying of the bladder.

The bladder and urethra are a peculiar organ system. Although it is innervated largely by the autonomic nervous system, it is – or should be – under complete cortical control. This control is exerted by the suppression or facilitation of spino-bulbar micturition reflex circuits involving the pelvic nerves, the pontine micturition centre and the sacral branch of the parasympathetic nervous system (de Groat 1975). Simplified, it can be stated that storage is a mainly sympathetic and micturition a mainly parasympathetic phenomenon.

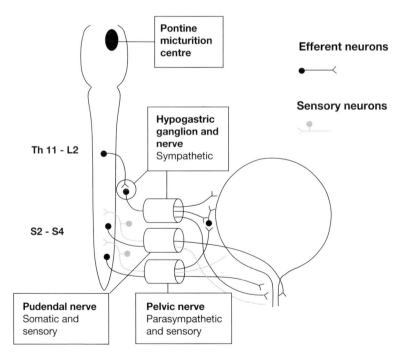

Fig. 3.1 Innervation of the lower urinary tract. Central nervous pathways are omitted in this highly schematic illustration.

11

STORAGE

During storage of urine the smooth muscle of the internal sphincter is tonically contracted through alpha-adrenergic stimulation in the urethra (Nergårdh and Boréus 1972, Raz et al 1972). The spinal motoneurons innervating the striated muscle of the external sphincter are also tonically active. At the same time a reflex arc, involving the pelvic nerve and the sympathetic fibres of the hypogastric and pelvic plexa, tonically inhibits excitatory input to the detrusor muscle via beta-adrenergic receptors in the corpus and fundus of the bladder (de Groat and Lalley 1972, Saum and de Groat 1972). The parasympathetic input to the bladder is quiescent during urine storage.

MICTURITION

During voluntary micturition input from the frontal cerebral cortex (Bradley et al 1974, Blok et al 1997a, Blok and Holstege 1998) inhibits the spinal storage reflexes and activates the parasympathetic excitatory outflow to the bladder. The crucial link between volition and micturition is the pontine micturition centre (PMC), or Barrington's nucleus (Barrington 1921), which is located in the rostral pons and has been shown to elicit or inhibit detrusor contractions when stimulated (Noto et al 1989).

The signals for initiating micturition are transmitted from the pontine micturition centre to the sacral motoneurons innervating the external sphincter (Kuru 1965, Blok et al 1997b), and to the parasympathetic neurons innervating the detrusor (de Groat and Booth 1980). These cholinergic fibres inhibit urethral smooth muscle and initiate detrusor contractions (Kuru 1965). Recent research has shown that extracellular adenosine triphosphate (ATP) is a cotransmitter on the cholinergic synapses on the detrusor and acts as a sort of 'initiator' while the acetylcholine maintains the contraction (Theobald 1995).

At the bladder level, voiding starts with relaxation of the sphincter and pelvic floor, immediately followed by reflex detrusor contraction (Tanagho and Miller 1970, Jonas and Tanagho 1975, Holstege et al 1986, de Groat 1993). The presence of urine in the urethra then facilitates continuing detrusor contraction and sphincter relaxation, so that emptying will be complete (de Groat and Booth 1980, Jung et al 1999).

Conscious interruption of micturition is accomplished in the following way. Signals originating from the motor cortex, probably via the so-called L area in the pontine tegmentum (Blok and Holstege 1998) and then the pudendal nerve, elicit the forceful contraction of the striated muscle of the external sphincter and the pelvic floor, and this contraction initiates a spinal reflex that inhibits further bladder contractile activity. The voluntary inhibition of involuntary detrusor contractions is a similar process.

NORMAL MICTURITION BEHAVIOUR

Micturition habits are highly variable among normal, continent children. Studies involving home measurements have shown voiding frequencies between 2 and 8 times daily (Hellström et al 1990, Mattsson 1994b), with a peak around 5–6 (Bloom et al 1993, Hansen et al 1997) and no gender or age differences during childhood (Hellström et al 1990, Bloom et al 1993).

The prevalence of nocturia – i.e. the need to wake up and micturate at night – in the normal population is not fully known. Approximately 80 per cent of 5 to 12-year-olds have

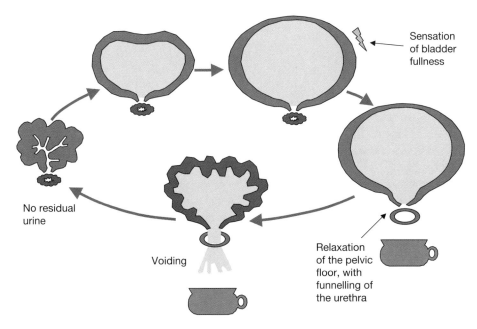

Fig. 3.2 Normal bladder function. Contracted muscle and relaxed muscle shown in dark and light shades of grey.

'occasional' nocturia (Bower et al 1996), whereas about 12 per cent need to get up and micturate at least once every week (Nevéus et al 1999a). When asked to complete a 24-hour micturition diary approximately 6 per cent of children aged 7 to 8 years reported nocturia (Hansen et al 1997).

Bladder volume is both easy and difficult to measure. Many different measurement strategies and a confusing number of definitions have been used, reflecting the fact that:

1 Cystometric volume measurements are acquired during highly unnatural conditions and are of limited clinical relevance.
2 The bladder is a distensible organ with no fixed diameter (how do you measure the size of a balloon?).
3 Children void when it suits them and not on attaining a specified magnitude of bladder filling (Mattsson et al 2003). Asking the child to postpone micturition maximally will yield highly variable volumes, since the sensation of bladder filling is very subjective.

The most sensible, clinically relevant way to measure bladder volume is to pick the largest voided volume from a voiding diary that has been completed by the family during a few days when the child has been drinking and voiding *ad libitum*. With this strategy it will be found that the largest voided volume will usually be the first morning void, but that many voidings will be less than half that volume (Mattsson et al 2003). Normal values, to which the measured volumes can be compared, can be derived from the classic formula (Koff 1983, Hjälmås 1988):

Expected bladder capacity in ml $\quad = 30 + (30 \times \text{age in years})$

or: $\quad = (\text{age} + 1) \times 30\,\text{ml}$

(up to the age of 12 years)

DEVELOPMENT OF BLADDER CONTROL

Several lines of evidence suggest that the micturition reflex is already under higher central nervous system control at the foetal and neonatal stage (Mevorach and Kogan 1995). For instance, intrauterine micturition seems to occur almost exclusively while the foetus is awake (Wlodek et al 1989, Ohel et al 1995). Furthermore, animal studies have shown that the central neural pathways controlling micturition in the adult can be detected in the newborn, before the micturition reflex has become functional (Sugaya et al 1997). The development of functional voiding and storage reflexes involves the selective suppression and stimulation of synapse proliferation in different pathways of the evolving nervous system (Araki and de Groat 1997).

Incomplete coordination of the detrusor and sphincter muscles is not uncommon in the infant (Hjälmås 1976), and it has been convincingly shown that – in contrast to what was previously believed – the infantile detrusor tends to be silent during storage, and the infant usually only voids while awake (Yeung et al 1995).

The first step towards social continence is usually taken during the second or third year, when the child becomes somewhat aware of bladder distension. By this time voiding is usually fully coordinated and leaves no residual urine. With the child's increasing awareness of bladder filling and increasing ability to postpone micturition and suppress reflex detrusor contractions, continence is gradually achieved, first during the day and then during the night as well. The final steps are taken when, around the age of 4 or 5, the child is able to initiate micturition even when the bladder is not full.

Bowel

EMBRYOLOGY

All three embryonic layers are involved in the formation of the gut. The most primitive gut is formed in the fourth gestational week by incorporated *entoderm*, of which the distended distal part is the so-called cloaca. The *mesoderm* forms the peritoneum and interstitial tissues. An intrusion of *ectoderm* is the precursor of the anal canal. At this time, the cloaca and the anal pit are not connected, but separated by the cloacal membrane. In other words, the primitive gut is not yet connected with the amniotic cavity. In subsequent development, the distal parts of the gut have no mesenterium, but remain in a retroperitoneal site. In contrast, the sigmoid has a shortened mesenterium and is located intraperitoneally.

By the sixth week, the cloaca is divided by the urogenital septum, which merges with the cloacal membrane, into two parts. The urogenital sinus, the precursor of the distal urogenital system, is located ventrally. The dorsal parts of the divided cloaca will form the rectum and the proximal anal canal. Finally, in the seventh week, the anal and urogenital membranes open, so that the gastrointestinal tract is connected with the amniotic sac (Moore 1980).

This complicated embryological development, involving all three layers, is responsible for the wide variety of often severe anorectal malformations. In its most severe form, a primitive cloaca can persist. The anal canal can be stenosed or covered by a persistent anal membrane. An ectopic opening of the gastrointestinal tract can occur by ano-perineal, recto-vaginal or recto-urethral fistulas. Finally, a variety of different rectal atresias can occur if ectoderm and entoderm are not connected (Moore 1980).

ANATOMY
Starting distally, the anatomical anal canal extends from the external anal ring (linea anocutanea) to the linea dentata. In contrast, the surgical anal canal is nearly twice as long and extends from the anus to the haemorrhoidal plexus, which is, in fact, where ectoderm and entoderm merge in embryological development. The walls are closely opposed with mucosal folds.

The rectum is not as straight as the Latin name (*rectum* = straight) implies. The rectum emerges proximally out of the sigmoid, has no mesenterium and is located retro- and extraperitonially. Functionally, the rectal ampulla, where stool accumulates before defecation, is located between the sacral and the perineal curvatures.

The most important muscle in the region is the internal anal sphincter (IAS), an elongation of the smooth ring muscles of the rectum. This involuntary muscle is innervated over the pelvic ganglion and over the hypogastric and pelvic nerves. It is under both excitatory (sympathetic L1–L2) and inhibitory (parasympathetic S2–S4) control.

The striated external anal sphincter (EAS) muscle consists of different muscles including the profound, superficial and subcutaneous external anal muscles, as well as the levator ani muscle. These voluntary sphincter and pelvic floor muscles are innervated via the sacral plexus by the levator and pudendal nerves.

As outlined in Chapter 9 (see page 230), the innervation of the gastrointestinal tract is especially closely connected to the central nervous system (CNS) over the enteric nervous system (ENS), also called the 'minibrain of the gut'. The connections are mainly afferent, i.e. receptors of the gut project to the ganglion nodosum, over the nucleus tractus solitarius to the brainstem, hypothalamus, limbic system and cortex (Frieling 1993).

NORMAL BOWEL FUNCTION
Normal defecation involves synchronized autonomic and voluntary functions in a complicated pattern (Hatch 1988). The rectum is distended by a descending faecal bolus, which stimulates sensory receptors in the bowel and pelvic floor. Parasympathic nerves (plexus myentericus), sympathic modulation and conscious awareness via ascending sensory fibres are all involved. The voluntary striated external anal sphincter muscle and the puborectalis sling contract transiently, initiating the so-called 'inflation reflex' (Hatch 1988). Distension of the sigmoid and rectum lead to a relaxation of the internal anal sphincter (the

15

'rectosphincteric relaxation reflex'). This relaxation occurs proportional to the volume and rate of rectal distension.

If defecation is desired, then the descending colon, sigmoid colon and rectum (especially the longitudinal muscles) contract and the external anal sphincter and puborectalis muscles relax, allowing widening of the anal rectal angle, producing an unobstructed anal pathway (Hatch 1988). Increased abdominal pressure then initiates defecation.

If defecation is not desired, the anorectal muscles contract reflexively. The relaxation of the internal sphincter decreases and the rectum adapts itself to the amount of retained stool. The intraluminal pressure and desire to defecate both diminish.

The structure and function of the anorectum change with growth and maturation (Hatch 1988). The rectum increases in length, rectal valves appear and forward angulation of the anal-rectal junction occurs. The internal anal sphincter relaxation reflex occurs approximately at term, but is not present in preterm infants. Before voluntary control is achieved, rectal distension leads to relaxation of the external anal sphincter (inhibition reflex).

By 2.5 years of age, maturation is associated with persistence of external anal sphincter contraction, which allows the normal inflation reflex and conscious control of defecation. Once continence is established, it remains a function of stool consistency, anatomic integrity of the bowel and the coordinated action of the smooth and striated muscles (Hatch 1988). In contrast, continence is not dependent on the function of the external anal sphincter. Maintenance of the anorectal angle in a normal range by the puborectalis muscle sling is far more important. In contrast to continence of solid stools, continence of flatus and liquid is a function of the closed anal canal maintained by the internal anal sphincter.

4
GENERAL PRINCIPLES: ASSESSMENT

The aim of this chapter is to provide an in-depth and at the same time practical approach to the evaluation of children with voiding disorders. Specific points related to the various different types of voiding disorders are covered in the chapters dealing with those disorders.

History taking, charts and questionnaires

APPROACH TO ASSESSING THE CHILD

General, sound principles of professional child-care and of how to communicate with children certainly apply to children with voiding disorders. Here we will focus on a few points that are of special relevance when dealing with these children.

First, we are dealing primarily with the *child's* problem, which only indirectly becomes also a parental problem. We are concerned first and foremost with the child's wetting or soiling, and the consequences for his or her health and self-esteem. The parental stress and the family's washing bills are secondary, although not unimportant, issues. Thus, it is imperative that we involve the child and talk to the child, not just the parents. This is important for therapeutic reasons as well. In the majority of the therapeutic approaches used in voiding disorders – voiding charts, alarm treatment, urotherapy (bladder control therapy), etc. – the active participation of the child is crucial for therapeutic success.

From this it follows that one needs to talk to the child in a language that he or she understands. The words for urine, faeces, anus and genitalia should, for instance, be replaced by expressions in more common usage in the family. If one uses words that the child understands, even though they might seem inaccurate or embarrassing, the child will not be embarrassed to use them and it will be possible to get a good case history directly from the child.

Furthermore, it is important to be aware that the child may have rudimentary or erroneous conceptions about urogenital and gastrointestinal anatomy and physiology. Children may believe that the urinary tract is just a straight tube between the mouth and the genitalia, or that the poo that leaves them at lunchtime is the food they ate for breakfast. Obviously, there is a need for teaching here, and this is also a part of therapy. The child who knows how his or her excretory organs work will have a greater chance of taking command over them.

Needless to say, the approach when dealing with a 5-year-old child will be different from that with a teenager. Both the language and the explanations need to be adapted to the child's age and developmental level. Keeping this in mind, it is also desirable to try to make the visit interesting for the child, using play, stories, pictures or cartoons to gain and sustain their attention.

Usually, all the history taking and the physical examination should be done together with both the child and the parent. The child will feel more secure when their mother/father is there, and the family needs to be involved anyway. But there are exceptions to this rule. Sometimes the doctor may get the impression that the child and the parents are hiding something from each other – in which case both parties need to be interviewed separately. Most importantly, this strategy is needed if there is any suspicion of sexual abuse, or if it is suspected that the child is being punished for his or her wetting/soiling accidents; but it may also reveal relevant family problems and conflicts that would not have been mentioned with everybody present. Furthermore, when dealing with teenagers it is a good rule to always have a few words with them privately. This demonstrates to the young person that he or she is the central person and that they are being taken seriously, which may help in building up a good relationship. And in the case of teenage girls with urinary tract infections it is important to know whether the girl is sexually active or not, which is something that she might not disclose with a parent in the room.

By talking to the child and not just to the parents, and by explaining things in an appropriate, interesting and child-oriented way, the doctor is more likely to gain the child's confidence. During the physical examination and/or subsequent therapy, it is important to explain to the child what is going to happen. For example, before the rectal examination, the procedure should be explained. Most children, when properly prepared, will not consider the examination painful, but some will. Things that are embarrassing – genital inspection, for instance – may have to wait until the child feels more comfortable with the doctor. It is also important not to make promises that cannot be kept – for example, telling the child that this or that treatment will certainly make their problems go away. There are always a few children who do not respond to therapy, and they will feel deceived. Above all, the child should always be prepared for what is to happen. No child will trust the person who exposes him or her to unpleasant surprises.

BACKGROUND

All medical handbooks stress the importance of a good case history and this inevitably needs time. It is the authors' experience that at least 30 minutes – sometimes a full hour – is needed for the first consultation, even in seemingly uncomplicated cases of, say, monosymptomatic nocturnal enuresis. But it is time well spent. With a full knowledge of the child's symptoms and a good therapeutic relationship with the child and family there is no need to waste time on unnecessary investigations and fruitless therapeutic attempts, and the next visit can be much shorter or may even be managed by phone.

It is important to get at the hard facts and to avoid vague estimations such as 'sometimes', 'slightly', etc. When asking about wetting frequency and wetting amounts, it is a good idea to get the informant to specify, for example, how many times per day/week/month. Is it a spot on the underpants or a puddle on the chair?

MICTURITION SYMPTOMS

Micturition symptoms will, of course, be the main area to scrutinize in children with wetting problems, but even in children with encopresis some basic micturition data are needed. The parents of the encopretic child with occasional daytime urinary incontinence may consider the latter symptom of minor significance and not spontaneously mention it, but it is of prime importance that the doctor knows about it. Thus, *all* children with *any* voiding disorder should be asked specifically about micturition symptoms.

From micturition history alone many specific kinds of bladder disturbances can be discerned (see Table 4.1) and an individualized diagnostic and therapeutic strategy can be delineated.

Daytime incontinence

Daytime incontinence should be specifically asked about even in the child whose presenting complaint is enuresis or encopresis (for example, incontinence in an enuretic child is an indicator of detrusor overactivity, a clue that has therapeutic implications). Some parents do not regard the leakage of small amounts of urine as incontinence, but it is still important to know about it. Incontinence, when present, must be described in some detail. The reason for this is that different kinds of incontinence present in different ways and require vastly different diagnostic and therapeutic approaches. The child with urge incontinence due to overactive bladder needs little diagnostic work-up and should be treated with urotherapy or anticholinergics, whereas the child with an ectopic ureteric orifice needs X-ray examinations and surgery. These are the questions that need to be asked:

1 *How often* does it happen?
2 *How much* urine? I.e. are the clothes just damp or soaking wet? Can the wet spot be seen? How big is it usually?
3 *When* does it happen? When feeling a sudden need to go to the toilet or totally without warning? Continuously dripping or in discrete amounts? Only after a visit to the toilet? Only when laughing? When the child has not been to the toilet for a long time or even if he/she goes regularly?
4 Has it *always* been this way? Has the child been dry for at least six months before?

Enuresis

Enuresis is a much simpler symptom to describe, but one still needs to know the frequency of the bedwetting and whether it is a new symptom or not, since these data have therapeutic and diagnostic importance. The child who wets his bed once every other week is not a suitable candidate for the enuresis alarm, and the enuretic child who had been dry between 3 and 8 years of age before starting wetting may have diabetes. The approximate amount of urine voided in bed is also a valuable piece of information; small wet spots are indicators either of detrusor overactivity or that the child wakes up and interrupts the voiding; whereas if the sheets are soaking wet it is likely that nocturnal polyuria is a pathogenetic factor.

TABLE 4.1
Types of incontinence that can be suspected from micturition history data alone

Typical micturition symptoms	Suspected aetiology
Leakage of small or large amounts of urine, sometimes without warning and sometimes with urgency symptoms. Increased micturition frequency. May have been dry before	Detrusor overactivity
Leakage of small or large amounts of urine, with increasing urgency. Low micturition frequency and habitual holding manoeuvres. May have been dry before	Voiding postponement
Straining, interrupted flow of urine	Dysfunctional voiding
Continuous leakage of urine in small amounts. Never been dry	Ectopic ureter
Continuous leakage of urine, worsened by straining or coughing. May have been dry before.	Neuropathic bladder with sphincteric incompetence
Girl wetting small to moderate portions a short while after normal micturition	Vaginal reflux
Apparently complete voiding occurring consistently during laughing, but not during coughing or straining	Giggle incontinence
Leakage of small amounts of urine during laughing, coughing, increased abdominal pressure	Stress incontinence
Large volumes voided, interrupted urine stream	Detrusor underactivity
Leakage of small or large amounts of urine in a child who was previously dry. Dysuria. Possibly increased micturition frequency and/or foul-smelling urine	Cystitis
Nocturnal enuresis, primary or secondary, with urgency symptoms	Non-monosymptomatic enuresis due to detrusor overactivity
Nocturnal enuresis, primary or secondary, with voiding postponement, interrupted voiding and or other symptoms of bladder dysfunction	Non-monosymptomatic enuresis due to other types of bladder dysfunction
Nocturnal enuresis, primary or secondary, without daytime incontinence/urgency symptoms	Monosymptomatic enuresis due to nocturnal polyuria and/or insufficient inhibition of the micturition reflex and/or inhibited arousal
Secondary enuresis with increased thirst, night-time drinking and gradually evolving general symptoms (tiredness, weight loss)	Diabetes mellitus

Micturition frequency

Micturition frequency is a crucial piece of information, at least in incontinent children. Normally, and provided the fluid intake is not excessive or minimal, a child should need to urinate between five and seven times per day (Hellström et al 1990). A high micturition frequency is an indicator of detrusor overactivity and a low frequency should raise a suspicion of voiding postponement. The only reliable way to get these data is through a voiding diary. One important question is to ask how long parents can be out driving (or shopping) before their child has to void.

Urgency, meaning the sudden and unexpected feeling of an imminent need to void, is the hallmark of detrusor overactivity (Allen and Bright 1978, Bauer et al 1980, Griffiths and Scholtmeijer 1983). Furthermore, the sensation of urgency is accompanied by the forceful contraction of the external sphincter and pelvic floor (van Gool and de Jonge 1989). Consequently, this is a symptom that should be specifically enquired about in all children with any voiding disorder. To find out if the child experiences urgency, one can ask whether, when the child senses the need to urinate, he or she has to go immediately – as an imperative urge – or whether it can wait for a while. One way to make the family specify the degree of urgency is to ask them how long, after the child has expressed a need to urinate, they can drive the car before having to stop.

Holding manoeuvres
Holding manoeuvres, such as squatting with the heel pressed against the perineum – the curtsey sign, or Vincent's sign (Vincent 1966) – holding the abdomen or penis, standing on toes with legs crossed, or tripping and swaying back and forth while trying to postpone micturition, are signs that indicate that the child is trying to suppress a detrusor contraction. Often children appear to daydream or be absent-minded during holding manoeuvres. This is often very obvious to parents; they see that the child is trying to postpone a micturition impulse but when they ask the child to go to the toilet the answer might be that they do not need to. Holding manoeuvres are common among children with urge incontinence and voiding postponement, and should be enquired after in all children with incontinence or suspected constipation.

Symptoms of disturbed micturition
Incontinent children should be asked about how they micturate. Do they have to strain to get the micturition going? Does he or she pass urine with a single good stream? Does it take a long time? Does it all come in one amount? It is important not to miss the child who needs to strain to expel urine or the child who cannot void in a single amount, since in both these cases neurogenic bladder disturbance may be the underlying mechanism.

DRINKING HABITS
The importance of fluid intake history in children with voiding disorders is often under-estimated. Many constipated children drink too little (which decreases the hydration of the faeces) and many incontinent or enuretic children have very inappropriate drinking habits (Spehr and De Geeter 1991). Drinking large amounts of fluid in the evening is obviously not a good idea for children with enuresis, since it increases the risk of wet nights. Still, many children with overactive bladders, and symptoms such as incontinence and/or enuresis, get into the habit of drinking very little during the morning and at lunchtime – presumably in order to reduce bladder filling and the risk of wetting accidents – and thus have to drink a lot in the evening. The child may also consume too much of diuretic- or stimulant-containing drinks, such as Coca-Cola or coffee, in the evening, which may increase the risk of bedwetting (clinical experience, not evidence-based). Meanwhile, the family are unaware that drinking habits are an important issue.

The only reliable way to assess fluid intake is to ask the family to complete a voiding chart with drinking data included (see below). While awaiting the results of this, however, it is a good idea to at least ask the enuretic child whether he or she is more thirsty than other children. The reason for this is that polydipsia (often with nocturnal drinking as well) is present in diabetes or renal tubular disorders, diseases that can have enuresis as a presenting symptom.

BOWEL HABITS

The bowel and the bladder are anatomically, neurologically and functionally interrelated organs. It seems obvious, but the bladder affects the bowel, and vice versa. If the child suffers from encopresis, it is clear that several bowel questions have to be asked, but even in the enuretic or incontinent child – especially the latter – one should at least ask about symptoms suggesting constipation. Questions 1, 2 and 3 below would be a minimum in such cases, since hard stools and/or infrequent emptying are indicative of constipation, and soiling of the underpants is a symptom that is not always spontaneously disclosed. Note, however, that even the child who goes to the toilet every day and produces faeces of normal consistency can still be constipated, and suffer from incontinence of urine and stomach pains, because of faecal impaction.

1 How often does the child go to the toilet?
2 Are the stools hard or soft?
3 Does encopresis occur? If yes: How often? How much (full amounts or only staining of the underpants)? When?
4 Are defecations painful or unpleasant?
5 Is there stomach-ache? If yes: How often? When?
6 Has there been blood on the stools?
7 Has it always been this way?

SLEEP

It is now, finally, recognized that sleep and arousal mechanisms are central to the pathogenesis of nocturnal enuresis: enuretic children usually sleep more 'deeply' than their dry peers (Wolfish et al 1997). It is thus natural to ask the parents of a bedwetting child if their son/daughter is difficult to arouse. In the majority of cases the answer will be affirmative. In these cases the main point of posing the question is to acknowledge and confirm the family's observation. However, in a minority of cases the parents will report that the arousability of the child varies from night to night or that he or she is, in fact, quite easy to awaken from sleep. In these cases the alarm treatment will have a very good chance of curing the child. The question 'What do you have to do to make your child wake up at night?' is a good way of getting some sort of quantification of the arousability.

It is informative to ask about the child's reactions when he or she is forcefully woken in the middle of the night. It is useful to know if the freshly awoken child is at all communicative or if he or she is still just semi-conscious and can be led to the toilet without remembering a thing the next morning. In the latter case, alarm treatment will be difficult to perform.

In enuretic children who sleep deeply it may also be interesting to enquire about other parasomnias, such as somnambulism, night terrors, etc., since their presence is another indication of a disorder of arousal (Stores and Wiggs 2001).

The presence or absence of nocturia (i.e. waking up with a need to urinate) in an enuretic child is also a useful piece of information, since it indicates that (a) the child is not *extremely* difficult to arouse from sleep (thus, the alarm may be useful); (b) nocturnal polyuria may be the pathogenetic mechanism behind the enuresis; and (c) the enuresis may be about to resolve spontaneously.

Obviously, sleep data are not relevant in the child with just daytime incontinence or encopresis.

GENERAL HEALTH, CONCOMITANT SOMATIC DISEASES
Just as no physical examination of a child is complete without measuring height, weight and head circumference, every first consultation with a child should include at least a rudimentary assessment of the general health of the child. We need to know if he or she has grown and developed in a normal way and if there has been any significant health problem besides the voiding disorder. Thus, severe diseases such as ulcerative colitis or pyelonephritis should not be missed. The list below can be used as a short guide to what to look for – apart from growth – in the previous health history of children with different micturition and bowel complaints.

1   *Enuretic children.* The simplest case is the child with monosymptomatic nocturnal enuresis; here it would suffice to check if growth has been within normal parameters and whether or not the child is generally more tired and less energetic than his or her peers. If the child has previously been dry but now suffers from enuresis we also need to know about excessive thirst, recent loss of weight, past UTIs, nausea and stomach pains (diabetes mellitus? diabetes insipidus? polyuric renal failure? renal tubular disorder?).

2   *Daytime incontinent children.* Most importantly, we need to know whether there have been any UTIs in the past, including during infancy. Children with disturbed bladder function are overrepresented among those with vesico-ureteral reflux and pyelonephritic scarring.

3   *Children with encopresis* need to be asked about allergies, especially food allergies, and particularly cow's milk allergy. Earlier problems related to the stomach or bowel, such as infant colic, gastrointestinal infections, episodes of diarrhoea, etc., should also be enquired after.

J., 7-year-old boy
Diagnosis: Primary non-monosymptomatic nocturnal enuresis

J. has had normal growth and general development and is very seldom ill. There have been no dry periods longer than a week or so. His father became dry at night at age 6. J. is a very deep sleeper and wets his bed most nights. He is dry during the daytime but admits that sometimes he has to rush to the toilet. Sometimes he needs to urinate but is too occupied with play to note it himself until the need becomes very urgent. J. has good peer relations and no significant school problems, but his enuresis is becoming an increasing burden and he is afraid that his friends will find out about it. He is not hyperactive or easily distracted. The physical examination is unremarkable and a urinalysis is negative. The frequency-volume chart shows three to six voidings daily, with an average volume of 100 ml, a low fluid intake and a tendency towards long voiding intervals when he is at school.

J. is given advice about increased fluid intake and regular voiding habits. The alarm is considered first-line treatment and is explained to J. and his parents, who are motivated to give it a try. Follow-up and encouragement during treatment are provided. During the first week of treatment everybody in the house except J. wakes to the alarm, so the father has to sleep in the same room as his son and wake him up. In the second week, J. manages to wake up without assistance. After four weeks, dry nights start to occur and after two months J. has gone two consecutive weeks without any wetting accident at all.

GENETICS – GENERAL PRINCIPLES

Without a doubt, heredity plays an important role in the aetiology of many syndromes of voiding disorders. On the other hand, even a marked genetic disposition can be modulated by environmental factors. Basically, the question is no longer 'heredity or environment' but how the two factors interact specifically. In some syndromes of enuresis and incontinence, heredity plays the decisive role, as can be seen in Table 4.2. These are all types of nocturnal enuresis and urge incontinence with positive, highly significant linkage results in molecular genetic studies. Also, heredity is clearly evident in families with giggle incontinence.

In other syndromes, such as in voiding postponement, environment plays the major role. Voiding postponement is considered to be an acquired habit in some children and a manifestation of a psychological disorder in others. In other subtypes, such as dysfunctional voiding, the issue is still being debated. Dyscoordinated bladder emptying has been shown early in life in infants and can occur in several members of the same family (Hjälmås 1995a). It is not clear, however, if this is due to heredity or mutual family habits.

Clinically, questions regarding heredity should be part of every history taking. It is advisable to start with an open question such as 'have any other members of your family

TABLE 4.2
Association of genetic and environmental factors

		Definition	Prevalence	Genetics	Environment
	NOCTURNAL ENURESIS				
1	Primary monosymptomatic nocturnal enuresis	NW, dry interval <6 months, no bladder dysfunction	+++ common	+++ sporadic (1/3) aut. dominant (chromosomes 4, 8, 12, 13, 22)	–
2	Primary non-monosymptomatic nocturnal enuresis	NW, dry interval <6 months, bladder dysfunction	+++ common	++ ditto	+ psychiatric disorders more common, signs of 4, 5, 6
3	Secondary nocturnal enuresis	NW, dry interval >6 months (with and without bladder dysfunction)	++ common	+++ ditto	+++ life events, psychiatric disorders
	DAYTIME WETTING/ FUNCTIONAL URINARY INCONTINENCE				
4	Overactive bladder	DW, detrusor instability, urgency, frequency	++ common	++ sporadic and aut. dominant (chromosome 17)	++ UTIs
5	Voiding postponement	DW, postponement of micturition and urine retention	++ common	–	+++ psychiatric disorders, acquired behaviour
6	Dysfunctional voiding	DW, dyscoordination of detrusor and sphincter	(+) rare	–	++ psychiatric disorders, acquired behaviour
7	Underactive bladder	DW, detrusor decompensation	(+) rare	–	+++ development from 5 and 6
8	Stress incontinence	DW with increase of intra-abdominal pressure, insufficiency of sphincter	– very rare	– ?	+ ?
9	Giggle incontinence	DW, complete emptying of bladder through laughing, cataplexy	– very rare	+++ female transmission	–

25

TABLE 4.2 continued

	Definition	Prevalence	Genetics	Environment
ENCOPRESIS				
10 Encopresis with constipation	retention of faeces, constipation, soiling	++ common	++	+++ somatic and psychogenic triggers
11 Encopresis without constipation	Soiling without retention	++ common	–	+++ aetiology unsolved
12 Toilet refusal syndrome	Defecation in diaper, not toilet	++ common	–	+++ toilet training, interaction
13 Toilet phobia	No defecation or micturition in toilet	(+) rare	–	+++ simple, acquired phobia

NW: night wetting
DW: daytime wetting

wetted during the day or at night – currently or in the past?' Then, one could ask specifically if parents or siblings of the child are wetting or have had problems in the past.

If time allows, the optimal procedure would be to draw up a full family tree over three generations and enquire, for every family member, if they have ever had wetting problems (see Fig. 4.1). The type of wetting, as well as the age at which dryness was achieved, should be noted. Experience has shown that due to recollection biases, emotional distress and social stigmatization many parents are not well informed regarding their family history. In such cases it can be helpful to ask parents to procure further information from their own parents or other relatives. This new information can then be added and the family tree modified accordingly.

PSYCHOLOGY AND LIFESTYLE
Even though it is now clear that voiding disorders are not usually psychogenic in origin, they do affect the psyche and the mental well-being of the patient, and there is a subgroup of children with significant psychiatric or psychological comorbidity. For instance, child psychiatric conditions such as ADHD are overrepresented among enuretic, incontinent and encopretic children (Baeyens 2005). In cases of secondary enuresis or incontinence significant family events often coincide with the (re-)emergence of the wetting (Järvelin et al 1990a). Also, compliance with treatment and outcome are worse in children with psychiatric comorbidity (Crimmins et al 2003). As *some* patients do need professional psychiatric evaluation, *all* children should be screened for behavioural and emotional disorders, as physical and behavioural factors are especially closely interrelated in voiding disorders.

'Is this a big problem for you?' is a very good question to ask any child with a voiding disorder. Another good question is: 'how do you feel when the bed or your trousers are

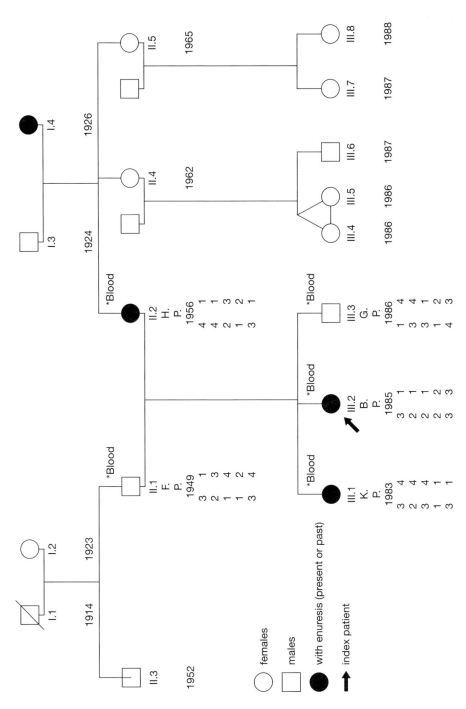

Fig. 4.1 Family tree compatible with an autosomal dominant mode of inheritance (numbers under date of birth refer to results from linkage studies) (von Gontard et al 1998).

wet?' Apart from showing concern for the child, such questions will elicit answers which give a good indication of whether the child will be able to comply with treatments requiring high motivation, such as urotherapy or alarm treatment. The 7-year-old child who does not regard his/her monosymptomatic enuresis as a problem should probably not start any treatment at all, while his/her 5-year-old sibling with the same condition who is very ashamed and concerned about the problem maybe should.

It is very informative to let the child and parents give their views on the problem. How is the wetting/soiling perceived by the child? What do the parents believe is causing it? Do they think that it is the child's fault, that he or she is doing it on purpose, or do they make other erroneous assumptions? This background information is indispensable before starting treatment.

In the case of children who feel troubled by their condition, it is useful to know whether they keep their problem secret or if their closest friends know about it. It is also helpful to know if the wetting/soiling affects the lifestyle of the child, e.g. if he or she still goes to camps, sleeps at friends' homes, etc. This information is important since one of the doctor's tasks, apart from curing the patient, is to give sound advice about how to handle the problem before it is solved (e.g. 'tell your friends', 'don't let it rule your life').

If any suspicion of significant psychological distress or psychiatric comorbidity is aroused, more questions need to be asked. In these cases, families are then asked to describe in some detail other aspects of the child's behaviour that worry them. The following questions can be used to explore whether the child has *externalizing problems*:

Is your child restless or constantly moving?
Is your child easily distracted?
Does your child act impulsively, without thinking?
Can your child be aggressive towards other people?
Does your child obey rules or does he display oppositional behaviour?

Internalizing problems can be assessed with questions such as:

Is your child sad or unhappy?
Has your child lost interest in play or in seeing other children?
Does your child often worry?
Are there problems with sleeping or eating?
Are there fears and anxieties towards certain objects, persons or situations?
Has your child developed peculiar habits or narrow interests?
Does your child act ritually or tend to repeat things in the same way?

Positive answers to the questions above – depending on the severity of the symptoms – may indicate that the child and family need professional psychiatric help or assessment, in addition to treatment of the child's voiding disorder.

The personal and developmental history of children with suspected psychiatric comorbidity is explored with general and specific questions regarding pregnancy, birth, and subsequent motor, cognitive and social development. Motor and language milestones are assessed, and the presence of feeding or sleeping difficulties during early infancy is enquired after. Problems at kindergarten, school and during leisure activities are probed, and specific attention is given to how the child has interacted with family, teachers and other children.

Finally, we need to know about the family situation and significant life events of these children. Are the parents divorced or living together? Are there many conflicts? Are both parents present or is one, or both, mostly absent? Has the family moved several times? Has the child lost significant relatives? What is the material/financial situation of the family? Are there cultural or ethnic differences between the family and the surrounding community?

In some circumstances it may not be possible to carry out a full evaluation of a child's symptoms, and in this situation one needs to ensure that certain essential questions are asked – see Tables 4.3, 4.4 and 4.5. The family should also be given a standard voiding chart to complete at home. Also, questionnaires (see Appendices 3–5 for examples) can be a great asset in obtaining information in a short time. With these data at hand, the cases that need further evaluation can be identified, and it will be clearer what action needs to be taken with the rest.

MICTURITION CHARTS

The micturition chart (or voiding diary) is a crucial tool both diagnostically and therapeutically when dealing with children with voiding disorders (Abrams and Klevmark 1996). After history and physical examination it is the third most important part of assessment. Often a seemingly clear-cut diagnosis – such as monosymptomatic enuresis – changes after the micturition chart data have arrived, or a confusing case history is clarified (McCormack et al 1992, Palnaes Hansen and Klarskov 1998).

TABLE 4.3
Essential questions: for the child who seeks attention for the first time for *nocturnal enuresis*

Question	Why ask this question?
Is this a new problem?	If yes, consider diabetes or kidney disease
How often does it happen?	If seldom or intermittently, then the alarm may not be the first-line therapy
Is there daytime incontinence or urgency?	If incontinence, then this needs to be addressed first, and additional bladder and bowel data (see Table 4.5 below) need to be obtained
	If urgency, then detrusor overactivity is probably the cause, and desmopressin is not first-line therapy
Is the general health and growth of the child within the normal range?	If no, consider kidney disease (or other medical causes)
Is this a problem *for the child*?	If no, perhaps treatment can wait
Are there other problems you are worried about? Have there been changes in the child's environment?	Look for comorbid behavioural problems, stressful life events

29

TABLE 4.4
Essential questions: for the child who seeks attention for the first time for *daytime incontinence*

Question	Why ask this question?
Is this a new problem?	If yes, consider UTI*
When do the wetting episodes occur?	Continuously dripping urine indicates ectopic ureter. Incontinence in girls shortly after normal micturition indicates vaginal reflux. Wetting after prolonged postponement of voiding indicates that the child needs to go to the toilet more often. Wetting concomitant with urgency implies urge incontinence/detrusor overactivity and basic urotherapy will be first-line therapy
Are there urgency symptoms?	If yes, detrusor overactivity is probable and basic urotherapy will be first-line therapy
How often does the child need to go to the toilet? (a micturition chart gives a more accurate answer to this question)	Frequent micturitions indicate detrusor overactivity. Infrequent micturitions indicate voiding postponement or detrusor underactivity. Basic urotherapy will be first-line treatment
Does the child usually try to postpone micturition?	Voiding postponement entails a risk of residual urine and UTI, and indicates that therapy should be directed at increasing micturition frequency and that anticholinergics may be harmful
Does the child strain to initiate micturition? Does he or she urinate in one stream?	These two signs are indicative of dysfunctional voiding
Are there signs of constipation (infrequent bowel movements, encopresis, hard stools)?	Constipation should be eradicated before treatment of the bladder can start (and it may not be needed)
Is the neurological development of the child normal?	Neurologically disabled children with incontinence may suffer from neurogenic bladder disturbances
Is this a problem *for the child*?	If no, compliance with treatment may be low
Are there other problems you are worried about? Have there been changes in the child's environment?	Look for comorbid behavioural problems, stressful life events

* more specific questions regarding symptoms of UTI are certainly useful, but a urine sample will be taken anyway

A micturition chart is used to record observations regarding measured urine volumes, fluid intake and other aspects of bladder (and bowel) function at home. Usually, data for two consecutive days are recorded. For practical reasons, a weekend without other obligations is best, as the process does require cooperation from the child and family. Also, measurements are not feasible during school days. There are many types of charts that can be used (see Appendices for a few examples). Different charts are used for different purposes; for example, the initial *diagnostic chart* usually contains more data than the *therapeutic chart* which is used to monitor treatment progress.

The *diagnostic* benefits of a micturition chart are obvious. First, one obtains hard data regarding micturition frequency, bladder volume, urine production, wetting accidents, fluid intake, defecation frequency and so on. Strictly speaking, a diagnosis such as monosymptomatic nocturnal enuresis can only be made after micturition chart data have been included. Second, one gets a good impression of the cooperativeness and expected compliance with

TABLE 4.5
Essential questions: for the child who seeks attention for the first time for *encopresis*

Question	Why ask this question?
Is this a new problem?	Secondary encopresis may be triggered by stressful life events. Primary encopresis may indicate underlying organic disease or abnormal toilet training
Is the general health and growth of the child within the normal range?	If no, consider organic causes (inflammatory bowel disease, gluten enteropathy, intestinal neuropathies, etc.)
How often do you pass faeces?	If less than three times per week, then constipation is very likely
Are the stools hard or soft?	Hard stools indicate constipation
Are defecations often painful or uncomfortable?	Painful defecations indicate constipation
Are there frequent stomach pains?	Abdominal pains indicate constipation
Is the appetite reduced?	Reduced appetite indicates constipation
Have there been urinary tract infections?	A history of UTIs indicates that further questions regarding the bladder will have to be asked and that an ultrasound examination may be needed
Is the neurological development of the child normal?	Neurologically disabled children with encopresis may suffer from neurogenic bowel disturbances
Is this a problem *for the child*?	If no, compliance with treatment may be low, and psychiatric comorbidity may be present
Are there other problems you are worried about? Have there been changes in the child's environment?	Look for comorbid behavioural problems, stressful life events

treatment of the patient and his or her caregivers. A family that is too chaotic or uninterested to fill in a standard micturition chart will probably be difficult to lead through urotherapy as well. Third, using the charts may even save time. The information obtained via a well-completed voiding diary would take a long time to get by just asking questions.

There are *therapeutic* benefits of charts when they are used over a longer time. Usually, for practical purposes, only direct incidences (of voiding, wetting, urgency, etc.) are recorded, without measuring volumes. The completing of a voiding diary makes the child conscious of the excretory organs and how they work, and helps him or her to see the link between sound micturition habits and treatment success. The child with voiding postponement, for instance, can see for him or herself that 'when I go more often to the toilet I don't wet my pants so much'. It is thus crucial that the chart is completed with the active participation of the child. If treatment effects are slow and the family or child are losing faith, even slight positive therapeutic effects that are visible on the chart can be used by the caregiver to boost morale: 'See, two months ago you had three accidents per day, but now you're down to two, so keep at it!' Not surprisingly, the repeated use of micturition charts is one of the mainstays of the treatment of voiding disorders.

The suggested minimum data to be included in a standard diagnostic chart to be used in enuretic or incontinent children are shown in Table 4.6. Additional data could and should be included in specific cases. In cases of *encopresis* or if *constipation* is suspected (which

TABLE 4.6
Data to be included in a standard micturition chart for the incontinent or enuretic child

First 48 hours	Type of data	Normal values
Micturitions	Volume and timing	5–7 times daily maximum volume: 30 + (30 × age) ml
Fluid intake	Volume and timing	70–100 ml/kg/day Fluid intake evenly distributed during the day, no nocturnal drinking
Enuresis	Yes/no	–
Incontinence	Timing, damp/wet/soaking	–
Micturition symptoms (urgency, holding manoeuvres, straining, interrupted micturitions) Additional parental observations	Timing	Occasional urgency
Rest of the week (or two weeks)		
Enuresis	Yes/no	–
Incontinence	Number of times daily	–

is often the case), bowel movements and encopretic episodes should be included in the chart for one week. Furthermore, in children with *daytime incontinence* it is often desirable to record the timing – though not necessarily the volume – of every micturition and every wetting episode for one whole week. This is important at least during therapy, and should certainly be included in the therapeutic chart; as noted above, the recording and observation of bladder behaviour are a major part of the treatment.

QUESTIONNAIRES
Questionnaires are often used in research. In the clinical setting questionnaires cannot compensate for poor history taking, but they can certainly be a valuable adjunct to the history. Also, they are very economical in that they provide a large amount of information in a short time.

Thus, questionnaires should be seen as a *complement* to history taking and as a *checklist* to ensure that nothing important is forgotten. Discrepancies between questionnaire, history and voiding chart data may also point out issues that may need to be scrutinized more closely. Pre-filled questionnaires may even serve to reduce the time that needs to be spent with the family, but it is still important that the doctor talks to the child and establishes a therapeutic relationship. It should also be underlined that a questionnaire can *never* give a diagnosis. A diagnosis is made after clinical appraisal of the patient.

Within the field of child psychiatry scientifically validated questionnaires are often used in order to obtain a strict and unbiased assessment of predefined behavioural variables. Comparison with norm values is also made in the clinical setting. These issues will be dealt with later in this chapter.

The Appendices give examples of a variety of questionnaires. These can be photocopied and used. They differ in length, ranging from short, screening questionnaires to more detailed instruments. Some follow a 'yes–no' format; others require answers regarding severity on a 0, 1, 2 scale; some have been validated, others not. The choice of questionnaire will depend on the clinical setting (or scientific questions) – therefore several have been included in this book.

Physical examination

It is our opinion that every child with enuresis, incontinence or encopresis should be examined by a doctor at least once. In uncomplicated cases most or all of the treatment and follow-up can then be handled by other professionals, such as school nurses or urotherapists.

Younger children may feel more at ease during embarrassing examinations – such as genital inspection or rectal palpation – if they sit on their mother's or father's lap; teenagers, on the other hand, may want the parents to leave the room. For legal reasons, if a teenage girl is examined without the presence of the parents, a nurse should also be in the room.

The examination will in all cases include height, weight, head circumference, and the simple but important observation of how the child moves and behaves; the rest is dictated by history with specific points delineated below.

CHEST ORGANS, EAR, NOSE, THROAT

Examination of these parts of the body seldom gives any relevant information in children who suffer from voiding disorders, provided the general health is good. But most parents rightly feel that the medical examination of their child is not complete if the doctor does not get out his/her stethoscope; and there is also the issue of cardiac arrhythmias which may interfere with medication. *Blood pressure* should be measured in any child with enuresis or in whom there is even the slightest suspicion of kidney disease.

ABDOMEN

The abdomen should be palpated in all children with voiding disorders. There are several reasons for this: faecal impaction can often be felt as a general abdominal distension or as palpable scybala (most often in the left iliac fossa); bladder distension can also be discerned and suprapubic tenderness might indicate cystitis. In the cases where urine may be expressed by applying manual pressure on the (usually distended) bladder, neuropathic bladder with some degree of sphincteric incompetence should be strongly suspected. Hydronephrosis may be felt via the abdomen and percussion of the flanks may reveal kidney tenderness in cases of pyelonephritis.

NEUROLOGICAL EXAMINATION

All voiding disorders, with the possible exception of purely monosymptomatic nocturnal enuresis, can in a minority of cases be presenting symptoms of underlying malformation of the nervous system, most often the spinal cord.

Thus, it is recommended that the doctor:

1 inspects the lower back to look for dimples, hairy area, gluteal asymmetry or leg length differences – possible tell-tale signs of occult spina bifida or tethered cord;
2 tests the reflexes in the lower limbs and checks for Babinski's sign. Hyperreflexia, reflex asymmetry or a positive Babinski may indicate spinal cord disorder.

Scoliosis, which is most easily seen from behind as thoracic asymmetry when the child leans forward, is also a feature of spina bifida – where it can be severe – but as an isolated finding without any of the above-mentioned signs it is usually not indicative of spinal dysraphism. Flattening of the upper buttocks is a sign suggesting sacral agenesis.

If suspicion of neurological malformation or disease is aroused by history or this simple examination, a full neurological examination should be performed, including fundoscopy, tests for perineal sensitivity, muscular strength and ataxia, inspection of gait (walking on toes and heels, jumping on one leg, etc.), and so on.

It is rarely necessary to elicit the bulbocavernous reflex. If it is present – that is, if manual compression of the glans or clitoris results in instant contraction of the anal sphincter – then the spinal neural pathways are intact, which is obviously a very useful piece of information. The problem here is that the examination may be a very unpleasant breach of the patient's privacy, especially in girls. Provided that you look carefully for the signs of spinal dysraphism mentioned above and make sure that children who show such signs are further evaluated with spinal MRI and/or cystometry (see below), then the testing of the bulbocavernous reflex can be dispensed with. It should definitely not be part of the routine neurological examination.

Neurological 'soft signs' that may be noted during physical examination are more common in children with enuresis or incontinence than in the general population. This includes findings such as general clumsiness, dyscoordinated movements, apparent slight (but symmetric) ataxia, or supination of the hands during the Fog test (walking on the lateral aspects of the feet) that is inappropriate for the child's age.

GENITAL EXAMINATION
The genitalia of every wetting child should be inspected. The child will usually comply with the examination if the reasons are explained. In the rare case of a child who refuses, one should not rush things: genital examination can usually wait until the child has understood that you are a gentle and respectful person, and if the complaint of the child is monosymptomatic enuresis it may perhaps even be omitted. All children with daytime incontinence must, however, sooner or later undergo a genital examination.

In the enuretic child the findings are usually completely normal, but in the child with daytime incontinence several relevant abnormalities may be found. Continuous seepage of urine in the vulva or from the vagina may rarely be observed in girls with ureteral ectopia. The urethral orifice and introitus of girls with the urogenital sinus anomaly or epispadias look highly abnormal. Reddening and oedema of the vulva or perineum can be seen in vulvitis; a purulent discharge may be seen in vaginitis; and perigenital eczema can often be seen in girls who have dysuria or urgency for local reasons. Synechiae of the labia minora is common in small girls and can cause vaginal reflux. Evidently, if there is any indication of sexual abuse one must look closely for bruises, bleeding or hymenal damage. In boys, the finding of balanitis or a tense, narrow prepuce is obviously relevant, as is the presence of epispadias, hypospadias or undescended testes.

ANAL AND RECTAL EXAMINATION

Anal and rectal examinations in children with incontinence or encopresis are indicated in many circumstances but should be approached with caution, particularly in a frightened child who might be withholding. With this reservation, these examinations are desirable in (1) any child with suspected constipation, (2) any child with suspected neurological causes behind the wetting/encopresis, and (3) any enuretic or incontinent child who proves to be resistant to standard first-line treatment.

Rectal examination is usually more uncomfortable or embarrassing than actually painful. One can reduce the discomfort of the child by: (1) ensuring that the child is relaxed and has both legs fully flexed at the hip and knees; (2) placing a gloved and lubricated little finger on the child's anus for a few seconds before palpating, in order to let the reflex sphincter spasm abate; and then (3) palpating quickly.

Inspection of the anus reveals any fissures, bruises and traces of faeces. Rectal palpation gives the opportunity to evaluate sphincter tone and, above all, to detect stools in the rectal ampulla. As will be discussed later, the presence of rectal stools in a child without present sensation of a need to go to the toilet is one of the signs indicative of constipation.

Laboratory investigations

URINE TESTS

A *urine dipstick test* for albumin, erythrocytes, leukocytes, bacteria and glucose is inexpensive, rapid and can, if negative, rule out UTI, glomerulonephritis and diabetes mellitus. Therefore, such a test should be performed once, at the first consultation, in *every* child with enuresis or incontinence. If the test turns out negative for glucose then diabetes mellitus is ruled out as a cause for polyuria. If the test is negative for erythrocytes, leukocytes and bacteria then UTI is (with a high degree of security) ruled out and a bacterial culture is not needed.

A *urine culture* should be taken when the dipstick test turns out positive for leukocytes, erythrocytes or bacteria. Since one of the main points of taking a urine sample is to rule out UTI, it is of utmost importance that the urine be acquired under as sterile conditions as possible. Luckily, the children we are dealing with are old enough to provide a clean catch specimen, at least with parental assistance. This means that the child voids after cleaning the urethral orifice with an antiseptic, and a midstream urine sample is caught from the stream and immediately put into a sterile container. This diminishes but does not abolish the risk of bacterial contamination from the skin.

Note, however, that UTI is an unlikely cause underlying primary nocturnal enuresis. In these cases, two urine cultures should be obtained before antibiotics are considered. Furthermore, it should be remembered that asymptomatic bacteriuria (ABU) is not uncommon; if antibiotic treatment does not lead to prompt relief of symptoms, then the bacteria were not the cause of the symptoms.

A *urine sediment* examination – the microscopical evaluation of a centrifugated urine sample – is called for when glomerular pathology is suspected. Thus, in children who provide repeated urine samples with proteinuria and/or erythrocyturia, who do not have UTI, examination of urine sediment is indicated. If red or white cell casts, hyaline cylinders or fragmented erythrocytes are found, further nephrological evaluation is mandatory.

BLOOD TESTS

Analyses of the blood are very seldom helpful in the evaluation of children with voiding disorders. They only become relevant if history, physical examination or urine tests give reason to suspect an underlying medical condition such as diabetes, celiac disease or kidney disease. We will mention these tests when these differential diagnoses are discussed below.

STOOL CULTURES

Stool cultures and/or microscopy are routine whenever bacterial gastroenteritis or infection with a bowel parasite are suspected. These children seldom present with constipation, but may have encopresis of the non-retentive kind.

Urodynamic studies

INDICATIONS

Uroflowmetry, always combined with assessment of residual urine, is a simple, non-invasive way to assess a child's detrusor and sphincter function during voiding (Hjälmås 1988). This makes the examination extremely useful when dealing with children with voiding disorders. With a good case history, a diagnostic voiding chart and the proper use of uroflowmetry the caregiver can quite easily identify (1) the children who need special biofeedback training, and (2) the small minority of patients who may need X-ray or cystometry. The only problem is that the equipment is not available everywhere.

We suggest that at least the following groups of children be evaluated with uroflowmetry and measurement of residual urine:

1   Patients with signs or symptoms of neurogenic bladder
2   Patients with signs or symptoms of dysfunctional voiding
3   Boys after their first UTI
4   Girls after their fourth UTI
5   Children with enuresis refractory to the alarm and desmopressin treatment
6   Children with daytime incontinence refractory to basal urotherapy
7   Whenever anticholinergic treatment is considered (to rule out residual urine)

If uroflowmetry is not available, which is the case in many countries, then simply listening to the sound of the child voiding does give similar, albeit more subjective, information.

The uroflowmeter was first described in the 1950s (von Garrelts 1956, Kaufman 1957). There are presently various models in use (Abrams 1997):

1   The weight transducer flowmeter simply measures the weight of the urine continuously as it is voided into a vessel.
2   The rotating-disc flowmeter measures the power needed by a small servomotor to keep a disc rotating at a constant speed while being hit by the urine stream.
3   The dipstick or capacitance flowmeter measures the changing capacitance of a vertical metal strip capacitor which is inserted into the urine collection vessel as it is gradually filled with urine.

Regardless of the method chosen, most commercially available flowmeters have acceptable accuracy. Small battery-operated flowmeters for home use are also available.

Uroflowmetry can be performed from about 4 years of age, and the practical aspects are simple: the child, who has been given something to drink, is asked to wait until he or she feels moderate bladder fullness and then to void sitting (boys too) on the uroflowmeter toilet. The room should be warm and the atmosphere relaxed, and the process should be clearly explained to the child. Privacy is also important: the child will often want a parent to be by his/her side, but not the doctor. This is an examination that cannot be rushed.

It should be noted on the flowmetry report whether the child was feeling intense urge, normal bladder fullness or no need to void at the time. If possible, it is best to do an ultrasound of the bladder before and after micturition for optimal comparisons. One can check if the bladder is sufficiently filled for uroflowmetry (volumes of 100 ml or more are required for reliable results). Immediately after voiding, residual urine is assessed with ultrasound apparatus, which may be of the simple Bladderscan® type or similar. Note that the diagnostic value of uroflowmetry is much diminished if measurement of residual urine is not included.

The addition of a non-invasive EMG assessment, via two perineal surface electrodes, is a quite simple and completely painless procedure which gives valuable extra information, especially when neurogenic bladder or dysfunctional voiding is suspected, since there is a high correspondence between the activity of the external sphincter and the muscles of the pelvic floor.

EVALUATION
The following data are obtained with a standard examination: the flow-curve appearance – with information about maximal flow, duration of micturition, duration of entire voiding, time until maximal flow – voided volume and residual volume. The different curve types are illustrated in Fig. 4.2. Table 4.7 shows the typical uroflow results in different bladder conditions. Note that there is no universal agreement regarding reference values for curve characteristics such as maximal flow, voiding duration, etc., and it is more informative to look at the shape of the curve than just the numerical values (Hjälmås 1988). As a rule of thumb, provided that the child empties a volume of at least 100 ml, then a maximum

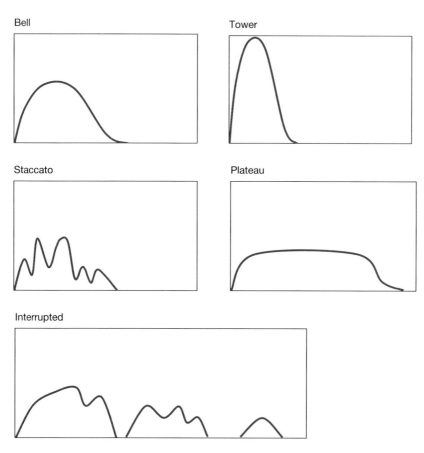

Fig. 4.2 A simplified depiction of the five basic uroflow curve types.

TABLE 4.7
Typical uroflow results in different micturition disorders

Condition	Typical uroflow curve	Voided volume	Residual
Normal bladder function	Bell-shaped, sometimes tower-shaped or plateau	Normal	No
Bladder overactivity	Tower-shaped, sometimes bell-shaped with an early peak	Small	No
Voiding postponement	Normal, sometimes plateau	Large	Sometimes
Dysfunctional voiding	Staccato curve	Normal, small or large	Yes
Detrusor underactivity	Interrupted curve	Large	Yes
Anatomical outlet obstruction	Plateau-shaped	Normal, small or large	Yes

TABLE 4.8
Approximate reference values for maximum urine flow in relation
to voided volumes (adapted from Szabo and Fegyvernski 1995)

Age (years)	Voided volume (ml)	Maximum urine flow (ml/s)	
		5th percentile	95th percentile
3–7	50	8	20
	150	12	24
	300	15	26
8–13	50	8	24
	150	13	28
	300	17	35
>13	50	6	28
	150	11	38
	300	14	44

flow below 10–15 ml/s on repeated testing should be considered low and prompt further investigation (Kaufman 1957, Scott and McIlhaney 1959, Palm and Nielsen 1967, Szabo and Fegyvernski 1995). Table 4.8 can be of some use when evaluating maximum flow rate. Note that values are approximate and that the difference between boys and girls – school-age girls void 1 or 2 ml/s faster than boys (Szabo and Fegyvernski 1995) – is not taken into account.

When evaluating these curves it should, however, always be kept in mind that uroflowmetry gives the opportunity to assess the emptying phase only, not the storage phase. Disorders of the storage phase, such as bladder overactivity, may result in completely normal uroflow curves.

The *bell-shaped curve*, with a smooth unimodal outline and rounded shape (maximum flow usually between 15 and 25 ml/s), is typical for the bladder with a neurologically and urologically normal emptying phase, especially when there is no residual urine. This curve does not, however, rule out detrusor overactivity during the storage phase. A bell-shaped curve is found in more than 90 per cent of normal children (Gutierrez Segura 1997).

The *tower-shaped curve*, with high urine flow (more than, say, 25 ml/s) and short duration, is very common among patients with urge incontinence and should raise the suspicion of detrusor overactivity. The peak often occurs early, in the first third of the micturition. It is not necessarily pathological, however, and some authors see this as a subtype of the bell curve.

The *plateau-shaped curve*, with a protracted but fairly smooth outline and a reduced maximum flow (below 10 ml/s or so), is indicative of outflow obstruction. The suspicion is strengthened if residual urine is present. The plateau-shaped uroflow pattern is an instance where the added information from perineal electrodes is very helpful: if EMG is silent during voiding then the obstruction is probably organic (phimosis, urethral valves or strictures); if not, then the obstruction is functional (dysfunctional voiding or neurogenic bladder with detrusor sphincter dyssynergia). Note, however, that in boys this type of uroflow can also be an artefact due to penile erection.

39

The *staccato curve*, with a ragged mountain-range profile including two or more discrete peaks, although the flow does not reach zero until the voiding is completed, usually indicates that sphincter and pelvic floor contractions occur during voiding, i.e. that dysfunctional voiding is present. It might also just indicate that the child is tense and nervous. EMG confirms the sphincter contractions. Residual urine is common in children with this curve.

The *interrupted curve*, when voiding is split into several discrete amounts with zero flow in between, is a clear indicator that the detrusor is underactive and the child needs to strain to expel urine. Large voided volumes as well as residual urine are usually present. EMG may show continuous or intermittent contractions or be totally silent. This curve, if consistently present during repeated examinations, is highly pathological.

From each uroflow curve one measurement of voided volume (or bladder capacity, in older terminology) can be obtained. Multiple measurements, such as are acquired from a voiding chart, are of course more reliable. For reference ranges see Hjälmås (1988).

A pathological amount of *residual urine* has been variously defined by different authors (Hjälmås 1988, Nørgaard et al 1998). Our suggestion is that the presence of residual urine amounting to more than 10 per cent of the just voided volume – or more than 10 ml in the case of small voidings – on repeated occasions constitutes significant residual urine.

Detection of residual urine is important diagnostically because (1) it represents a risk for UTIs, (2) it indicates acquired retention as a part of the syndrome of voiding post-ponement, and (3) it strengthens the suspicion of outflow obstruction, dysfunctional voiding or detrusor underactivity in children with pathological uroflow curves. But we are treating children, not laboratory measurements – if the child is symptom-free after treatment and gets no UTIs, then a lingering small amount of residual urine is *per se* no reason for follow-up. There are a few pitfalls that one should be aware of when evaluating flowmetry results:

1 *Major decisions should not be based on just one examination.* Any child can produce highly pathological curves or residual urine when nervous or tense (or if the room is not heated). Thus, if the curve looks abnormal, the child should be asked to go away and have something to drink, and then the examination should be repeated once or twice. Or better still, it should be done again another day.

2 *Uroflowmetry can only be reliably evaluated with a reasonably full bladder*, with a volume of at least 80–100 ml, since otherwise straining artefacts will appear.

3 *Abnormal conditions yield abnormal curves.* If the child is overambitious and has waited longer than he or she usually does before going to the toilet, the curve and residual urine may give a false impression of detrusor underactivity, dysfunctional voiding or obstruction. And if the child voids with an unusually small volume the curve will also be very difficult to judge. Flow rate is a function of voided volume (Szabo and Fegyvernski 1995) and cannot be reliably measured if the volume is less than 100 ml.

4 *Severe vesico-ureteral reflux may be mistaken for residual urine.* In these children, urine may empty into the bladder from a dilated ureter as the child moves from the uroflow toilet to the berth for residual measurement.

5 *Artefacts can be induced voluntarily*: some children deliberately interrupt the urine flow (they like the sound this makes, play 'fire-engine' with their urine, etc.).

Ultrasound

The decision whether to undertake ultrasound evaluation of the kidneys and urinary tracts *routinely* in children with voiding disorders is a matter of debate.

Ultrasound can provide a variety of important information and complement the physical examination. Kidney size, medullocortical differentiation, number and position can be determined and anomalies of the upper urinary tract such as hydronephrosis, megaureter and ureterocoele can be detected or ruled out. In the lower urinary tract, bladder wall thickness can be assessed – a thick bladder wall indicating detrusor overactivity (or sphincter overactivity, or cystitis) (Cvitkovic-Kuzmic et al 2002) – provided the bladder is full and measurements are made in the dorsal part of the bladder close to the trigone. Residual urine is readily detected.

Last, but not least, ultrasound can sometimes be useful in the diagnosis and follow-up of constipation. The impression of a filled rectal ampulla bulging retrovesically and displacing the bladder can be seen in constipated children. Rectal diameter can be measured and the course of treatment may be monitored via these variables.

In some countries, such as Germany, an ultrasound assessment is recommended for every child with any voiding disorder. This strategy has many advantages, given the information that can be drawn from the procedure, and makes it very unlikely that structural causes for incontinence are missed, but it requires that every (or almost every) doctor caring for these children is well acquainted with the investigation and has the equipment readily at hand.

In other countries, such as Sweden, the availability of and experience with ultrasound are more or less restricted to radiologists, and the above strategy is not feasible. This situation is still acceptable due to the high awareness and good follow-up of children with UTIs, who are routinely examined with ultrasound.

So the choice of strategy will partly be dependent on availability and regional practices. It should also be remembered that ultrasound is an examiner-dependent examination. If the doctor is not familiar with the procedure he or she might miss important details that a skilled sonographer would detect.

Our recommendation, then, if ultrasound is *not* undertaken routinely, is that it should still be used in the following situations:

1 Children with a history of UTI (even if it was a long time ago)
2 Children with incontinence resistant to standard first- and second-line therapy
3 Whenever urological malformations, such as hydronephrosis, urethral valves or megaureter, are suspected
4 Whenever kidney disease is suspected

Radiology and imaging

MICTURITION CYSTOURETHROGRAM (MCU)

The MCU is a routine examination in infants and young children with pyelonephritis (at least this is the case in Sweden, but traditions differ in some other countries), in order to

41

detect vesico-ureteric reflux (VUR). VUR, as a risk factor for pyelonephritis, is much less common in the child who first develops pyelonephritis after the first two to three years of life (Jodal 2000, Nuutinen and Uhari 2001). Thus, an MCU is only rarely indicated in the older child.

Before the MCU a transurethral catheter is inserted, in surroundings as calm and comfortable as possible, by a well-trained professional. The child, who should be allowed to sit in mother's or father's lap, may, if needed, safely be sedated with midazolam before the procedure (Stokland et al 2003). Radio-opaque contrast is then infused via the catheter

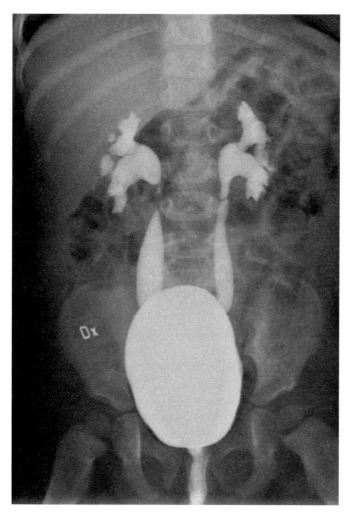

Fig. 4.5 Bilateral dilated vesico-ureteric reflux (grade IV), as visualized by micturating urethrocystography.

and several anteroposterior pictures are taken during filling and voiding. Steep oblique or true lateral views, as well as a picture after the removal of the catheter, are also needed if posterior urethral valves are to be detected or excluded.

Since catheterization during the MCU procedure may introduce virulent bacteria and cause UTI, all children undergoing MCU should receive at least one dose of antibiotic prophylaxis during the hours before or after the examination (with the exception of children who are on clean intermittent catheterization). If the child is already on regular antibiotic prophylaxis one dose of *another* antibiotic should be given in conjunction with the MCU, as the selection pressure from the ongoing prophylaxis will have caused resistant strains to proliferate in the child's perineum or lower urethra.

There are really only two groups of children relevant for this book in whom an MCU is mandatory: (1) children with suspected bladder outlet obstruction (except phimosis) – in which case the MCU will be needed to detect a posterior urethral valve or urethral stenosis; (2) children with cystometrically confirmed neurogenic bladder disturbance.

Incontinent children with a history of febrile UTIs who have dilatation of the upper urinary tract visible on ultrasound may also need an MCU – in this case in order to detect VUR – but it is then the history of pyelonephritis that provides the indication for the examination, not the incontinence.

UROGRAPHY

Urography is of very limited value in children with voiding disorders. It has often been used to detect pyelonephritic kidney scarring, but renal scintigraphy (see below) is a much more reliable technique in such cases. Urography is mandatory in the rare cases of incontinence due to ureteral ectopia. It is also sometimes indicated for the detection of unilateral ureteral duplication when renal scintigraphy has disclosed kidneys of unequal size. The advantage of the technique is that it delineates the anatomy of the (functioning) upper urinary tract in excellent detail. Drawbacks are the irradiation burden and the lack of good kidney visualization (Costello and Cook 2004).

Standard urography includes:

1   A view of the entire area of the urinary tract before contrast injection
2   A film three minutes post-injection, limited to the renal areas
3   A full-length radiograph after 15 minutes

Further, delayed pictures are needed in cases of upper urinary tract obstruction.

MAGNETIC RESONANCE IMAGING (MRI)

Magnetic resonance imaging of the kidneys and urinary tract is developing fast and may in the future play an important role in paediatric nephrology and urology. Advantages of the technique, in addition to the detailed morphological information it gives (Chan et al 1999), are the absence of ionizing radiation and the possibility of assessing function as well as anatomy. Drawbacks are the cost, the time required and the need for the patient to be absolutely immobile during the process. In wetting children the importance of

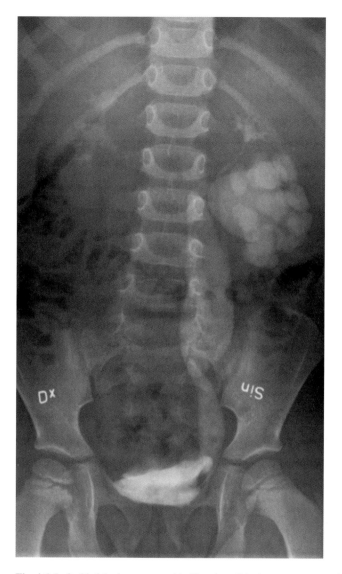

Fig. 4.6 Left-sided duplex ureters with dilatation of the lower system, as visualized by urography.

MRI is, and will probably remain, quite minimal. In encopretic children the same is true – at least for the time being – of MRI of the bowel, with the possible exception of children who have been operated on for congenital anorectal malformations (Hettiarachchi et al 2002).

MRI of the spinal canal, on the other hand, is a routine examination in every child with neurogenic bladder (as indicated by history and uroflowmetry and confirmed by cystometry), or if the physical examination has given rise to the suspicion of spinal dysraphism (Pippi

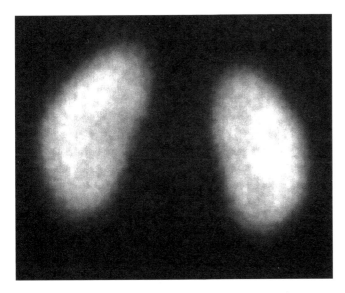

Fig. 4.7 Normal DMSA scintigram.

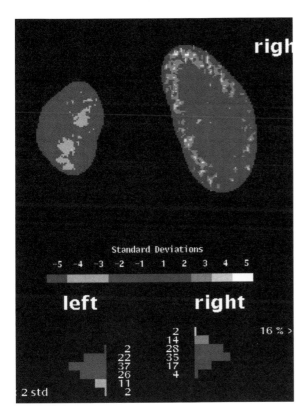

Fig. 4.8 Left-sided kidney damage or hypoplasia, as detected by DMSA scintigraphy.

Salle et al 1998). Suspicions of tethered cord or a spinal tumour are, of course, also indications for spinal MRI.

DIMERCAPTOSUCCINIC ACID (DMSA) SCINTIGRAPHY

The technetium-labelled radioactive marker DMSA is selectively taken up, but not excreted, by the cells of the renal tubules, and therefore provides a good way of visualizing functional renal parenchyma. DMSA scintigraphy has therefore become the criterion standard for assessing and following pyelonephritic renal scarring, but it gives no information about the urinary tract.

The substance is injected intravenously, the adult irradiation dose of 80 Mbq reduced according to the weight of the child, and the images are obtained two hours after the injection. Sedation is not usually required since the time the child needs to be immobile is short (about 10 minutes), repeated scanning attempts can be made, and modern software can usually correct for some degree of moving.

The pictures obtained give good anatomical detail, but it has to be remembered that the function of the kidneys is shown in relative, not absolute, values. Thus, in cases where one small and one large kidney, both with a smooth general contour, are shown, the scintigram cannot reveal whether the larger kidney has ureteral duplication or the smaller kidney is hypoplastic. This situation may call for intravenous urography.

Renal uptake defects on DMSA scintigraphy during the weeks following acute pyelonephritis represent areas of potentially reversible kidney malfunction, and this is in fact a very good instrument to diagnose pyelonephritis in uncertain cases. When used as a means of detecting congenital hypoplasia or irreversible renal scarring – a more common use of the method – DMSA scintigraphy should not be undertaken until six months have elapsed since the latest pyelonephritic episode (Jakobsson et al 1994).

Scintigraphy is indicated when looking for renal scars or renal hypoplasia in children with known urological malformations (VUR, hydronephrosis) or a history of febrile UTI. The latter indication is less strict than the first, with traditions varying between regions and centres; we propose that scintigraphy be undertaken at least in children who have had recurrent pyelonephritis, severe pyelonephritis or a delay in therapeutic response. Needless to say, voiding disorders as such are not an indication for scintigraphy.

One potential problem with DMSA scintigraphy is not that it cannot detect all kidney scars, but that it detects them too well. Small 'scars' with a reduction of the ipsilateral relative kidney function of, say, 5 per cent are easily seen, but are probably of little or no clinical significance (Wennerström et al 2000). One good rule of thumb is to follow up the children, with yearly measurement of blood pressure and albuminuria, if (1) scars result in a relative reduction of kidney function of 10 per cent or more, or (2) if scars are bilateral.

RENOGRAPHY

Dynamic diuresis renography, using technetium-labelled dimercaptoacetyltriglycine (MAG3), is partly similar to DMSA scintigraphy, but the radioactive marker in this case is excreted via tubular secretion and can thus be followed downstream in the upper and lower

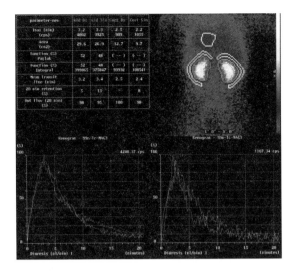

Fig. 4.9 Normal MAG3-renogram. Lower curves represent pelvic (left) and parenchymal (right) detection of the radionuclide.

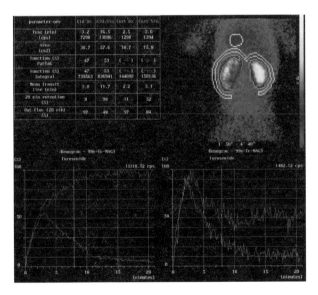

Fig. 4.10 Left-sided hydronephrosis without obstruction, as detected by MAG3-renography. Lower curves represent pelvic (left) and parenchymal (right) detection of the radionuclide. Note the delayed elimination of the nuclide from the left renal pelvis (the upper curve in the lower left diagram), but the basically normal parenchymal curves.

47

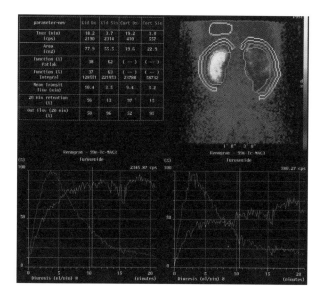

parameter-new	Kid Dx	Kid Sin	Cort Dx	Cort Sin
Tmax (min) (cps)	18.2 2190	3.7 2314	19.2 410	3.0 557
Area (cm2)	77.9	55.5	19.6	22.9
Function (%) Patlak	38	62	(--)	(--)
Function (%) Integral	37 128551	63 221953	(--) 23788	(--) 58732
Mean Transit Time (min)	10.4	3.5	9.4	3.2
20 min retention (%)	96	13	97	15
Out flow (20 min) (%)	50	96	52	95

Renogram - 99m-Tc-MAG3
Furosemide
2345.87 cps
Diuresis (ml/min) 8 (minutes)

Renogram - 99m-Tc-MAG3
Furosemide
580.27 cps
Diuresis (ml/min) 8 (minutes)

Fig. 4.11 Right-sided hydronephrosis and obstruction, as detected by MAG3-renography. Lower curves represent pelvic (left) and parenchymal (right) detection of the radionuclide. Note the delayed and diminished parenchymal uptake in the right kidney (lower right diagram) and the delayed elimination from the renal pelvis of the same side (lower left diagram).

urinary tract by repeated imaging and by continuous detection of irradiation from various anatomical fields of interest. MAG3 renography also allows for the calculation of approximate absolute renal function, i.e. the estimation of glomerular filtration rate, for each kidney. By analysing time–activity curves during the excretory phase, obstructive and non-obstructive hydronephrosis can often be distinguished. An additional bonus of the technique is that indirect cystographic images can be obtained in children who are able to micturate when asked to. In this way VUR may be detected, although not graded, in older children without the need for an indwelling urethral catheter. The main drawback, compared to DMSA scintigraphy, is that MAG3 gives poorer anatomical detail of the kidneys. Diethylenetriamine pentaacetic acid (DTPA) is an alternative but slightly inferior marker which is used in the same way as MAG3.

MAG3 is injected intravenously in the normally hydrated child, the irradiation dose calculated from the child's surface area, and the loop-diuretic furosemide is injected after 16 minutes to increase diuresis. Several images are taken and time–activity curves are followed over the renal areas (and bladder if indirect cystography is needed). The images and curves are interpreted together. Renal scarring is detected in the first images, representing the nephrogenic phase before excretion of the marker, whereas the following images and curves, especially after furosemide injection, give information about obstruction, dilatation and reflux.

The main indication for MAG3 renography is in the investigation of suspected supravesical obstruction detected by ultrasound. As mentioned above, it may also be used to screen for VUR in older children. Bladder or bowel disturbances *per se* do not constitute indications for MAG3 scintigraphy.

Table 4.14 shows the relative value of various imaging techniques.

X-RAY EVALUATION OF THE BOWEL

In children with voiding disorders we often need to look for constipation. We are then faced with the problem that examinations are either cumbersome or unvalidated, or both.

Plain X-ray of the abdomen is straightforward in cases of outright coprostasis but of limited use in the detection of 'ordinary' constipation. Various techniques have been developed to evaluate the degree of faecal impaction (Barr et al 1979, Blethyn et al 1995, Leech et al 1999), mostly based on the quantification of sigmoid and left colon content, but none has so far gained universal acceptance (Fotter 1998). X-ray is therefore not recommended.

X-ray of the bowel using ordinary single- or double-contrast techniques is of limited use in voiding disorders. Colonoscopy with biopsy would be the first choice if inflammatory bowel disease is suspected, and computed tomography if an abdominal tumour needs to be excluded.

TABLE 4.14
The relative value of various studies in the evaluation of the kidneys and urinary tract

	Anatomy			Function		
	Kidney	Upper urinary tract	Lower urinary tract	Kidney	Upper urinary tract	Lower urinary tract
Ultrasound	+++	++	++	–	–	–
Plain abdominal X-ray	+	–	–	–	–	–
Urography	++	++++	+	++	++	+
Micturating cystourethrography	–	– (+++ if reflux)	++++	–	++	++
Computerized tomography	++++	+++	++	++	++	+
Magnetic resonance imaging	++++	+++	++	++	++	+
DMSA scintigraphy	+++	–	–	++++	–	–
MAG3/DTPA scintigraphy	++	+	+	++++	++++	+
Uroflowmetry & residual urine	–	–	–	+	–	+++
Cystometry	–	–	–	+	++	++++
Cystoscopy	–	+	++++	–	+	++
Micturition charts	–	–	+	++	–	++

COLONIC TRANSIT TIME

The measurement of *colonic transit time*, with either radio-opaque or radioactive markers, is a more logical approach, since by these methods the markers can be followed through the gastrointestinal canal and a true estimate obtained of transit time in different parts of the bowel (Arhan et al 1989, Papadopoulou et al 1994, Bouchoucha and Thomas 2000). A delay of the markers in the colon is fairly diagnostic of constipation. The drawbacks of this examination are radiation dose (several photos need to be taken) and the time and work that needs to be allotted to every examination.

The *corn test* is a logically appealing, though not scientifically validated, method of getting a rough estimate of gastrointestinal transit time and thus screening for constipation. The principle is simple: the child is asked to swallow ten kernels of sweetcorn and the time that elapses before they come out again is then measured – 36 hours or more indicates constipation. Future research will determine if this examination has a role in the evaluation or follow-up of constipated children.

Cystoscopy and colonoscopy

CYSTOSCOPY

Cystoscopy is indicated when there is suspicion of urethral obstruction, or in the few cases where the bladder or urethra needs to be observed or operated on. In many children with ectopic ureters, double ureters and ureterocoele, operative correction is performed at the time of diagnosic cystoscopy. See also below regarding endoscopic treatment of VUR. Boys with urethral valves are obvious candidates for cystoscopy, as are children with suspected bladder haemorrhages, but these children are not the subject of this book.

Cystoscopy may also be considered in some children with severe, recurrent and painful cystitis. In these cases, follicular cystitis, or a bladder lumen which is irritated for other reasons, may be observed. Obviously, cystoscopy is more commonly required in the adult population in whom diagnoses such as interstitial cystitis, neoplasia or bladder stones may need to be excluded. Incontinence or UTIs (including haemorrhagic cystitis) *per se* do not constitute indications for cystoscopy, if they are not caused by obstruction in the lower urinary tract.

COLONOSCOPY

Colonoscopy is the examination of choice whenever inflammatory bowel disease – such as Crohn's disease or ulcerative colitis – is seriously considered. As mentioned above, patients with Hirschsprung disease should also undergo this examination. *Gastroscopy* is often performed in the same session, since inflammatory bowel disease can involve the upper as well as the lower gastrointestinal tract. Gastroscopy with a duodenal biopsy is still part of the evaluation of children with celiac disease.

Physiological examinations

Four-hour Micturition Observation

Four-hour micturition observation is a useful urodynamic screening method in children who are too young to urinate on the uroflow apparatus. Briefly, the child is observed on the ward for four hours, the diaper (nappy) is checked every ten minutes and residual urine (via ultrasound) and diaper weight are measured after every voiding. With this now scientifically validated procedure (Hanson et al 1995, Holmdahl et al 1996, Sillén et al 1999) cystometry may not be necessary in many children and those who need to be further evaluated with cystometry and/or MRI can usually be detected. It is mostly used in infants, and the relevance for this book is thus limited.

Cystometry

Cystometry is the only method by which bladder function can be evaluated directly and in detail. With continuous assessment of detrusor pressure and sphincter activity during filling and voiding a precise diagnosis can be arrived at for most disturbances of the lower urinary tract. Consequently it is the standard examination for detecting and following up children with neurogenic bladder disturbances. Given the fact that the normal detrusor is silent during filling and active during voiding, and the normal sphincter has the opposite function, cystometry can give a limited number of primary diagnoses: normal bladder function, detrusor overactivity during storage, acontractile/underactive detrusor during voiding, urethral incompetence during filling, or inappropriate obstruction during voiding. The compliance, or distensibility, of the bladder during filling can also be assessed during the filling phase, and various measurements of bladder volume can be made (maximum volume, volume at first bladder sensation, etc). For a simplified scheme of cystometrically detectable pathology, see Table 4.15.

During cystometry intravesical pressure is measured with a catheter inserted either via the urethra or suprapubically (in the latter case under general anaesthesia), while intra-abdominal pressure is estimated with a catheter placed in the rectum. The detrusor pressure curve is acquired by electronically subtracting the intra-abdominal pressure from the intravesical pressure. Whilst detrusor function can be assessed directly by looking at the detrusor pressure curve, urethral function must be inferred from pressure changes

TABLE 4.15
Simplified abnormalities detectable by cystometry

	Storage phase	Voiding phase
Detrusor	Detrusor overactivity Low bladder compliance	Detrusor underactivity Acontractile detrusor
Urethra	Incompetence (with leakage with or without raised intra-abdominal pressure)	Functional obstruction (detrusor–sphincter dyssynergia) Anatomic obstruction

within the bladder and by measuring urine flow and leakage. Just as was the case with uroflowmetry, additional sphincter information can be obtained by using surface electrodes to record pelvic floor muscular activity. This is of value especially in children with dysfunctional voiding or neurogenic detrusor–sphincter dyssynergia. In cooperative children it is standard practice to test sphincteric competence several times during filling by asking them to raise intra-abdominal pressure by straining or coughing. For more technical and practical details about how to perform cystometry the reader is referred to specific handbooks such as Abrams (1997).

Basically, cystometries can be of two kinds: *standard cystometry*, during which water or physiological saline is infused into the bladder via a catheter (either a separate catheter or a second lumen of the one used for measurement of intravesical pressure); and *ambulatory* (or natural-fill) *cystometry*. During the latter investigation the bladder is only filled with the patient's own urine and detrusor pressure is measured, via a suprapubic catheter, over one or several days and nights while the patient goes about his or her daily activities, the pressure data being fed into a small box that can be carried on the belt or in a rucksack. This also gives the child or parents the opportunity to note the time of events such as incontinence, bladder cramps or urgency symptoms, which can then be correlated with data from the recording box.

If cystometry were a simple examination that was comfortable for the patient and did not take lots of time it would be performed as a standard, second-line assessment in children with therapy-resistant incontinence or enuresis, since it would certainly give useful information regarding the nature of the underlying bladder disturbance. Sadly, this is not the case. Cystometry is often painful or at least uncomfortable for the child and it demands a lot of time and effort from both nurse and doctor. Artefacts are not uncommon and skill is needed to evaluate the recordings. And if the probably superior ambulatory natural-fill technique is to be used, the child will have to be admitted to hospital for suprapubic catheter insertion under general anaesthesia. These drawbacks, and the scarcity of findings in, for instance, enuretic children, have limited the indications for cystometry in children with voiding disorders to those cases in which neurogenic bladder disturbance is suspected. This means that cystometry should be considered in children who on repeated uroflow measurements provide staccato, interrupted or plateau-shaped curves, especially when combined with residual urine, or if urotherapy does not ameliorate the situation. In the case of the plateau-shaped curve, obstruction should be suspected and cystoscopy and MCU may be indicated prior to cystometry.

The main indication for ambulatory cystometry outside the research setting is to confirm the incontinent patient's history if standard cystometry has turned out normal, and to detect whether detrusor overactivity or sphincter incompetence is causing incontinence in a patient who may suffer from both disturbances. It is also of great value in infants, since urethral catheterization in this group often gives results that are difficult to interpret. It can also be used in children who have attacks of suprapubic pains or bladder spasms which may or may not be caused by detrusor contractions. When evaluating cystometric data the correlation with subjective symptoms is crucial, and especially so in the ambulatory setting. This is illustrated by the finding that 41 per cent of adult volunteers without any subjective urinary complaints exhibited involuntary detrusor contractions on ambulatory cystometry (Heslington and Hilton 1996).

VIDEOCYSTOMETRY

Videocystometry is the combination of cystometry and micturating cystourethrography. It is used in many patients with neurogenic bladder disturbance to explore bladder/urethral anatomy and the presence or absence of vesico-ureteric reflux as well as bladder/sphincter function (Hoebeke et al 2001). Two catheters – or one double-lumen catheter – are inserted urethrally or suprapubically to permit simultaneous filling of radiographic contrast and registration of intravesical pressure. A rectal balloon catheter records intra-abdominal pressure which is then subtracted from the intravesical pressure to obtain intrinsic detrusor pressure.

ICE-WATER TEST

The *ice-water test*, or *bladder cooling reflex*, in which cold water is instilled into the bladder to detect the presence or absence of uninhibited detrusor contractions, is sometimes used in the differential diagnostic evaluation of neurogenic bladder disturbance. It has been likened to Babinski's sign and the other neonatal reflexes in that it is normally positive in neonates, turns negative during growth (at approximately 2 to 4 years of age) and becomes positive again in cases of central neuropathology (Geirsson et al 1999, Gladh et al 2004). The sensitivity and specificity of the procedure as a tool in the detection of neurogenic bladder disturbance, 65 per cent and 85 per cent, respectively, are not high enough to make it clinically very useful (Petersen et al 1997). The greatest role for the ice-water test is perhaps in the research setting.

THIRST PROVOCATION, DESMOPRESSIN TEST

These are examinations that are indicated when there is a suspicion of central or nephrogenic diabetes insipidus, i.e. in the evaluation of children with excessive thirst who have no glucosuria. There are various ways to perform a thirst provocation test (Miller et al 1970, Czernichow et al 1979) – and the reader is strongly advised to consult nephrological or endocrinological handbooks before choosing which method to use – but what they have in common is that plasma and urine osmolality are followed closely over a period of time (usually 12 to 24 hours) during which the child is denied fluid intake. Measurements of vasopressin in plasma or urine may be added, but the tests are costly and time-consuming and values are often hard to interpret (Zerbe and Robertson 1981). Furthermore, although short, ambulatory thirst deprivation tests have been proposed as alternatives to the strategy outlined above (Dunger et al 1988, Shimura 1993), it has to be pointed out that fluid restriction in a child with full-blown diabetes insipidus is potentially dangerous, with a definitive risk for hypernatremia and cerebral oedema, if the electrolyte balance of the child is not checked at short time intervals throughout the provocation.

In the presence of sufficient vasopressin secretion *and* intact renal response to the hormone, urine osmolality will rise and plasma osmolality will remain normal throughout the thirst provocation. This rules out diabetes insipidus. If, however, the results are the opposite, then the next step should be to see whether the polyuria responds to exogenous hormone administration or not – i.e. if it is a case of central or renal diabetes insipidus. This is easily done: urine osmolality is tested before and after desmopressin administration; if it rises, then central diabetes insipidus is the likely cause; if not, then a renal defect is probable (see below). One way to do this in practice is to give the child desmopressin 0.4 mg orally or 40 μg intranasally in the evening, let him or her sleep at home with permission to drink if thirsty, and then test the osmolality of the first urine sample the following morning.

The simple measurement of urine osmolality after an overnight thirst provocation has been used in enuresis research and has shown that children with enuresis responsive to desmopressin therapy tend to concentrate urine more poorly than non-responders (Nevéus et al 1999b, 2001b). However, the clinical usefulness of this procedure as a way of predicting therapy response is meagre, since there is a wide overlap in the urine osmolality of responders and non-responders (Eller et al 1997, Nevéus 2001), and a simpler way to test therapy response is to just test the therapy.

ANAL MANOMETRY
Anal manometry was previously often used in constipated or encopretic children, but recent studies have shown that the diagnostic value in this situation is not satisfactory. Only in children with Hirschsprung's disease is manometry useful, but then a colonoscopy is needed as well to obtain biopsies. And patients with Hirschsprung's disease (before surgery) are only rarely faecally incontinent. Children with encopresis due to earlier anorectal surgery may also be candidates for manometry (Hettiarachchi et al 2002).

Psychological and psychiatric assessment

REASONS FOR ASSESSMENT
There are two major reasons why it is important to address psychological issues in children with voiding disorders:

1   As can be seen in Table 4.9, the rate of comorbid behavioural and emotional disorders is much higher than for possible organic causes. Thus, even paediatricians and urologists should have a basic understanding of psychological principles if they are to treat their young patients adequately.
2   In functional voiding disorders, provision of information, cognitive therapy and behavioural modification are the most effective, first-line approaches to treatment. Medication can be helpful in many cases, but is usually not the mainstay of treatment. Surgery is rarely indicated.

RATE OF BEHAVIOURAL DISTURBANCES
The rate of clinically relevant behavioural disorders in children and adolescents lies between 12.0 per cent (ICD-10 criteria) and 14.3 per cent (DSM-IV criteria) (Bird 1996). This overall rate is around the same in most cultures. Epidemiological studies have also shown that children with wetting problems are more prone to develop comorbid psychological problems.

One practical way to differentiate psychological problems is to divide them into manifest child psychiatric disturbances of clinical relevance, and subclinical symptoms such as sad affect, social withdrawal and lower self-esteem, which can be extremely distressing for children and parents, but are often understandable reactions to the wetting problem and not a disorder *per se*.

COMORBIDITY

In this context, it is most practical to focus on comorbidity, i.e. the coexistence of wetting and psychological disturbances and symptoms. Dealing with questions of causality can often be confusing and speculative, as basically four different associations of psychological symptoms and wetting can be differentiated:

1   Behavioural disorder can be a consequence of the wetting problem.
2   Behavioural disorder can precede and induce a relapse when a genetic disposition for enuresis is present, for example in secondary nocturnal enuresis.
3   Wetting and behavioural disorder can both be due to a common neurobiological dysfunction (such as in nocturnal enuresis and ADHD).
4   Finally, with such common disorders, there may be no causal relationship and the two may coexist by chance.

Therefore, it is wise to adopt a descriptive approach and report the empirical facts available regarding the comorbidity of enuresis/urinary incontinence and psychological disorders.

CLINICALLY RELEVANT PSYCHIATRIC DISORDERS

There are no good general definitions for psychiatric disorders. Synonyms that are in use include 'psychiatric', 'psychic', 'psychological' or 'mental' disorder or disturbance. All

TABLE 4.9
Organic causes and comorbidity of clinically relevant psychological disorders or symptom scores*

Nocturnal enuresis	
Organic causes	< 1%
Behavioural comorbidity*	20–30%
Urinary incontinence	
Organic causes	< 10%
Behavioural comorbidity*	20–40%
Encopresis with constipation	
Organic causes	< 5%
Behavioural comorbidity*	30–50%
Encopresis without constipation	
Organic causes	< 1%
Behavioural comorbidity*	30–50%

* comparable norms: 10%

55

these terms indicate that there is 'a clinically significant behavioural or psychological syndrome or pattern (not a variant of normal behaviour) that occurs in an individual, that it is associated with present distress, disability or impairment and carries a risk for the future development of the individual' (DSM-IV, APA 1994).

METHODS OF ASSESSMENT: CATEGORICAL AND DIMENSIONAL
Clinically relevant disorders can be assessed by two basic methods: the categorical and the dimensional. The categorical method is based on a detailed diagnostic process (including history, observation, exploration, mental state examination, questionnaires, testing, physical examination and other procedures) and is a professional diagnosis according to standardized classification schemes: ICD-10 (WHO 1993) or DSM-IV (APA 1994). Dimensional assessment is based on symptom scores from questionnaires. Cut-offs are then defined to delineate a clinical (and subclinical) range. A widely used cut-off for the clinical range is the 90th percentile. Symptom scores are never a diagnosis, but reflect the view of the informant. The best-known parental questionnaire is the CBCL (Child Behavior Checklist, Achenbach 1991).

One can differentiate externalizing or behavioural disorders with outwardly-directed visible behaviour (examples include conduct disorders, ADHD, etc.); internalizing, i.e. inwardly-directed, intrapsychical disorders such as emotional disorders (examples include separation anxiety, social anxiety, phobias, sibling rivalry, depressive disorders, etc.); and other disorders that do not fit into these two categories, such as anorexia nervosa, tic disorders, autistic syndromes, etc.

Children with voiding disorders show a higher rate of comorbid behavioural and emotional problems than non-wetting children. The rates in epidemiological and clinical studies are approximately the same: 13.5 to 40.1 per cent of all wetting children have clinically relevant behavioural problems (according to questionnaires such as the CBCL and psychiatric diagnoses). The relative risk is 1.3 to 4.5 times higher (von Gontard 2002).

In general, children with day wetting problems have a slightly higher rate of behavioural disorders than children with nocturnal enuresis. The results of our own study (von Gontard et al 1999a) are shown in Table 4.10: 40 per cent of children fulfilled the criteria for at least one ICD-10 diagnosis, and more day-wetting (53 per cent) than night-wetting children were affected.

Regarding the specific comorbidity of the different forms of wetting, children with primary nocturnal enuresis have the lowest rate of psychiatric problems. The rate in the subgroup with monosymptomatic primary nocturnal enuresis is no higher than in the general population. Of the day-wetting children, those with urge incontinence have a low rate of comorbidity; those with voiding postponement syndrome, in contrast, a high rate. The highest rate of comorbid psychiatric disorders can be found among the children with secondary nocturnal enuresis. Children with encopresis have much higher rates of behavioural and emotional disorders than children with wetting problems – and if children soil and wet, the rates are even higher (von Gontard and Hollmann 2004). Details will be presented in the individual chapters.

TABLE 4.10
ICD-10 diagnoses (multiple diagnoses possible) in 167 children aged 5–11 years with nocturnal enuresis and functional urinary incontinence (von Gontard et al 1999a)

Type of diagnosis	Day wetting (n=57)	Night wetting (n=110)	Total
Externalizing disorders	28.1%	17.3%	21.0%
Hyperkinetic syndrome	10.5%	9.1%	9.6%
Conduct disorder	17.5%	8.2%	11.4%
Internalizing (emotional) disorders	19.5%	8.2%	12.0%
Encopresis	24.6%	5.5%	12.0%
Others	3.5%	7.3%	6.0%
At least one ICD-10 diagnosis	52.6%	33.6%	40.1%

IMPACT ON CHILDREN

Most children are distressed by enuresis and urinary incontinence. For example, in one study (40 children aged 5–15 years, Morison et al 2000), 35 per cent said that they felt unhappy, 25 per cent even very unhappy, about wetting at night. In a Finnish population-based study (Moilanen et al 1987), 156 day- and night-wetting children (from 3375 7-year-olds) showed significant differences ($p < .01$) compared to 170 controls regarding the following personality traits: they were more fitful (vs. peaceful), more fearful (vs. coura-geous), more impatient (vs. calm), more anxious (vs. does not worry) and had more inferiority feelings (vs. feels equal).

The results of our own study (Sonnenschein 2001) of 165 day- and night-wetting children aged 5 to 11 years are shown in Table 4.11.

TABLE 4.11
Disadvantages described by children with enuresis/urinary incontinence in a structured interview (n=165) (Sonnenschein 2001)

Consequences of wetting	
DISADVANTAGES	70.3%
Social: I can't sleep at friend's house, friends can't stay overnight	32.1%
Affect: I feel sad, ashamed, annoyed	16.4%
Isolation: I feel like a baby, nobody is allowed to know about it, I feel different from other children	6.7%
Sensation: It feels unpleasant, cold, wet, itchy, nasty	32.1%
Direct consequences: I have to take a shower, sleep in pampers, I won't get a bicycle	17.6%
ADVANTAGES	
I like the wet feeling; get more attention from mother	4.9%

Behavioural and psychiatric assessment

SCREENING

Due to the high comorbidity of behavioural symptoms and disturbances, every child should be screened for coexisting psychological problems as part of the routine assessment. Those risk groups mentioned should of course undergo an especially careful screening and assessment.

The best screening instrument is still a good history and careful clinical observation. Studies have shown that paediatricians are not experienced in picking up behavioural disorders in children and tend to overlook them (Chang et al 1988). The same probably holds true for paediatric urologists and surgeons as well, while many urotherapists, who work very closely with their families, have often acquired greater skill in dealing with psychological issues.

The second best approach is the use of screening questionnaires (see Appendices 3–5 for examples). These are simple, yes/no questionnaires. If the screening questionnaire flags up areas that need further investigation, a standardized, validated questionnaire such as the Child Behavior Checklist (CBCL, Achenbach 1991) should then be used. If it is possible as part of the clinical routine, it is preferable to start with the CBCL questionnaire as a screening instrument in the first place.

If the child has no or only subclinical symptoms, the voiding disorder should be treated with a symptom-oriented approach. Once a child stops wetting or soiling, many of these symptoms will recede and disappear. If, however, a behavioural or emotional disorder is suspected, a full child psychiatric assessment should follow.

CHILD PSYCHIATRIC ASSESSMENT

As in other medical fields, this is a professional procedure with the goal of coming to a categorical decision: to see if a diagnosis is possible or not. In contrast, all questionnaires, even the standardized ones, reflect the view of the informant and can never produce or replace a professional diagnosis. The diagnostic assessment of behavioural problems in children is a procedure that requires time and cannot be rushed. A minimum of 60 to 90 minutes is required for the first contact, which usually takes place with parent(s) and child together.

The first step is a detailed developmental, behavioural and family history, with much greater detail than provided in the outline in Appendix 1. The next step is to observe the child as well as the parent–child interaction. An interview with the child follows, in which the child is asked directly regarding his or her views, thoughts, emotions and behaviour. Some problems, such as suicidal ideas or depressive emotions, cannot be assessed sufficiently merely by observing the child or by asking the parents. The child (or adolescent) needs to asked, skilfully and directly. Children are usually relieved if they are asked about things they are worrying about. If the symptoms are not there, they will let you know.

The information gained from history, observation and exploration form the basis of the mental state examination. This is a descriptive, phenomenological assessment of cognitive and behavioural signs and symptoms. Mental state examinations have been adapted to the specific developmental stages of children and adolescents. They often follow a checklist principle for easier use in clinical practice. The severity of signs and symptoms is simply ticked off on a four-point scale. A glossary with examples is provided for training and research purposes (CASCAP-D, Döpfner et al 1999).

QUESTIONNAIRES

Questionnaires are an essential part of child psychiatric assessment. They are a time-economical way to gather information from different informants. They can contribute towards but do not provide a diagnosis. Different types of questionnaires can be used: specific questionnaires for voiding disorders and behavioural questionnaires.

Some of the specific voiding questionnaires appear in the Appendices and will be referred to in the text. In addition, voiding questionnaires addressing specific aspects have been developed, for example by Butler (1994), to assess the subjective views and attributions of parents and children. These can be important in special cases – for example, in children with low self-esteem and motivation. Also, if parental intolerance is suspected, these questionnaires are of great use. Parental intolerance was described by Butler (1994) and denotes a risk factor for interactional problems and parental aggression towards the child – even culminating in punishment and physical maltreatment. It develops if parents believe that children are wetting or soiling on purpose to provoke the parents. Nocturnal enuresis is never volitional, while day wetting and soiling can, in rare cases, have a voluntary component. In any case, the mere assumption that the child is doing it on purpose is detrimental to the treatment process. In these cases, special wetting questionnaires can be of great help, although they are not necessary in routine assessment (Butler 1994).

Behavioural questionnaires can be divided into general and specific questionnaires. The best-known, most widely used general parental questionnaire is the Child Behavior Checklist, which has been translated into many languages (CBCL/4–18, Achenbach 1991). Also, local norms exist in many countries. This questionnaire can be used in three different ways: it can be employed in a purely clinical fashion by looking at the marked items and discussing these with the parents. In more refined clinical use, the scales can be evaluated and compared to population-based norm values. Finally, the CBCL can be used in research, as shown in the later chapters on the specific disorders. The advantage of an internationally established questionnaire is that results across studies and countries can be compared.

The CBCL consists of two parts. In the first part, the child's competences, abilities, interests and positive aspects of behaviour are assessed. This is of great interest clinically, but, unfortunately, the psychometric quality is often not sufficient for research. The second part consists of 113 empirically derived behavioural items. These are checked on a three-point scale and are formulated using simple wording, so that parents of even a low educational background have no problems in filling out the questionnaire. From these items, eight specific syndrome scales and three general scales can be calculated. Examples include 'anxious/depressed' and 'delinquent behavioural problems'. The general scales allow calculation of a total behavioural score, as well as specific internalizing and externalizing problems. After adding up the raw scores, the T-values based on the normative population can be calculated. By allowing a comparison with children in the normal population,

59

clinically relevant information can be gained – for example, it can be seen that children show behavioural problems that are clearly in the clinical range, in the borderline range or in the normal, subclinical range. For the specific syndrome scales, the clinical range is defined by a cut-off at the 98th percentile (i.e. 2 per cent of children in the population would be clinically deviant), and the borderline range at the 95th percentile (i.e. 5 per cent would be borderline or clinically deviant). For the general scales (internalizing, externalizing, total score), the cut-offs are different: at the 90th percentile for the clinical range (i.e. 10 per cent clinically deviant), and at the 85th percentile for the borderline range (i.e. 15 per cent borderline or clinically deviant).

Achenbach and co-workers have also produced a whole 'family' of questionnaires for different age groups (infants, children, adolescents, young adults) and different informants (parents, teachers, and children themselves starting from age 11) (see Table 4.12). The advantage of using same-format questionnaires is that comparisons across age groups and informants are possible. Of course, other good questionnaires exist, but the CBCL family has become the 'market leader' in this field.

In addition, other specific questionnaires address circumscribed areas or constructs. For example, questionnaires addressing depressive syndromes or ADHD problems can be very useful in addition to the CBCL if these disorders are suspected.

One construct of special interest in children with voiding disorders is that of 'self-esteem' or self-worth. This is thought to be an important construct in mental health and denotes the subjective appraisal of symptoms by the children themselves. Well-known self-esteem questionnaires include the Piers–Harris Children's Self-concept Scale (Piers 1984) as well as others (Butler 2001). Although self-esteem is not always lower in children with voiding disorders, it has been shown repeatedly that self-esteem increases when children achieve dryness (Longstaffe et al 2000).

Another important construct is that of health-related quality of life (HQOL). This is a complex construct which tries to assess health-related well-being in different domains of daily life. Generic HQOL questionnaires allow comparisons between children with different medical disorders (Eiser and Morse 2001, Matza et al 2004). They range from short screening to longer, more detailed questionnaires (such as the KINDLR questionnaire,

TABLE 4.12
Achenbach questionnaires for different age groups and different informants

Ages (years)	Parent	Self	Teacher
1½–5	CBCL 1½–5		C-TRF
4–18	CBCL 4–18		TRF
11–18		YSR	
18–30	YABCL	YASR	

C-TRF: Caregiver-Teacher Report Form
TRF: Teacher Report Form
YSR: Youth Self Report
YABCL: Young Adult Behavior Checklist
YASR: Young Adult Self Report

Ravens-Sieberer and Bullinger 2000). Thus, it could be shown that high 'quality of life' correlated positively with adaptive everyday and illness-related coping strategies (Stauber et al 2005). Recently the first specific quality of life questionnaire for children with wetting problems was developed by Bower et al (2004). This has the advantage that the specific, voiding-related effects on daily life can be assessed. It has the disadvantage that comparisons with other disorders are no longer possible. Another potentially useful questionnaire addresses aspects of the everyday burden of enuresis (but not specifically quality of life) on children and their families (Landgraf et al 2004).

In general, questionnaires can be used reliably in children aged 8 years or older. In younger children methodological problems in assessment have to be considered in order to gain reliable information. Some younger children will require assistance in filling out the questionnaires. In other children, a structured interview would be preferable. In contrast to questionnaires, psychological testing is time-consuming as it has to be performed by a professional. Thus, it needs a special indication and is not performed routinely even in child psychiatric clinics.

STRUCTURED INTERVIEW

Structured interviews can be performed even in very young children and enable an assessment of their subjective view. If children are interviewed alone, without their parents, conflicts of loyalty or effects of social desirability can be avoided. A structured interview for children with nocturnal enuresis was developed by Butler (1987) and has been adapted for specific clinical settings, even for day-wetting children (von Gontard and Lehmkuhl 2002). Table 4.11 reveals information gained from structured interviews.

Another useful technique is to let the children draw how they feel after a wet night (Butler 1987). In an adaptation of this technique, children are asked to draw how they feel after both a dry and a wet night (von Gontard and Lehmkuhl 2002). Most of the children will produce a sad or distressed expression of their feelings following a wet night. These pictures can be a useful starting point for exploring the child's subjective distress (see Fig. 4.3).

Also, children can be asked about what they know about body image and function (see Fig. 4.4). In one study (von Gontard et al 1999b), 44 per cent of children aged 5 to 10 years expressed the view that fluids passed through a 'tube' from their mouth to their genitalia (see Table 4.13). Two-thirds had no idea that they had a bladder. This means that children usually do not have sufficient knowledge of the anatomy or physiology of the bladder and need this information for treatment to be successful.

COGNITIVE TESTS

An intelligence test is not routinely indicated in the assessment of children with voiding disorders, as IQ is in the normal range for most children with wetting and soiling problems. However, the rate of voiding disorders is clearly increased in children with general developmental disorders with cognitive and physical disability (Roijen et al 2001, Van Laecke et al 2001). The rate of wetting increases with the degree of mental retardation.[1] In

---

[1] Equivalent UK usage: learning disability.

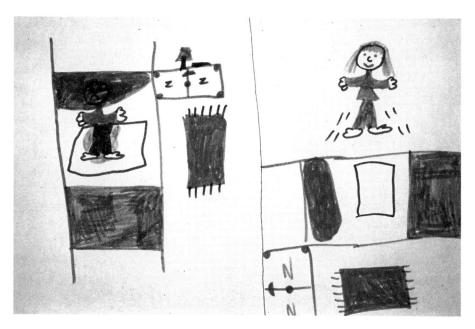

Fig. 4.3 Feelings after a wet night (left) and a dry night (right): the emotions expressed differ greatly. (Reprinted with permission from von Gontard 2001.)

a population-based study of 7-year-old children, the rates for nocturnal (and daytime) wetting were: for mild mental retardation 11 per cent (17 per cent), for moderate 44 per cent (40 per cent), for severe 33 per cent (38 per cent), and for profound 100 per cent (100 per cent) (von Wendt et al 1990).

If lower intelligence is suspected, one can perform either a general screening test, such as the one-dimensional Culture Fair Intelligence Test (CFT1-20, Catell et al 1997), or the CPM and SPM Raven tests (Becker et al 1980). On the other hand, multidimensional intelligence tests will provide a differentiated cognitive profile with specific individual weaknesses and strengths. Therefore, if time allows, multidimensional tests, such as the Kaufman Assessment Battery for Children (K-ABC) (Kaufman and Kaufman 1983) or the Wechsler tests, are to be preferred.

Specific Developmental Tests
Specific developmental disorders are also associated with higher rates of wetting and soiling problems. These are defined by marked, circumscribed deficits in certain areas, compared to general abilities in a normal range. Specific developmental disorders can affect areas such as reading and writing (dyslexia), arithmetic (dyscalculia), speech and language, as well as motor abilities. In the cases of dyslexia and dyscalculia, specific tests for spelling and arithmetic are required in addition to an intelligence test. If the results of the two differ significantly, by 1.5 standard deviations, a diagnosis is possible.

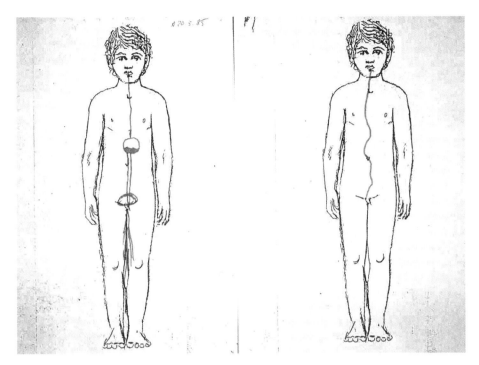

Fig. 4.4 Body concept: children were asked to draw where they believed urine came from; the most common concept was one of a tube leading from the mouth to the genitals (right); a more differentiated view (left) included stomach and bladder; both illustrate that children are not aware of basic anatomical facts, which have to be taught for urotherapy to be effective.

TABLE 4.13

Children's concepts of body function (where does the urine come from? – questions and drawings) (von Gontard et al 1999b)

Children's concepts of where urine comes from	Percentage (n=165)
No idea	10.3%
Tube	44.2%
Any additional organ involved	45.5%
Genitals	35.2%
Bladder	33.9%
Kidneys	6.1%
Other organs	1.8%

Disorders of speech or language (such as articulation, expressive and receptive speech disorders) require a detailed assessment by an audiologist and speech therapist.

Motor disorders can be assessed clinically by including 'soft' neurological signs in the physical examination of children. For research, a standardized assessment of motor abilities can be used, such as the Zurich Motor Tests (Largo et al 2001a, 2001b).

In addition to intelligence and specific developmental tests, projective tests can be useful for assessing the child's subjective view of his or her family. In the Family-as-Animals test (Brem-Gräser 1995), children are asked to draw the members of their family as animals. Although the psychometric properties are low, this clinically useful, easy to perform test is in widespread use in many child psychiatric departments.

More differentiated family diagnostic tests include the Family Relations Test (Anthony and Bene 1957). Children are asked to assign positive as well as negative messages to their family members. These can be calculated and compared to norms (Flämig and Wörner 1977). The test enables an assessment of the subjective view of children regarding the feelings they perceive towards and from family members.

OTHER TESTS IN CHILD PSYCHIATRY

As in other areas of medicine, each child is examined physically and an EEG is often performed as a general screening instrument to exclude seizures, as well as focal abnormalities in CNS function. If indicated, CT, MRI and other laboratory tests including chromosome and molecular genetic analyses are performed.

CHILD PSYCHIATRIC DIAGNOSES

After the diagnostic process has been completed, the child's disorder is diagnosed according to standardized classification schemes. The two standard classification systems are the ICD-10 (WHO 1993), which is widely used in Europe and in other parts of the world, and the DSM-IV (APA 1994) which is used in the United States. For some disorders, the two classification schemes are remarkably similar, while for others, such as ADHD, they differ greatly.

In contrast to diagnosis in paediatrics, psychological disorders cannot adequately be described by one diagnosis only. Therefore, a multiaxial classification scheme has been developed. Based on ICD-10 criteria, six different axes denoting different domains are classified. These include:

1   Clinical psychiatric diagnosis (such as anorexia nervosa, depressive episodes, etc.)
2   Specific developmental disorders (such as dyslexia)
3   Intelligence (such as dyslexia, speech and motor disorders)
4   Somatic diagnosis (such as epilepsy and other paediatric diagnoses)
5   Psychosocial risks occurring within the last six months (such as distorted intrafamilial interaction, isolated family and other stressful life events)
6   Global severity of a disorder (ranging from mild incapacitation to disorders requiring constant supervision and guidance)

Only after the diagnostic process has been completed and discussed with parents and children should therapeutical interventions be planned.

5
GENERAL PRINCIPLES: TREATMENT

The aim of this chapter is to provide a general approach to therapy – including those treatments with and without medication. Therefore, the basic principles will be outlined. Detailed aspects will be covered in the chapters dealing with specific conditions.

Non-pharmacological approaches

CREATING A RELATIONSHIP WITH CHILD AND PARENTS

The first step in any diagnostic and therapeutic process is to create a good relationship with both the child and the parent. It can be helpful to recall the specific situation many children and parents are in. Many children are distressed and ashamed, they have low feelings of self-worth and are insecure and anxious, and some have even been stigmatized by peers and teachers. Some children have behavioural problems at home and at school. Many parents are concerned about their children and have feelings of guilt; some are also angry and annoyed with their children. The first step therefore is to accept the child and parents as they are, make them feel at ease and reduce all stress. It is helpful to approach voiding disorders in an open, neutral, matter-of-fact way and to treat them as medical disorders.

One should enquire and talk about all relevant facts, signs and symptoms openly. It is also important to take into account the educational level and previous experience of the parents, and the developmental stage of the children, when asking about subjective meanings and connotations. Knowledge of the basic principles of developmental psychology can be very helpful, such as the cognitive constructs at different ages researched and described by Jean Piaget (1896–1980) (Piaget 1975). One has to remember that even school-aged children can retain elements of 'magical thinking' from the preoperational stage. Examples are a lack of clear causality, i.e. some children will not believe that one thing causes another, but that there is a 'circular causality'. Another example is 'egocentricity', i.e. children will continue to believe that they are the centre of events. Another is 'animism', i.e. the belief that non-living objects have a life of their own. Finally one should always bear in mind that children have not studied medicine and that their idea of anatomy differs greatly from one's own (see Table 4.13 and Fig. 4.4). All of these aspects have to be considered in order to really understand what children mean and think.

The next step is to clarify the context, i.e. who has referred the family, what do the child and parents really want? In other words, what are their expectations and wishes? These may differ greatly between child and parent. Thus, treatment will be especially difficult if parents have higher expectations than their child. The likelihood that the child will not cooperate, but oppose treatment recommendations, will be greatly increased. Another difficult situation arises when parents think that their child is wetting or soiling on purpose ('parental intolerance'). Again, a dysfunctional interaction can ensue – sometimes with harsh punitive reactions (Butler 1994).

Expectations can also differ greatly between family and experts. If one does not understand the subjective views of the family, one will not gain the full trust of the family. Compliance will be low, effectiveness will be reduced and working with patients and families will be less rewarding and enjoyable. Therefore, it is of great importance to create a good therapeutic relationship right at the beginning. This will be the basis of all further work – especially when difficulties arrive. Carl Rogers, the founder of person-centred psychotherapy, and Virginia Axline, who adopted the principles of play therapy (Axline 1947), were the first to empirically identify the three most important factors in all therapeutic relationships:

1   Unconditional acceptance: accepting the child and the family exactly as they are and not how one would like them to be.
2   Empathy: trying not only to understand but to put oneself into the situation of the patients and feel as near as possible what they might feel.
3   Authenticity: trying to act in congruence with one's own personality, staying true to oneself and not acting out a role that is not genuine (e.g. the omnipotent doctor) – no matter how tempting it may be.

PROVISION OF INFORMATION

The provision of information is essential, because parents and children are ignorant of many of the facts. Their ideas can be based on misconceptions and misinformation. Even if parents have tried to inform themselves, they may have embarked on the wrong track. Books can provide general information, but cannot specify the relevance of this information for the individual child. Some parents tend to selectively pick out information that will strengthen rather than mitigate their own preconceptions. Information gained via browsing the internet is often not very helpful either. Although such information is available to everyone, it is not weighted as to practical relevance and scientific value.

Examples of misinformation are that parents think that their child should be dry by the age of 2.7 years, on average, instead of the defined age of 5 years (Shelov et al 1981). Also, many parents think that emotional factors are the cause of nocturnal enuresis and forget that they might instead be the effect of the wetting problem (Haque et al 1981). Some parents are even given wrong information by experts. For example, even though it is not effective, some experts still advise not letting children drink in the afternoons and evenings (Haque et al 1981, Shelov et al 1981).

Therefore, one should allow plenty of time for the provision of information, a process that has also been called 'demystification' (Levine 1991). Information has to be provided actively. It is not enough to wait for questions. The information has to be presented individually – sometimes it is better to start with the basics first and provide more detail later on. Information is not processed reliably in an emotionally distressing situation. So sometimes it has to be repeated again and again. To ensure that it has been understood it can be checked by asking direct questions or by using questionnaires and charts.

It is often forgotten that not only parents but also each child needs information as well. This should be provided using words and concepts that a child can understand and in a format that is attractive and not boring. Thus, picture books, comics, diagrams and illustrations to colour in, and illustrated charts can be useful tools. Again, not only the objective facts but subjective meanings should be included. Wishes and anxieties need to be explored. Basic knowledge of developmental psychology can be helpful in understanding cognitive and emotional processes in children of different age groups.

COUNSELLING

Counselling, or 'psycho-education', as it is called, is part of the treatment process. It therefore follows that it should be provided only after assessment and diagnosis: one has to know what the problem is before endeavouring to change things. Counselling is an active process engaging both parents and children. It is defined as 'the provision of assistance and guidance in resolving personal, social, or psychological difficulties, especially by a trained person on a personal basis' (*New Oxford Dictionary of English* 2001).

Counselling is part of everyday paediatric practice and many doctors are well acquainted with giving advice regarding feeding, sleeping patterns, clothing, handling of the child, etc. Counselling itself is not too difficult, but sometimes it is not easy to get parents to actually do what one would like them do. Therefore, again, consideration and knowledge of the entire family situation is essential. Advice should be followed up and checked. If it has been followed, this should be reinforced positively. If it is not put into practice, possible intervening factors should be identified. Sometimes it can be helpful to enhance the counselling process by using other techniques. One simple technique is that of 'demonstration', e.g. actively showing how an alarm works. In 'coaching', parents and children take an even more active role, e.g. they set and activate an alarm themselves. They can be observed and corrected. Other techniques might include 'modelling' and 'role-playing'. The learning effect is much greater in these active forms of teaching than in solely verbal counselling.

BASELINE AND OBSERVATION

These are effective techniques used in cognitive-behavioural therapy. They are based on the observation that children (and parents) are often not aware of their feelings, thoughts and actions. They are therefore advised to observe a defined symptom. Different parameters such as frequency (how often it occurs), severity (how marked it is), symptomatology (in what form it occurs) and situation (associated factors) can be registered. To enable awareness and insight, one has to concentrate on and register these symptoms in a systematic way, e.g. using an observation chart. Experience has shown that the mere observation and registration actually have a therapeutic effect. Tics, depressive symptoms and anxiety can diminish if they are observed – as can the wetting problem in some children.

Baseline means the starting point or basis, but actually it is already part of the therapeutic process – e.g. in nocturnal enuresis children are asked to simply register if the nights were dry or wet using symbols such as 'stars' or 'suns' for dry nights and 'clouds' for wet nights.

Several studies have shown that 15 to 20 per cent of all children will become dry within four to eight weeks of baseline observation (Devlin and O'Cathlain 1990). In other words, for 15 to 20 per cent of all children, these simple methods, combined with provision of information and counselling, will be completely sufficient – no other specific intervention will be necessary.

COGNITIVE-BEHAVIOURAL THERAPY

Cognitive-behavioural therapy (CBT) is a subtype of psychotherapy which has been shown to be effective for many disorders. As the name implies, it consists of two components that are usually combined, but can be employed separately: cognitive therapy and behavioural therapy.

Cognitive therapy focuses on irrational, dysfunctional conditions, thoughts and beliefs. These dysfunctional cognitions need to be identified first before changes can be initiated. Cognitive therapy encompasses a whole variety of techniques. These include 'self-monitoring' (observation and registration), 'activity scheduling' (organization of activities), 'labelling' (using positive suggestive statements) and 'bibliotherapy' (use of books and written instructions).

Behavioural therapy concentrates on observable behaviour, which it aims to modify with a variety of techniques. These include 'classical conditioning', based on the co-appearance of a stimulus and a certain behaviour. One technique of classical conditioning is 'systematic desensitization', which is highly effective in the treatment of phobias. 'Operant conditioning' basically means learning by success, which can be achieved by different strategies using punishment versus reinforcement. In 'contingency management', behaviour is modified by social (praise) as well as material (rewards) reinforcement. 'Shaping' means that changes are achieved step by step. In 'extinction', reinforcement of an undesired behaviour is withdrawn. In 'time-out' techniques, the child is withdrawn from a social environment and placed in an isolated room when an undesirable behaviour occurs. In 'exposition', children are exposed to situations in which symptoms usually appear. They are guided and accompanied by the therapist, so that they learn to endure these situations without symptoms – a technique called 'response prevention'. Finally, 'social learning' includes techniques such as 'modelling' (learning from the success of a model) as well as basic interactional skills.

CBT is therefore a specific type of psychotherapy. Although most of the non-surgical treatments of voiding disorders contain cognitive-behavioural elements, the term CBT should not be used indiscriminately. It should be used only when referring to a specific type of technique or treatment.

ALARM TREATMENT

Alarm treatment is, indeed, a type of cognitive-behavioural therapy. It works through positive reinforcement, as well as aversive, negative experiences, and has been shown to be highly effective. The basic principle of alarm treatment lies in converting afferent sensations of the full bladder either into arousal (waking up) or into an inhibition of a micturition reflex (sleeping through without emptying the bladder).

Alarm treatment was introduced by Mowrer and Mowrer (1938), who developed a special type of mechanical bed. After wetting, the bed was tilted to one side and the child was rolled out onto a mattress on the floor (Mowrer 1980). Although very effective, it was too complicated to be used elsewhere, so the basic principle of an alarm attached to a pad via a cable was introduced. This simple technique has been in use for nearly 70 years, although the exact way it works is not known. Mowrer and Mowrer (1938) believed that it was a type of classical conditioning. This is not logical, as the alarm is not activated by the full bladder, but essentially too late, after the wetting has occurred. Also, alarm treatment is equally effective if the child is woken by the alarm directly or by his or her parent indirectly (Azrin et al 1974). The decisive component for successful treatment is a short time interval between wetting and awaking, as well as the ensuing therapeutic steps. These include positive elements, such as praise, as well as aversive elements, such as getting up, going to the toilet and remaking the bed afterwards: in other words it is an 'operant' and not a 'classical' type of 'conditioning'.

Recently, new types of alarms have been constructed based on a classical conditioning paradigm. A small ultrasound sensor is strapped to the child's abdomen; it is programmed so that the alarm is activated once the bladder is filled to 80 per cent of its expected functional capacity. It has been demonstrated to be effective – but not more effective than classical alarm treatment (Pretlow 1999).

UROTHERAPY (BLADDER CONTROL THERAPY)
Urotherapy is an umbrella term for all non-surgical measures used for treatment of enuresis and functional, as well as organic, urinary incontinence. Urotherapy is established as a profession mainly in the Scandinavian countries, so far, but it is not established in the UK and in many other European countries. In essence, urotherapy is a

> type of training which makes use of cortical control of the bladder, teaching children to recognize and employ conscious command over their lower urinary tract. Its main ingredients are information about normal lower urinary tract function and the specific dysfunction in the child, instruction about what to do about it and support and encouragement to go through with the training program.
>
> (Hellström et al 1987)

In other words, it uses a wide array of cognitive and behavioural techniques (including alarm treatment), although, of course, it is not CBT in a stricter sense. Urotherapy is performed by different professionals such as nurses, educators and physiotherapists.

BIOFEEDBACK
Biofeedback is defined as a variety of techniques by which physiological activity is registered, enhanced and presented to the patient in real time using visual and acoustic signals (Kjolseth et al 1993). By this means, information regarding physiological processes is registered, enabling active, conscious self-control of physiological activity one has not

previously been aware of. Biofeedback has been shown to be effective in some voiding disorders such as dysfunctional voiding (Kjolseth et al 1993), while it is no more effective than standard behavioural techniques in functional faecal incontinence (encopresis) both with (Cox et al 1996) and without (van Ginkel et al 2000) constipation.

OTHER FORMS OF PSYCHOTHERAPY

For most children with voiding disorders, a symptom-oriented approach is sufficient. If, however, a co-occurring child psychiatric disorder is present, additional types of treatment will be necessary. In these cases, a differential indication for therapy is mandatory. The question is: which treatment is most effective for this child in this family at this moment?

It has been estimated that over 500 different types of psychotherapy exist in the USA for children and adolescents alone (Kazdin 2000). Of those that have been evaluated, four basic schools of psychotherapy can be differentiated:

1 Depth psychology (or psychoanalysis), which addresses and works with unconscious aspects of the psyche.
2 Client- (or child-) centred psychotherapy, which focuses on the current conscious experience of the child and the healing aspects of the therapeutic relationship.
3 Family therapy, which focuses on the interaction between family members but not the individual person.
4 Cognitive-behavioural therapy, which focuses on cognitions and observable behaviour.

N.N., 5-year-old girl
Diagnoses: urge incontinence; primary nocturnal enuresis; recurrent UTIs;
VUR grade III left, grade II to III right; duplication of the ureter;
articulation disorder (ICD-10: F 80.0); emotional disorder (ICD-10: F 93.8)

N. had never been dry and wetted every night and day. She was operated on successfully at the age of 3 to 4 years for vesico-ureteric reflux. Recurrent urinary tract infections were treated with antibiotics and antibiotic prophylaxis was instituted. In the family, the father had also had nocturnal enuresis as a child. There were overt marital conflicts. N. was the only child.

The paediatric examination was normal. Ultrasound showed duplication of the left ureter. Bladder wall thickness was 2.8 mm, residual urine 25 ml. There was a staccato uroflow curve with EMG contractions, initially. The frequency-volume chart showed 11 micturitions per day with volumes between 20 and 100 ml as well as imperative urge symptoms. N. was shy, insecure, anxious, dysphoric and unhappy. Intelligence was above normal (IQ 118).

N. was treated with a toilet regime and 7.5 mg of oxybutynin per day. She became completely dry during the day and showed a reduction of the nocturnal wetting. She refused alarm treatment and was a non-responder on desmopressin. Then she experienced a complete relapse during day and night. At the same time, depressive and anxiety symptoms increased dramatically, and so analytical play therapy was started. At this time, her parents separated and this loss was one of the main topics of the therapy. The emotional symptoms were completely cured by psychotherapy. Also, day wetting stopped and she was willing to try a round of alarm treatment, becoming completely dry within seven weeks.

In this case, analytical play therapy was indicated because of the severe emotional disorder. In the course of this therapy, symptom-oriented treatments such as the alarm, which she had refused beforehand, became possible.

EFFECTIVENESS OF PSYCHOTHERAPY

There can be no doubt that psychotherapy in children is effective. Psychotherapy has been defined as 'any intervention intended to alleviate psychological distress, reduce maladaptive behaviour through counselling, structured and unstructured interaction, a training program, or a predetermined treatment plan'. In one of the best and largest meta-analyses of 150 studies, Weisz et al (1995) conclude that 'psychotherapy with young people produces positive effects of respectable magnitude'. The effect sizes are in the medium to large range, but there are important differences between groups.

Generally, in meta-analyses, behavioural therapy (BT) is more effective than non-BT (such as insight-oriented therapy), but differences are less prominent, if instruments, which had been used during treatment, are excluded for measuring outcome (Weisz et al 1995). There are great differences among components of BT – ranging from a maximum for systematic desensitization to a minimum for multiple operant methods. Also, person- (child-) centred psychotherapy is less effective than insight-oriented psychotherapy. There are good effects for mixed approaches, i.e. combining different types of psychotherapy.

Also, there are no differences in the treatment of undercontrolled (externalizing) versus overcontrolled (internalizing) disorders. This means that even externalizing disorders can be treated well with psychotherapy. The psychotherapy of adolescents (>12 years) is more effective than that of children (<12 years). And girls can be treated with greater success than boys. Therefore, psychotherapy generally shows the best effect among female adolescents. Another point is important to remember: paraprofessionals (trained parents and teachers) have higher effect sizes (0.71) than professionals (0.55) and students (0.43). This means that 'indirect' treatment of the child by training parents and caregivers can be more advantageous than 'direct' treatment of the child in individual psychotherapy by a professional.

DIFFERENTIAL INDICATION FOR PSYCHOTHERAPY

Before initiating any psychotherapy, the first question should be: is treatment needed at all? In many cases counselling of parents and child is all that is required. In other cases, changes in the child's environment (such as changing school) or help from social services can be more useful than psychological treatment in the narrower sense.

The modality has to be considered. Although parents are nearly always included, the focus can be on individual, group or family therapy. The intensity and duration have to be addressed: is a short focal therapy focused on one specific problem needed, or a longer, more general treatment? The age of the patient plays an important role: while older children and adolescents can be reached verbally, younger children require play or other non-verbal media in their therapy.

Psychotherapies can be combined with other methods, such as pharmacotherapy, but also with speech, occupational, physio-, music and other types of therapies – if indicated. The decision should not be based on personal inclinations. Instead, empirically based 'practice parameters' or 'guidelines' have been developed in many countries (e.g. Schmidt and Poustka 2003).

OTHER CHILD PSYCHIATRIC INTERVENTIONS

If comorbid emotional and behavioural disorders coexist, other child psychiatric interventions can be indicated. In addition to the classical psychotherapeutic approaches, 'relaxation methods' can be used to reduce anxiety and relieve tension. 'Training techniques' can be of great use in children with specific developmental disorders such as dyslexia or dyscalculia. All therapies can be inducted in an individual or a group setting, depending on the type of disorder and the treatment goal. Thus, group therapies can be indicated in cases in which social learning is a main goal.

These interventions are usually performed on an outpatient basis. Day clinic treatment can be indicated in more severe disorders, which require a more intense approach and management. Finally, in-patient child psychiatric treatment, in which a more intense type of treatment is possible, is indicated in severe disorders. As a general guideline, children with voiding disorders should only be admitted to day clinic or in-patient treatment if outpatient approaches have failed or if in-patient treatment is needed for a coexisting psychiatric disorder.

ESTABLISHMENT OF SOUND DRINKING HABITS

This is a part of standard urotherapy that is often forgotten. Children with enuresis and incontinence may comply with all the interventions regarding regular voiding practice, voiding position, bowel habits and so on but still wet their bed because they drink half a litre of Coke before bedtime! This is another argument for the use of voiding charts – abnormal drinking habits are often missed if one goes by history alone.

Almost all parents of bedwetting children have tried to reduce enuretic accidents by reducing the child's fluid intake before going to bed. The therapeutic benefit of this intervention – which is often erroneously advocated by doctors as well – is usually very modest, and it is really off the point. The point is this: the child should drink enough during the *daytime* so that he or she (1) gets a good daytime diuresis and (2) does not become very thirsty during the evening. Fluid restriction in the evening is only necessary in extreme cases.

Many children with bladder disturbances habitually reduce daytime drinking to a minimum (Spehr and De Geeter 1991), perhaps in an attempt not to have to go to the toilet so often. This strategy does not help them very much during the daytime and has the additional drawback that they may become very thirsty in the evening and then drink a lot.

Thus, the proper advice to children with enuresis with or without incontinence is to increase fluid intake at breakfast and lunch, preferably plain water (not soft drinks), and only drink to quench thirst in the evening. It is a good idea for parents to provide the child with a bottle of water to bring to school. There is some scientific support for the clinical and parental observation that caffeine-containing drinks, such as coffee and Coca-Cola, increase the risk for subsequent incontinence or enuresis (Arya et al 2000). Furthermore, as will be discussed later, children who are on desmopressin treatment should avoid excessive fluid intake in the evening.

So what can be considered normal fluid intake for a child? The problem here is that published fluid intake recommendations are, almost without exception, based on the intravenous fluid needs of hospitalized children, often in the intensive care setting. The values are arrived at via calculations of minimum energy requirements, insensible losses and minimum urine production (Holliday and Segar 1957). The relevance of such data for basically healthy children, with or without nocturnal polyuria, is questionable.

When investigators have measured how much normal children actually drink when fluid intake is ad libitum, the results have invariably been lower than the recommended norms (Ballauff et al 1988, Fusch et al 1993). The conclusion usually drawn by the investigators, that the children drink too little, may not be wholly correct: if the children have no health problems, then they evidently drink enough, regardless of published norms. But for children with disturbances of the bladder or bowel it is certainly recommendable to increase fluid intake to the norms (see Table 5.1), since this will have positive effects on bladder function and diminish the risk of constipation.

CONSTIPATION TREATMENT

The basic approaches to the treatment of constipation are provision of information, psychoeducation and counselling. A pretreatment observation time ('baseline') can usually be omitted. Instead, a toilet regulation regime can be started directly. Children are asked to sit on the toilet three times a day, after mealtimes, in a relaxed mode for five to ten minutes.

TABLE 5.1
Recommended daily fluid intake, according to the Deutsche Gesellschaft für Ernährung (DGE 1989), compared with actual fluid intake (Fusch et al 1993)

Age (years)	Recommended fluid intake (ml/kg/day)	Actual fluid intake (+/- SD) (ml/kg/day)
4–6	100–110	55 (15)
7–9	90–100	47 (11)
10–12	70–85	40 (8)
13–15	50–60	35 (6)

This is documented on a chart and can be reinforced positively. If necessary, dietary changes (increasing fibre intake) and increasing oral fluids can be of help. In one study, 15 per cent of children were cured within six weeks by these simple methods (Van der Plas et al 1997).

If a large amount of faecal masses has accumulated, disimpaction with enemas will have to be performed at the beginning of treatment. To avoid reaccumulation of faecal masses, a maintenance therapy with oral laxatives is recommended for at least 6 and up to 24 months (Felt et al 1999). The preferred oral laxatives are osmotic laxatives such as polyethylene glycol (PEG).

CLEAN INTERMITTENT CATHETERIZATION
Clean intermittent catheterization (CIC), as established by Lapides in the 1970s (Lapides et al 1971), has revolutionized the treatment of children or adults with neurogenic bladder disturbances, and certainly saved innumerable kidneys and quite a few lives as well.

The principle is simple: patients who are chronically unable to void without significant residual urine are regularly catheterized, by their parents or by doing it themselves. In this way the kidneys are protected against damage due to relapsing UTIs or high intravesical pressure and reflux, and the bladder is protected against overdistension. As a bonus, the patient may become continent as well.

CIC is indicated in the majority of children with myelomeningocele or neurogenic bladder from other causes (trauma, tumour, occult spinal dysraphism), and may also be necessary in a few neurologically normal children who have relapsing, symptomatic UTIs due to residual urine that do not respond to intensive urotherapy. This is the case with a small group of children with underactive detrusor ('lazy bladder') or dysfunctional voiding.

To be effective, CIC should usually be performed about every three hours while awake. Sometimes catheterization once during the night is also required. The family and patient are instructed by a trained urotherapist or paediatric nurse until they feel comfortable with the procedure. This requires a lot of work and time, but it is usually successful in the end. Risks and side effects are remarkably few. It is interesting to note that although a non-sterile catheter is repeatedly introduced into the bladder, antibiotic prophylaxis is usually not needed. In fact, CIC administered properly often means that previous long-term antibiotic prophylaxis can be discontinued.

Pharmacological approaches
In this section the indications for and basic pharmacology and side effects of the various medications that may be indicated in voiding disorders will be considered. Dosage, practicalities regarding their use and evidence for their effectiveness will be handled in later chapters, which discuss the various conditions in which the drugs may be used.

DESMOPRESSIN
Desmopressin, or desamino-8-D-vasopressin, is an analogue to the neurohypophyseal hormone vasopressin (or antidiuretic hormone, ADH), with the hormone's antidiuretic but without its pressor effects. The drug has become one of the mainstays of enuresis treatment.

Desmopressin – and vasopressin – binds to the V2-receptors in the renal collecting ducts, making them permeable to water and resulting in an outflow of water from the tubuli into the hyperosmolar renal medulla. The net result is the production of less, and more concentrated, urine. The antienuretic effect of desmopressin is presumed to reside in these antidiuretic properties – a presumption that is logical given the fact that polyuria is probably a central pathogenetic factor in monosymptomatic enuresis.

However, some doubt has recently been cast upon this explanation, since it has been shown that the drug may be effective even in children with congenital absence of V2-receptors (Muller et al 2002). Central nervous system effects on arousal have been proposed as an alternative or complementary therapeutic action. This alternative explanation, on the other hand, is hampered by two circumstances: the first is the fact that the CNS effects of vasopressin, the parent hormone, are mediated via the V1-receptors (Ebenezer 1994), to which desmopressin has low affinity (Vallotton 1991). The second is the fact that desmopressin does not cross the blood–brain barrier of mammalians (Ang and Jenkins 1982, Stegner et al 1983), including humans (Sorensen et al 1984). But the issue is not settled by these arguments. Effects on memory or behaviour have been reported since early in the history of desmopressin (Anderson et al 1979, Beckwith et al 1987, von Gontard and Lehmkuhl 1996). Furthermore, the structures within the CNS gathered under the term circumventricular organs provide a 'window' in the blood–brain barrier through which much of the central neuroendocrine control of body fluid homeostasis is managed (Thrasher 1989). This is the window used by vasopressin (Jurzak and Schmidt 1998), and desmopressin has also been shown to bind to receptors in it (Jurzak et al 1995). Furthermore, other vasopressin receptors, apart from V1 and V2, have been found (Jurzak et al 1995, Saito et al 1997), and it cannot be excluded that such receptors provide desmopressin with a possibility of influencing the CNS. Last, and perhaps least, nasal administration of vasopressin or desmopressin may provide a more direct access to the brain (Lawrence 2002). So, more remains to be discovered about the CNS effects of desmopressin. However, in the majority of cases we believe that the central antienuretic action of desmopressin is its anti*diuretic* action.

Desmopressin is available as nasal spray and oral tablets. There are no major differences between the two preparations as regards safety and therapeutic effects (Fjellestad-Paulsen et al 1987a), but nasal administration has the disadvantage of a reduced effect in the presence of allergic or viral rhinitis (Feber et al 1993) – a notion that has, however, recently been questioned (Greiff et al 2002). The tablets may be crushed or dissolved in water (Argenti et al 2001). The bioavailability of the spray is 2–10 per cent (Fjellestad-Paulsen et al 1993a, Feber et al 1993) and the tablets 0.1–0.2 per cent (Fjellestad-Paulsen et al 1993a, d'Agay-Abensour et al 1993), thus the adequate oral dose is more than ten times the intranasal (Fjellestad-Paulsen et al 1987b). The full antidiuretic effect can be expected to be achieved two hours after administration (Hammer and Vilhardt 1985, Williams et al 1986, Fjellestad-Paulsen et al 1987b), and although the plasma half-life of the drug is approximately one hour (Vilhardt 1990, Fjellestad-Paulsen et al 1993a), the therapeutic effect can be expected to linger on for 8 to12 hours (Edwards et al 1973, Williams et al 1986, d'Agay-Abensour et al 1993). Recently a new tablet, which dissolves quickly on the tongue, has been registered for use in enuresis.

75

The bioavailability and half-life of the drug differ significantly between individuals (Robinson 1976, Hammer and Vilhardt 1985), but this has not been shown to have a major impact on therapeutic response (Robinson 1976). Likewise, the delayed and diminished bioavailability that has been observed with concomitant food intake seems not to affect the antidiuretic effects (Rittig et al 1998). Since the drug is eliminated mostly via the kidneys (Fjellestad-Paulsen et al 1993a), treatment with desmopressin is not appropriate in the rare case of renal failure, where enuresis is likely to be due to poor concentrating ability (Agersø et al 2004). Desmopressin pharmacokinetics does not differ between responders and non-responders to the drug (Nevéus et al 1999b).

Given the widespread usage of desmopressin and the scarcity of reported serious adverse effects, it must be considered a very atoxic drug (Hjälmås and Bengtsson 1993, Robson and Leung 1994). Although side effects such as headache are sporadically reported, the only real safety concern is that if desmopressin administration is combined with excessive fluid intake, hyponatremia with convulsions may occur, with a need for intensive care (Beach et al 1992, Yaouyanc et al 1992, Guillaud et al 1993, Kallio et al 1993, Schwab et al 1996). How to prevent this serious complication is outlined in the enuresis section below, but the important point is that desmopressin should not be combined with excessive fluid intake and that the child should not drink anything after taking desmopressin in the evening. Hyponatremia and/or convulsions after desmopressin medication but *without* excessive fluid intake is a very rare complication (Hamed et al 1993, Hourihane and Salisbury 1993, Bernstein and Williford 1997). Studies of long-term desmopressin administration have so far not given any serious concerns (Rew and Rundle 1989, Sukhai 1993). The endogenous vasopressin secretion seems not to be affected (Knudsen et al 1991).

TRICYCLIC ANTIDEPRESSANT DRUGS

Two or three decades ago imipramine was the most commonly prescribed medication in nocturnal enuresis, and related compounds such as amitryptiline, clomipramine and desipramine were also widely used. Sadly, in many countries imipramine is even today used as a first-line choice. Although this is to be deplored, imipramine still has a minor role to play in the treatment of severe, therapy-resistant enuresis (see the section on enuresis for details).

The mechanism(s) behind the documented antienuretic effect of imipramine is not clear, but there are several possibilities. First, it is well known that tricyclic antidepressants have anticholinergic side effects. They may thus diminish detrusor overactivity. Second, imipramine may increase sphincter tone, and it has for this reason been used in stress incontinence (Castleden et al 1981). Third, it has been shown in at least one study that imipramine may also decrease urine production (Hunsballe et al 1997). Fourth, sleep architecture (Rapoport et al 1980) and arousal mechanisms are probably affected by the drug via the reticular activating centre and the sympathetic branch of the autonomous nervous system. Of these mechanisms the fourth is probably the most important. Desipramine, the active metabolite of imipramine, binds highly specifically to the locus coeruleus – a noradrenergic nucleus in the upper pons that is pivotal in arousal from sleep. Tricyclics may act via correction of a central cathecholaminergic imbalance. Regardless of which mechanisms are responsible for the anti*enuretic* properties it is certain that they are distinct from the anti*depressant* effects. The antienuretic effects appear much earlier and at lower dosage than the antidepressant effects (Korczyn and Kish 1979).

Therapeutic response is slightly dose-dependent, but the overlap between the serum concentration of responders and non-responders is great (Jørgensen et al 1980, de Gatta et al 1984, DeVane et al 1984, Furlanut et al 1989, Fritz et al 1994).

As usual, knowledge of the pharmacokinetics stems mostly from studies in adults. There are, however, a few studies in children and adolescents, and they show no major differences from those in adults (Potter et al 1982, Preskorn et al 1989, Dell et al 1990). The oral bioavailability of imipramine is around 40 per cent and the time until maximum plasma concentration is reached approximately three hours. The interindividual variation of pharmacokinetic parameters is quite large (Fritz et al 1994) and the situation is complicated by the fact that the drug is partly metabolized to the active metabolite desipramine, and desipramine concentration rises disproportionately with increased imipramine dosage (Brosen et al 1986). This may have clinical implications, since more serious adverse events are reported with desipramine than imipramine usage in therapeutic dosage. The plasma half-life of imipramine and desipramine in adolescents is 1–6 hours and 4–12 hours, respectively (Dell et al 1990).

Concurrent use of imipramine and selective serotonin reuptake inhibitors (SSRIs) such as fluoxetine, fluvoxamine and sertraline should be avoided, since this may result in increased imipramine serum concentrations (Vandel et al 1992).

The main safety concern with tricyclic antidepressant drugs is the risk for serious cardiac arrhythmias. Fatal reactions with imipramine have been reported when the drug has been given in too high dosage or to patients with an underlying long QT-syndrome (Varley and McLellan 1997, Varley 2000). Fatal reactions with normal dosage have occurred with the related drug desipramine (Riddle et al 1991, 1993). With the higher dosage used for antidepressant purposes a few cardiac deaths have been reported with imipramine as well (Swanson et al 1997), but given the very widespread usage that the drug previously had in the treatment of enuresis this complication should be regarded as extremely rare. Less serious side effects, such as nausea, sweating, palpitations, constipation, dry mouth or affective changes are more common (Furlanut et al 1989) and may lead to a need to discontinue medication.

It should also be noted that imipramine has sometimes been used in the treatment of children with attention deficit hyperactivity disorder (ADHD) (Spencer et al 1996), and that quite a few enuretic children report that they become more calm and focused when taking the drug (Gepertz and Nevéus 2004).

Imipramine would be recommended as a good second-line treatment alternative in enuresis, were it not for the concern about cardiac risks. Given the pharmacological considerations above, it may be speculated that modern antidepressants with noradrenergic profile but without cardiotoxicity may prove to be useful in nocturnal enuresis. A pilot investigation of such a drug, reboxetine, has recently indicated that there may be some truth in such speculations (Nevéus 2006).

ANTICHOLINERGICS (ANTIMUSCARINICS)

Parasympatholytic drugs with detrusor-relaxant properties have for obvious reasons long been used in the treatment of various bladder disturbances. Several compounds have been tried, such as oxybutynin, tolterodine and propiverine, but most data are available concerning oxybutynin. In the adult population several other drugs are in use or have been used – e.g. flavoxate, trospium chloride, emepronium – but they will only be mentioned very briefly here.

Anticholinergics are indicated for neurogenic bladder, and also in urge incontinence, when urotherapy has failed. Furthermore, there are probably children with therapy-resistant enuresis due to detrusor overactivity (i.e. in most cases non-monosymptomatic enuresis) in whom anticholinergics are efficient, but this has yet to be proven in randomized controlled studies.

The anticholinergic drugs in use today for the above conditions act via blocking the muscarinic acetylcholine receptor of the parasympathetic nervous system. This, and direct analgesic and smooth muscle-relaxant effects, result in a varying degree of peripheral inhibition of detrusor contractions.

Oxybutynin, given orally, has a low bioavailability, usually below 10 per cent, and a plasma half-life of a few hours. The drug is, like most anticholinergics, eliminated via liver metabolism. For an exhaustive review of the pharmacokinetics of drugs used in the treatment of the overactive bladder the reader is advised to consult the review by Guay (2003).

Though anticholinergic drugs are not highly toxic they do entail some risks and a certain amount of monitoring is needed in all treated children. Quite a few children have to discontinue treatment or cannot reach therapeutic concentrations because of untoward drug effects. The most important side effect to know about is the risk for residual urine, which may lead to UTIs. The most common problem, however, is constipation. This may appear *de novo* or a subclinical concomitant constipation may be exacerbated during treatment, resulting in bowel symptoms and/or reduced therapeutic efficacy against the micturition disturbance. For the practicalities regarding constipation and/or residual urine monitoring during and before anticholinergic treatment, see the section on urge incontinence.

Anticholinergic drugs with low bladder specificity (oxybutynin, for instance) reduce salivation and thus increase the risk for caries, even if the child does not feel any oral discomfort. Other side effects, such as nausea, vertigo, flushing, tachycardia or accommodation disturbances, can also occur with varying frequencies. Unfortunately, psychic effects – mostly aggressivity – sometimes occur, at least when using oxybutynin. Side effects are dose-dependent and disappear upon dose reduction or discontinuation of the drug.

Due to side effects and pharmacokinetic considerations extended-release formulations may be more efficient than immediate-release tablets. This has been shown to be the case in the treatment of urge incontinence with oxybutynin (Nilsson et al 1997), for which the transdermal route of administration is also available, although not tested in children (Dmochowski et al 2002). Intravesical administration of oxybutynin has become routine practice in the treatment of children with neurogenic bladder disturbance who are on CIC, whenever there is significant detrusor hyperreflexia, since this mode of administration significantly reduces side effects (Madersbacher and Jilg 1991).

78

As mentioned above, oxybutynin is the most well-known anticholinergic drug for the paediatric population. The more bladder-selective drug *tolterodine* was developed with the aim of reducing side effects without reducing efficacy. This goal seems to have been achieved in the adult population (Ruscin and Morgenstern 1999), and side effects are few among children as well (Raes et al 2004), but randomized controlled studies in this age group have so far been disappointing as regards therapeutic effect, and it has not been given label use in the USA by the FDA. As with oxybutynin, the extended-release formulation of tolterodine may be superior to the immediate-release tablets (van Kerrebroeck et al 2001). The future role of tolterodine in children is, as yet, unknown.

Propiverine, an antimuscarinic drug with calcium channel-blocking properties (Haruno et al 1989), has been approved for use against bladder overactivity (Mazur et al 1995) and is commonly used in Germany, Austria and Japan. Its efficiency is probably comparable to that of oxybutynin, and safety may even be better, but more studies are needed before the proper place of this drug in detrusor therapy can be determined.

Trospium chloride is a non-selective antimuscarinic drug with low bioavailability (Schladitz-Keil et al 1986), which has gained widespread usage in the adult population, in which it has been shown to be better than placebo in increasing bladder volume and decreasing symptoms of detrusor overactivity (Stoher et al 1999, Cardozo et al 2000). It may also have a more benign safety profile than oxybutynin (Madersbacher et al 1995, Halaska et al 2003), but no studies on children have so far been conducted.

Terodiline is a calcium channel inhibitor with anticholinergic properties, which has been tested and has shown positive effects in a few studies in children with enuresis (Ishigooka et al 1992), detrusor overactivity (Hellström et al 1989) or daytime incontinence (Langtry and McTavish 1990). This drug has, however, been withdrawn after reports of cardiotoxicity in the elderly.

A summary of the pharmacokinetics of the most widely used drugs is provided in Table 5.2.

ADRENERGIC AND ANTI-ADRENERGIC DRUGS

Adrenergic agonists have for many years now been used in the pharmacological management of incontinence in adult women. Phenylpropanolamine is the drug most commonly used, and there are sufficient randomized, controlled trials to claim that it is probably better than either placebo or pelvic floor training alone in the treatment of stress incontinence in adults (Alhasso et al 2003). The drug has been tested in children with neurogenic bladder disturbance, in whom modest effects on incontinence and detrusor overactivity were observed (Åmark and Beck 1992). In one open, uncontrolled study phenylpropanolamine was quite effective in children with therapy-resistant enuresis (Penders et al 1984), but this finding has not been repeated.

There is a logical appeal in the use of anti-adrenergic drugs in patients with voiding dysfunction, neurogenic detrusor–sphincter dyssynergia or bladder outlet obstruction for other causes, since sphincter contraction is partly sympathetically mediated. Anti-adrenergic drugs have been used in children with disturbances of bladder function, but there are not enough studies for it to be considered an evidence-based therapy. The most widely studied

TABLE 5.2
Pharmacokinetics of some drugs used in the treatment of incontinence
(those drugs mainly used in children are shaded)

Drug	Oral bioavailability	t_{max}	Half-life	Elimination
Oxybutynin[ab]	2–11%, mean 6%	0.5–1.5 h[c]	1–5 h	Liver metabolization
Tolterodine[a]	10–74%, mean 33%	0.5–2 h	2–4 h	Liver metabolization
Propiverine	Mean 85%	2 h	3–5 h	Metabolization
Imipramine[bd]	27–42%, mean 38%	2.5–4 h	9–21 h	Liver metabolization
Trospium chloride	1–4%, mean 3%[f]	5–6 h	10–12 h	Renal elimination
Desmopressin[bdf]	0.1–0.2%	2 h	1 h	Renal elimination

[a] Extended-release formulation available. Table data are for the immediate-release formulation
[b] Paediatric data available
[c] Concomitant food intake delays absorption
[d] Adolescent data available
[e] Note that imipramine is partly metabolized in a first step to the active metabolite desipramine
[f] Concomitant food intake diminishes bioavailability

drug, *doxazosin* (Serels and Stein 1998), has shown some promising results in the treatment of voiding dysfunction (Austin et al 1999, Cain et al 2003, Yang et al 2003). Side effects are usually mild (Carruthers 1994), but it is not surprising that these drugs can actually cause incontinence due to urethral underactivity (Dwyer and Teele 1992, Marshall and Beevers 1996).

Thus, until randomized, controlled studies in children have been performed, the use of either adrenergic agonists or antagonists in children cannot be recommended, but an educated guess is that one fruitful approach in the future will be drugs of the latter kind in the treatment of therapy-resistant voiding dysfunction.

BOTULINUM TOXIN

The use of botulinum A toxin has shown promising results in the treatment of neurogenic bladder disturbance in children (Schulte-Baukloh et al 2003, Riccabona et al 2004) and detrusor overactivity for neurogenic or non-neurogenic causes in adults (Kuo 2004). The toxin is injected peri-urethrally in the case of detrusor–sphincter dyssynergia, or into the detrusor if detrusor overactivity is the main disturbance. The effects usually last for about half a year, after which treatment has to be renewed (Leippold et al 2003). There is presently too little data from children for general recommendations to be made, but the drug seems to represent a promising avenue for the future treatment of therapy-resistant cases.

ANTIBIOTICS

In children with voiding disorders the main problem with antibiotics is not their use but their overuse. The unnecessary prescription of antibiotics leads to increasing bacterial resistance in the community. The specifics about when and how to use antibiotics in a child with enuresis or incontinence are covered in Chapter 8 (see pages 200–213).

Table 5.3 gives basic information about dosage, side effects and antibacterial spectrum for antibiotics that may be used in children with UTI after infancy.

Trimethoprim and the combined *trimethoprim-sulfamethoxazole* share the same antibacterial spectrum but the combination is more bacteriocidal than trimethoprim alone. This means that trimethoprim-sulfamethoxazole is indicated in the treatment of pyelonephritis, whereas in the case of cystitis or UTI prophylaxis trimethoprim is a better choice. Skin reactions or unspecific gastrointestinal complaints are the most common side effects. The main problem with these drugs is that bacterial resistance is increasing because of overuse. In Scandinavia 15 to 20 per cent of E Coli has become resistant.

Nitrofurantoin is an old drug which occasionally produces serious adverse effects (lung fibrosis) in the adult population but is almost totally harmless when used in children. Its main

TABLE 5.3
Oral antibiotics commonly used against UTI in childhood

Drug	Indications	Dosage (mg/kg/d)	Antibacterial spectrum	Common side effects	Comments
Trimethoprim	Cystitis, prophylaxis	Cystitis: 6 in 2 doses Prophylaxis: 1 in 1 dose	E. coli resistance is increasing due to overuse Enterococci sensitive	Rash	
Trimethoprim-sulfamethoxazole	Pyelonephritis	Trim 10 and sulf 50 in 2 doses	Identical to trimethoprim	Rash, Stevens–Johnson syndrome	
Nitrofurantoin	Cystitis, prophylaxis	Cystitis: 5–7 in 2–4 doses Prophylaxis: 1 in 1 dose	Enterococci sensitive	Nausea, unpleasant taste	Ecologically favourable
Mecillinam	Cystitis	20 in 3 doses	Enterococci resistant		Carnitine supplementation needed if used for long time
Ampicillin, amoxicillin	Cystitis (?)	Ampicillin: 100–150 in 3–4 doses Amoxicillin: 25–50 in 3 doses	Enterococci sensitive. Many E. coli resistant		Not to be used unless offending bacteria are known
Cefadroxil	Cystitis, prophylaxis	Cystitis: 30 in 2 doses Prophylaxis: 10 in 1 dose	Enterococci resistant. E Coli often intermediately sensitive (OK in cystitis)		Oral mixture has limited durability
Ceftibuten	Pyelonephritis	9 in 1 dose	Enterococci resistant		

indications are UTI prophylaxis or treatment of cystitis. The bacteriostatic action of the drug makes it unsuitable for treatment of pyelonephritis. This is an ecologically attractive drug, since it more or less bypasses the gastrointestinal canal, is found in high concentration in the urine and, despite many years of use, has not resulted in significant development of bacterial resistance. But, as usual, there is one drawback: many patients need to discontinue treatment because of nausea or vomiting.

Among the *penicillins*, mecillinam can be recommended as a first-line alternative for the treatment of cystitis. The antibacterial spectrum is excellent, since it is quite selective to uropathogens, and side effects in short-term treatment are rare. The one concern about this drug is that long-term treatment (more than several weeks) may lead to carnitine deficiency (Holme et al 1989), which may possibly have deleterious effects on heart and skeletal muscle function. Thus, if mecillinam is to be used as UTI prophylaxis, carnitine supplementation should also be provided.

Ampicillin (or amoxicillin) has frequently been used, and is still often used in some parts of the world, in the treatment of UTI. It is not to be recommended, however, at least not in pyelonephritis, since bacterial resistance is now very common. If it is known that the bacteria in question are susceptible, however, then ampicillin may certainly be used, since side effects are rare.

Cephalosporins are frequently used, because of a generally favourable antibacterial spectrum and few side effects. Cefadroxil is a good antibiotic to use in cystitis or as UTI prophylaxis. The fact that E Coli strains often show intermediate resistance to the drug makes it unsuitable as a first-line therapy in pyelonephritis if the resistance pattern of the offending bacteria is not already known. But this is no problem in cystitis or UTI prophylaxis, since full bacterial susceptibility is not needed. One practical problem with using cefadroxil in UTI prophylaxis is that the durability of liquid oral preparations is limited to approximately two weeks.

The new cephalosporin ceftibuten has emerged as a good alternative to trimethoprim-sulfamethoxazole in the oral treatment of acute pyelonephritis. The antibacterial spectrum is, so far, good, although whether this situation will last remains to be seen. An additional bonus is that the drug needs to be given only once daily.

Cefotaxime is one of the standard drugs to use when intravenous therapy of pyelonephritis is deemed necessary.

Quinolones, such as norfloxacin or ciprofloxacin, are not routinely used in children since they have not, as yet, undergone enough clinical trials in this age group. However, in the few cases where a child needs to be treated or protected from infections with *pseudomonas spp*, ciprofloxacin has sometimes been used, since this is the only oral preparation with efficacy against those bacteria. The common clinical experience is that this drug is acceptable for use even in children, but until more studies have been done it should be given only after specialist evaluation.

URINARY TRACT ANTISEPTICS AND PROBIOTICS
Many parents provide children suffering from relapsing UTIs with *cranberry juice*, following claims in the press about its beneficial effects. Cranberries contain molecules

that inhibit adhesion of E Coli to the urothelium (it is possible that many berries do this), but the few controlled studies that have been undertaken to date have yielded ambiguous results (Reid et al 2001, Linsenmeyer et al 2004, Waites et al 2004) and no recommendation can so far be given. But the berries are certainly not harmful.

The same can probably be said about treatment with *probiotics*, i.e. introducing supposedly harmless bacteria via a pad in the underpants, or even orally, with the aim of establishing a more healthy bladder flora and thus keeping the virulent bacteria out. The concept is certainly appealing, but results so far have, sadly, not fulfilled expectations (Kontiokari et al 2004). Adult women with UTIs have been found to consume less bacteria-containing food (yoghurt etc.) than matched controls (Kontiokari et al 2003). This is a field in which more research is certainly needed.

The antiseptic drug *methenamine hippurate* is metabolized in acid urine into formaldehyde and hippurate, which acts bacteriostatically against most urinary tract pathogens. It has been used in adults for many years as UTI prophylaxis after eradication of bacteria with antibiotics, and there are studies to indicate that it is safe and useful in children as well (Petersen 1978). The drug is relatively harmless and can certainly be considered as an alternative to antibiotic prophylaxis, although more studies are needed before general recommendations can be given. It cannot, as yet, be considered an evidence-based therapy (Lee et al 2002).

METHYLPHENIDATE

Psychopharmacotherapy can be an important aspect of treatment in such disorders as obsessive–compulsive disorders, depressive disorders or ADHD. The main drug groups comprise neuroleptics, antidepressants, tranquillizers and stimulants. Due to the high comorbidity of nocturnal enuresis and ADHD, knowledge of stimulant prescription is useful and will therefore be covered in greater detail. Also, methylphenidate is indicated in giggle incontinence. The guidelines for the use of stimulants have been summarized in the 'Practice parameters for the use of stimulant medications in the treatment of children, adolescents and adults' (AACP 2002).

In the treatment of ADHD, stimulants are the preferred medication, with antidepressants or neuroleptics requiring special indications. Stimulants are indicated for only three disorders: ADHD, narcolepsy and giggle incontinence. The best-known stimulant is methylphenidate, which was developed in 1944 and has been prescribed for ADHD since 1964. It is one of the best-studied and -investigated medications used in childhood. Seventy per cent of children are responders, showing a reduction of hyperactivity, an increased attention span and other cognitive effects (such as improved short-term memory). A variety of secondary effects have also been shown, such as improving interactions with parents and peers by modifying aggressive and impulsive behaviour. In the famous multicentre MTA Cooperative Group study, stimulants were shown to be the most important component of treatment (MTA 1999).

Methylphenidate is absorbed quickly; the effects start 30 minutes after taking medication and last three to four hours. It is recommended to start with a low dose of 5 mg in the morning. Effective doses range between 0.3 and 0.8 mg per kg bodyweight per day in two doses (morning and midday). Methylphenidate is well tolerated – 4 to 10 per cent of children have mild side effects such as sleep disorders, reduced appetite, abdominal pain and mood changes, but these usually recede within the first few days. Tics can be induced by stimulants, psychotic symptoms are possible when overdosed and one should be careful in children with (untreated) epilepsy as the seizure threshold can be lowered. Also, body length can be reduced (MTA 2004). However, no tolerance or dependency develops. On the contrary, the risk of later substance abuse in children with ADHD can be markedly reduced by stimulants (Wilens et al 2003).

In addition to classical methylphenidate, which has a short half-life, several long-acting formulas have been introduced (Lopez et al 2003). In methylphenidate non-respondence, a switch to D-amphetamine can increase the response rate to 90 per cent. Recently, atom-oxetine, a presynaptic noradrenalin reuptake inhibitor, has shown effects in a similar range to those of stimulants (Michelson et al 2001).

As with all medication, stimulants require a professional diagnosis before prescription. Epidemiological studies in the USA have pointed to an alarming development: many children on stimulants (72 per cent) did not fulfil the criteria for ADHD (Angold et al 2000). On the other hand, only 25 per cent of children with ADHD were actually receiving stim-ulants (Jensen et al 1999). Overall, over 3.5 per cent of children in the USA (over 2 million) are currently being treated for ADHD (Olfson et al 2003).

While stimulants are highly effective in the treatment of ADHD, they do not have a specific antienuretic effect. Clinical observations of children becoming dry with stimulants could be explained by their secondary effect of increasing compliance. Children with nocturnal enuresis and AHDH had a higher rate of non-compliance (38 per cent) than children with nocturnal enuresis alone (22 per cent) in a retrospective analysis (Crimmins et al 2003). This shows that the wetting problems and comorbid child psychiatric disorders need to be addressed and treated individually. This dual treatment has a synergistic, positive effect with higher rates of treatment success.

Surgical interventions
Historically, meatotomy was once not infrequently performed in neurologically and anatomically normal children with incontinence. This is a practice that should now be strongly discouraged. We have neither a clear pathogenetic rationale for the proce-dure, nor evidence for its efficacy. We do, however, know that such a procedure may lead to decreased urethral closing pressure and stress incontinence in young adulthood (Kessler and Constantinou 1986). In children without malformations or neurogenic bladder disturbance, there is almost never an indication for surgery as a treatment of voiding disorders.

In children with neurogenic bladder disturbance, on the other hand, there is sometimes good reason to do bladder augmentation surgery or various forms of continent diversion of the urinary tract, but this is almost always done to protect the kidneys from damage caused by high intravesical pressure or relapsing infections, not just to make the child dry. But the dryness that may be achieved is, of course, an appreciated bonus.

The situation is slightly different in children with chronic constipation and faecal impaction due to neurogenic bowel dysfunction or as a long-term complication of anorectal surgery. In this group of children laxatives and the frequent need for enemas may cause considerable pain and distress and still not be completely successful. The situation for these children may sometimes be alleviated by providing a way to give the enemas anterogradely, directly into the transverse colon. This may be accomplished via the Malone antegrade continence enema (MACE) procedure (Malone et al 1990), whereby a continent stoma into the colon is created. This procedure has also been successfully employed in a few extreme cases of functional constipation (Youssef et al 2004).

Posterior urethral valves (see Chapter 8) are surgically ablated, usually via the endoscopic route, although this does not solve the many bladder- and kidney-related problems that are associated with this exclusively male congenital malformation.

Children who suffer from excessive polyuria due to kidney disease such as nephrogenic diabetes insipidus or polyuric renal failure may suffer from therapy-resistant nocturnal enuresis because of nocturnal polyuria. Some of these children need the surgical provision of a catheterizable urinary diversion in order to provide low-pressure urine drainage during the night. The indication for this operation is the protection of the kidneys from pressure-related damage caused by the polyuria, but the provision of nocturnal continence is an added bonus.

Artificial urinary sphincters are sometimes used, with varying degrees of success, in the management of adults with severe stress incontinence. Artificial *anal* sphincters have likewise been used, but systematic reviews of their usefulness have not given reason for optimism (Mundy et al 2004). Their indication in children with voiding disorders is negligible.

6
NOCTURNAL ENURESIS

Definitions and classification

The scientific term for bedwetting is nocturnal enuresis. In many texts the terms enuresis and incontinence are used interchangeably in a confusing way. We will consistently use the term *nocturnal enuresis* (or just enuresis) simply as denoting bedwetting, that is, the passing of urine in bed while asleep, in a child who has passed his or her fifth birthday – after organic causes have been ruled out. We will, furthermore, call it enuresis regardless of which of the various pathogenetic mechanisms is supposed to be operative and regardless of concomitant daytime symptoms (these would require a second diagnosis). This practice is in accordance with the new recommendations of the ICCS (Nevéus et al 2006).

The general diagnostic criteria according to the ICD-10, DSM-IV and ICCS classification schemes have been outlined in Chapter 2. The most relevant subdivisions of nocturnal enuresis are (1) *primary* and *secondary* types, on the basis of the presence or absence of a dry interval of six months or more, and (2) *monosymptomatic* and *non-monosymptomatic* types, depending on whether other micturition problems – daytime incontinence, urgency, holding manoeuvres or interrupted micturitions – are present or not (see Table 2.3). Note that in earlier terminology monosymptomatic enuresis denoted just nocturnal enuresis without daytime incontinence.

The relevance of differentiating between primary and secondary enuresis is that in the latter case concomitant psychological or psychiatric problems are not uncommon, and, although this seldom affects the choice of first-line treatment, compliance can be expected to be lower. The distinction between mono- and non-monosymptomatic enuresis is, however, of central importance, since the presence of daytime micturition problems in an enuretic child indicates significant disturbances of bladder function that often affect the assessment and treatment of the child.

Epidemiology

Enuresis is a common problem among children and adolescents. If a wetting frequency of at least one 'wet night' per month is used as the criterion, the prevalence of nocturnal enuresis is probably above 10 per cent among 6-year-olds (Hellström et al 1990), around 5 per cent among 10-year-olds (Alon et al 1992, Laberge et al 1996, Nevéus et al 1999a), and 0.5–1.0 per cent among teenagers and young adults (Alon et al 1992, Hirasing et al 1997a). The studies performed so far on enuresis prevalence in different age groups are summarized in Table 6.1.

Enuresis without daytime incontinence is 1.5–2 times as common among boys as among girls (Hellström et al 1990, Bower et al 1996, Nevéus et al 1999a). In children with combined

TABLE 6.1
Enuresis prevalence in different age groups (symptom frequency,
when stated in the study, is at least once per month)

Reference	N	<7 years	7–10 years	10–15 years	Adults
Cher et al 2002	7225		5.5%		
Bakker et al 2002	4332			5%	
Bower et al 1996	2292		7.8%		
Cayan et al 2001	5350		12.7%		
Devlin 1991	1806		13%		
Fergusson and Horwood 1994		9%	2.5%		
Foldspang and Mommsen 1994	2613				2.2% (women)
Gur et al 2004	1576		12.4%		
Gümüs et al 1999	1703		13.7%		
Hansen et al 1997	1557		7%		
Hellström et al 1990	3556		7%		
Hirasing et al 1997b	13081				0.5%
Järvelin et al 1988	3206		6.4%		
Jonge 1969	10000	10–15%	7%	2–3%	
Kalo and Bella 1996	640		15%		
Klackenberg 1981	212		9%		
Laberge et al 1996	2000			3.8%	
Marugan de Miguelsanz et al 1996	1300		13%	7%	
Nevéus et al 2001a	1300		8.2%		
Osungbade and Oshiname 2003	644		17.6%		
Ouedraogo et al 1997	1575		13%		
Power and Manor 1995	12537			5%	
Smedje et al 1999	1844	20%			
Söderström et al 2004	1478		7.1%	2.7%	
Swithinbank et al 2000	2075				5.8% (women)
Yeung et al 2004	8534				2.3%
Weighted summary		**10–20%**	**7–13%**	**3–7%**	**0.5–3.0%**

day- and night-time wetting, and among adults, this gender difference is not found
(Hellström et al 1990, Hirasing et al 1997b, Nevéus et al 1999a). There are no clear cultural
or ethnic variations in enuresis prevalence.

Aetiology and pathophysiology

The former notion of enuresis as a purely psychiatric disorder has now been abandoned.
Alternative – non-exclusive – pathogenetic explanations, with sounder scientific foun-
dations, have now emerged from the fields of endocrinology, urology, sleep research *and*
child psychiatry. It has become increasingly clear that enuresis is not one disorder but
several, and that different subgroups of enuretic children have different causes behind their
bedwetting (and require different treatment).

GENETICS

Nocturnal enuresis can be considered to be a common, genetically complex and hetero-geneous disorder. Without a doubt, genetic factors are the most important in the aetiology of nocturnal enuresis, while environmental factors (both somatic and psychosocial) exert major modulatory effects on the phenotype. The genetics of nocturnal enuresis has been studied by formal and molecular genetic methods (review: von Gontard et al 2001a).

Formal genetics

Empirical *family studies* have repeatedly demonstrated a high rate of relatives affected by enuresis: 39 per cent of fathers and 23 per cent of mothers (Hallgren 1957), and 46 per cent of parents (either parent) (Bakwin 1961). The recurrence risk for a child to be affected by enuresis is 40 per cent if one parent had been enuretic and 70 per cent if both parents had been enuretic (Bakwin 1973). In a clinical population, a positive family history was found in 63.2 per cent of the families – 22.2 per cent of the fathers, 23.9 per cent of the mothers and 16.5 per cent of the siblings being affected (von Gontard 1995). There were no differences in rates of affected relatives between primary and secondary types of enuresis. Within families, the phenotype was often not uniform: different members can show the same or different forms of wetting. Also, family history was the strongest predictor for the age of attaining dryness in a prospective, longitudinal epidemiological study (Fergusson et al 1986). In children with at least two first-degree relatives with a history of nocturnal enuresis, the development of nocturnal bladder control was delayed by 1.5 years. In another cross-sectional epidemiological study, the risk for enuresis was five to seven times higher if one parent had a history of enuresis. If both parents had been affected, the risk ratio was 11.3, in comparison to healthy families (Järvelin et al 1988).

Twin studies can assess the degree to which genetic factors contribute to the aetiology of enuresis by comparing concordance rates of mono- and dizygotic twins. The rates of different studies were: 79 per cent for MZ and 0 per cent for DZ twins (Hallgren 1960); 68 per cent for MZ and 36 per cent for DZ twins (Bakwin 1971); 81.8 per cent for MZ and 33.3 per cent for DZ twins (Abe et al 1984); and 46 per cent for MZ and 19 per cent for DZ twins (Hublin et al 1998). The proportion of total phenotypic variance attributed to genetic influence was 67 per cent in males and 70 per cent in females (Hublin et al 1998).

The aim of *segregation analyses* is to identify the specific mode of inheritance of enuresis. The most common mode of transmission is an autosomal dominant one with high penetrance (90 per cent) (Eiberg et al 1995). Most, but not all, families follow an autosomal dominant mode of inheritance. In a formal genetic analysis of 392 children with nocturnal enuresis, 45 per cent were compatible with an autosomal dominant and 9 per cent with an autosomal recessive mode of inheritance. The rate of sporadic cases was 44 per cent, if only first-degree relatives were considered, and 33 per cent with no other relatives affected (Arnell et al 1997). Similarly, in another study, 44 per cent were compatible with an autosomal dominant mode of inheritance with high penetrance, 23.3 per cent with low penetrance, and 4.4 per cent with an autosomal recessive mode of inheritance. The total 'true' sporadic rate was 28.3 per cent (von Gontard et al 1999c).

Molecular genetics: linkage analyses
Linkage analyses determine the relative position between known DNA-markers (microsatellite markers) and the locus of the defective gene. Linkage studies have defined different 'loci' or 'chromosome intervals' on several chromosomes: on chromosome 13 (Eiberg et al 1995), chromosome 12 (Arnell et al 1997) and chromosome 22 (Eiberg 1998, von Gontard et al 1999d). This phenomenon is known as 'locus heterogeneity', meaning that genes on different chromosomes can lead to the same disorder. There was no clear association with any type of enuresis with any of the identified loci (von Gontard et al 1998b). Also, all likely candidate genes for nocturnal enuresis have been excluded, so far.

These linkage analyses have been replicated in a Belgian study of 32 families with positive LOD scores to chromosome 22 (LOD score 3.63), chromosome 12 (LOD score 1.95) and chromosome 13 (LOD score 1.3) (Loeys et al 2002). Finally, three new loci were identified in multi-generational families from Denmark and the Faeroe Isles: on chromosomes 4 and 12 for nocturnal enuresis and on chromosome 17 for urge incontinence (Eiberg et al 2001). Urge incontinence is therefore the first syndrome of day wetting with a clear genetic aetiology proven even in molecular genetic studies.

In summary, molecular genetic studies have clearly shown that nocturnal enuresis is a complex disease with locus heterogeneity (different loci leading to the same phenotype) and no clear genotype–phenotype association. They do, however, underline the importance of genetic factors in the aetiology of nocturnal enuresis, which requires further elucidation in the future.

ENDOCRINOLOGICAL AND NEPHROLOGICAL FACTORS
The discovery that many enuretic children and adolescents have nocturnal polyuria secondary to a relative nocturnal deficiency of the antidiuretic neurohypophyseal hormone vasopressin has rightly been considered a breakthrough in enuresis research. It was shown that this group of bedwetting children lacked the physiological nocturnal peak of vasopressin secretion and had a nocturnal urine production exceeding their bladder capacity (Puri 1980, Nørgaard et al 1985b, Rittig et al 1989). This led to the formulation of the 'polyuria hypothesis' of nocturnal enuresis.

This finding has since been repeated (Aikawa et al 1998, Hunsballe et al 1998, Vurgun et al 1998), *and* contradicted (Steffens et al 1993, Eggert and Kühn 1995, Hunsballe et al 1995, Läckgren et al 1999). One explanation for the conflicting results regarding vasopressin values could be the fact that this hormone is released in a pulsatile manner (Weitzman et al 1977), and accurate measurements of circadian profiles would call for measurements every 15 minutes. Measurement of vasopressin in morning urine, as a way of overcoming this problem, did not show any differences between dry and enuretic children (Nevéus et al 2002). In addition, the inter- and intraindividual variability of vasopressin secretion is high, and the circadian vasopressin profile changes as the child grows. It has become increasingly clear that, although many enuretic children exhibit nocturnal polyuria, this is multifactorial and not necessarily always caused by vasopressin deficiency (Vurgun et al 1998, Natochin and Kuznetsova 2000, Nevéus et al 2000).

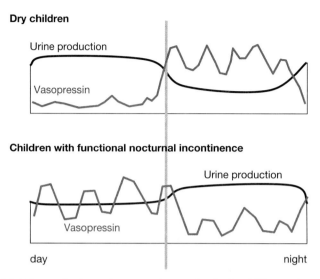

Dry children

Urine production

Vasopressin

Children with functional nocturnal incontinence

Urine production

Vasopressin

day   night

Fig. 6.1 Urine production and vasopressin secretion in dry children and a subgroup of children with enuresis due to nocturnal polyuria (adapted from Rittig et al 1989).

A problem with the polyuria hypothesis is the finding that nocturnal polyuria is not a phenomenon exclusive to bedwetters. It has been shown that 12 per cent of dry children produce more urine during the night than during the daytime (Mattsson 1994a), and the fact that nocturia is not rare among non-enuretic children (Bower et al 1996, Nevéus et al 1999a) suggests that nocturnal polyuria may be common as well. So, additional mechanisms are needed to explain why the bedwetting children do not wake up instead.

The finding of nocturnal polyuria in enuretic children provided an explanation for the antienuretic effect of the antidiuretic drug desmopressin. Not surprisingly, it seems that the children with nocturnal polyuria – those with, one might say, 'diuresis-dependent enuresis' (Nevéus et al 2000) – are those that are most likely to respond to desmopressin therapy (Hunsballe et al 1995, Nørgaard et al 1995a, Rittig et al 1997, Hunsballe et al 1998, Nevéus et al 1999b, 2001b).

An attractive way of testing the polyuria hypothesis is to induce nocturnal polyuria in dry children, with a fluid load and/or diuretics, and see if they then wet their beds. Results of such tests have, however, been conflicting. On the one hand, enuresis *has* by this method been induced in some children (Rasmussen et al 1996). On the other hand, nocturia was much more easy to provoke than enuresis; the children either wet small amounts, unrelated to bladder volume, or woke up. A study in children aged between 4 and 18 years with polyuria due to recently diagnosed diabetes mellitus showed that 46 per cent of them, mainly the younger children, did experience enuresis at the time of diagnosis (Alon et al 1992).

Notwithstanding the objections above, it is quite well established that nocturnal polyuria – with or without vasopressin deficiency – is one important pathogenetic factor in nocturnal enuresis, especially the kind that responds to desmopressin therapy. But it can only be a contributing factor, not the sole pathogenetic mechanism.

An Italian group has proposed that hypercalciuria may be a cause of polyuria and enuresis in a subset of bedwetting children (Valenti et al 2002, Aceto et al 2003), but this has been contradicted by authors who found no difference in nocturnal urinary calcium excretion between enuretic children and controls (Nevéus et al 2002), and it has so far not been shown that hypercalciuric children require specific treatment to become dry.

URODYNAMIC FACTORS
Given the prominent role of detrusor overactivity in the pathogenesis of daytime incontinence, and the great overlap between the groups of bedwetting and day-wetting children (Järvelin et al 1988, Hellström et al 1990, Bower et al 1996, Nevéus et al 1999a), it should come as no surprise that detrusor overactivity is a pathogenic factor in nocturnal enuresis as well, even when not accompanied by concomitant daytime incontinence.

Sleep cystometries in children with nocturnal enuresis without daytime incontinence have revealed frequent uninhibited nocturnal detrusor contractions in a substantial minority of the children although they had relaxed detrusors while awake (Watanabe and Azuma 1989, Cisternino and Passerini-Glazel 1995). Not surprisingly, in studies in which enuretic children both with and without daytime incontinence were included, the finding of urodynamic abnormalities was even more common (Broughton 1968, Hindmarsh and Byrne 1980). In a cystometric study in a group of children with therapy-resistant enuresis without daytime incontinence, *all* children examined were found to exhibit pathological cystometrograms during sleep, with nocturnal detrusor overactivity, dysfunctional voidings and/or obstruction (Yeung et al 1999). An interesting publication in the 1980s reported uninhibited *urethral* relaxations in therapy-resistant enuretic children, who subsequently became dry

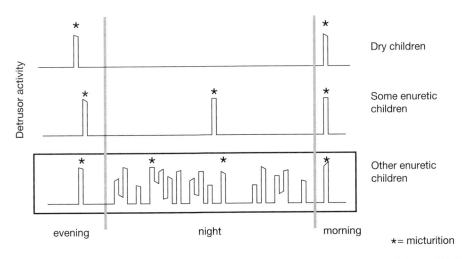

Fig. 6.2 Ambulatory cystometry in dry and enuretic children (adapted from Watanabe and Azuma 1989).

91

on sympathicomimetic treatment (Penders et al 1984). These findings, however, have not been repeated.

An overactive bladder is usually a small bladder. It has been noted for several decades that the voided volumes of enuretic children tend to be smaller than those of dry children (Vulliamy 1959, Starfield 1967, Yeung et al 1999, Nevéus et al 2001b). Further support for the detrusor overactivity hypothesis is also provided by the finding that children with enuresis go to the toilet more often (Esperanca and Gerrard 1969, Bloom et al 1993), and that urgency symptoms are more common in this group (Nevéus et al 1999a).

In analogy to the polyuria hypothesis, it seems reasonable to conclude that there is a subgroup of enuretic children in whom nocturnal detrusor overactivity is a crucial contributing pathogenetic factor. It can also be assumed that this group of children often have concomitant daytime micturition symptoms (frequency, urgency, etc.), which can be detected by the use of voiding charts.

SLEEP AND AROUSAL

Mammalian sleep is characterized by the cyclic alternation between rapid eye movement (REM) sleep, with the experience of dreams, and non-REM sleep without such imagery. The latter kind of sleep is further subdivided according to electroencephalographic criteria into deep non-REM, or delta sleep, and superficial non-REM sleep.

During sleep, the perception of extracerebral stimuli is more or less completely blocked on a thalamic level (Steriade et al 1969). To overcome this and wake up in response to urgent stimuli such as an alarm clock or a distended bladder the reticular activating system (RAS) is necessary (Moruzzi and Magoun 1949, Starzl et al 1951). This is a diffuse neuronal network extending all along the neuraxis below the telencephalon, organized so that it receives collaterals from all sensory pathways (Starzl et al 1951) and projects to more or less the whole cerebral cortex. The result is that sensory stimulation of any kind, provided it is strong enough, will, via the RAS, result in general cortical arousal (Moruzzi and Magoun 1949). Sensory input from the distended or contracting bladder is no exception to this rule (Bradley 1980). In terms of the autonomic nervous system, arousal from sleep is characterized by high sympathetic activity and parasympathetic inhibition (Horner 1996).

The arousal threshold is highest during delta sleep (Rechtschaffen et al 1966), and since this kind of sleep predominates during the early part of the night, this is also the time when the sleeper is most difficult to wake up (Rechtschaffen et al 1966, Keefe et al 1971). Regardless of this, two persons with the same amount and distribution of delta sleep and with the same sleep EEG may have enormously different arousal thresholds (Bonnet and Johnson 1978), i.e. person A may wake up when the cat walks through the room, while person B may not notice the bedside telephone ringing.

The idea that enuretic children are 'deep sleepers' is not new (Trousseau 1870). Many parents report that their bedwetting children are almost impossible to awaken from sleep at night. This subjectively low arousability has been reported in numerous epidemiological studies (Hindmarsh and Byrne 1980, Wille 1994, Kalo and Bella 1996, Yeung 1997, Nevéus et al 1999a). The common observation made by parents of children being treated with the enuresis alarm, that the whole family wakes up at the sound of the alarm *except* the child

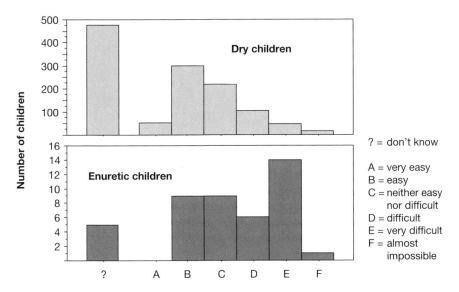

Fig. 6.3 Subjective arousal thresholds in enuretic and dry children. Answers to the question 'How easy or difficult are you to arouse from sleep at night?' (Nevéus et al 1999a)

who is using it, is also well known to clinicians in the field. It is noteworthy that this observation involves a 'control group' – i.e. the rest of the family – as well.

Studies on objective arousal thresholds of enuretic children have been scarce. The problem here is that the mere recording of the sleep EEG gives no information regarding differences in arousal thresholds between subjects. The fact that children generally sleep more soundly than adults (Busby and Pivik 1983, Busby et al 1994) and that the sleep EEG of enuretic children is not clearly different from that of dry children (Rapoport et al 1980) has often led to the erroneous conclusion that enuretic children do not sleep more 'deeply' than dry children. In fact, they do. In the well-designed study by Wolfish and co-workers (Wolfish et al 1997) it was quite clearly shown that children with severe enuresis were significantly more difficult to arouse from sleep than controls.

Furthermore, it seems logical for sleep to play at least a permissive role in the pathogenesis of enuresis, since both bladder distension and detrusor contractions are strong arousal stimuli (Bradley 1980, Page et al 1992).

The 'deep sleep' of enuretic children can also – and in some cases perhaps more accurately – be described as a lack of inhibition of the micturition reflex during sleep, i.e. their micturition reflex may be too quick or too strong rather than their arousal mechanisms being too slow or weak (Koff 1996).

CENTRAL NERVOUS SYSTEM

So, some consensus has now emerged around the view that the four most important pathogenetic factors in nocturnal enuresis are nocturnal polyuria, detrusor overactivity, low arousability and/or a lack of inhibition of the micturition reflex. Fruitful speculation has also

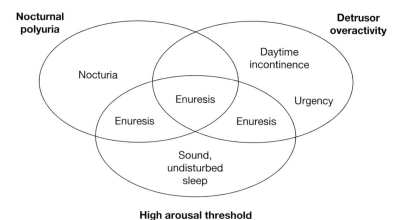

Fig. 6.4 Suspected major pathogenetic factors in nocturnal enuresis.

been growing that there must be central nervous system factors involved, and that a disturbance on the brainstem level may underlie the other pathogenetic mechanisms.

The locus coeruleus (LC) is a noradrenergic neuron group in the upper pons which has several functions that are relevant in this regard:

1   As the central brainstem nucleus of the RAS it is central for *vigilance* – i.e. the preparedness for new or sudden stimuli – and arousal from sleep (Foote et al 1983).
2   It is the main nucleus of the central nervous system portion of the sympathetic nervous system (Foote et al 1983).
3   It overlaps, anatomically and functionally, the pontine micturition centre which is essential for bladder control (Barrington 1925, Holstege et al 1986, Yoshimura et al 1988, Noto et al 1989).
4   It has direct and indirect connections to the hypothalamic nuclei which synthesize the vasopressin that is secreted by the neurohypophysis (Bowden et al 1978, Sawchenko and Swanson 1982, Lightman et al 1984).

Furthermore, as has been remarked above, the active metabolite of the antienuretic drug imipramine binds specifically to this neuron group. It is thus natural to hypothesize that a disturbance in the upper pons may be operative in nocturnal enuresis (Nevéus 1999).

Some evidence to support these speculations has recently been published. Studies of the so-called startle inhibition reflex have indicated that enuretic children have a disturbance at the brainstem level (Ornitz et al 1999), although the data are by no means clear-cut. A recent study showed that early acoustic evoked potentials, but not startle modulation, are altered, indicating a more general dysfunction of the brainstem (Freitag et al 2006). A Japanese group have made indirect measurements of sympathetic and parasympathetic tone in enuretic and non-enuretic subjects, using overnight measurements of heart rate variability

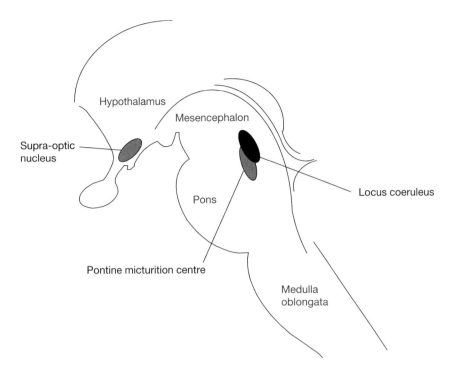

Fig. 6.5 Anatomy of the brainstem with structures relevant to enuresis pathogenesis.

(Fujiwara et al 2001). Their data indicate that bedwetters have more parasympathetic and less sympathetic activity than dry children – an observation that fits well with the hypothesis above and which has received some confirmation from a recent Turkish study (Unalacak et al 2004).

Psychological and psychiatric factors

OVERALL COMORBIDITY

Not all epidemiological studies on enuresis actually assess behavioural problems in a standardized way. Thus, the famous studies of Fergusson et al (1986) unfortunately do not address the question of comorbidity. Others report raw or mean T-values, which might not be easily understood if one is not familiar with the questionnaire used in the study. Only those studies that clearly define the group of clinically deviant children are reported in Table 6.2. If a control group is reported, the relative risk for a behavioural problem (relative risk) can be calculated; otherwise the normative data are used.

In the famous Isle of Wight study, the 31-item Rutter Child Scale, a standard instrument at the time of the study, was filled out by parents (Rutter et al 1973). At the defined cut-off, between 25 per cent and 28 per cent of enuretic children were reported by their parents to show problematic behaviour – three to four times the incidence reported among the controls.

TABLE 6.2
Epidemiological and clinical studies: percentage of children with clinically relevant
behavioural problems in comparison to controls, and their increased relative risk

Study	Age (years)	N	Type of wetting	Enuretic children	Controls	Higher risk (relative risk)
Epidemiological (population-based) studies						
				Rutter Child Scale; cut-off >13		
Rutter et al 1973	5–14 (7)	4481	NW/DW	Boys: 25.6%	7.9%	3.2
				Girls: 28.6%	7.8%	3.7
McGee et al 1984	7–9 (7)	1037	NW	Primary: 30.8%	21.6%	1.4
				Secondary: 51.9%		2.4
				DSM-III diagnoses		
Feehan et al 1990	11–15 (11)	1037	NW	Total: 23.4%	9.5%	2.5
				Primary: 0%		4.5
				Secondary: 42.3%		
				CBCL total >90th percentile		
Liu et al 2000	6–18	3344	NW	30.3%	9.1%	4.3
Hirasing et al 1997b	9	1652	NW	23.0%	10.0%	2.3
				BPI >90th percentile		
Byrd et al 1996	5–17	10960	NW	16.5%	10.2%	1.6
Clinical studies						
				Rutter A questionnaire, cut-off >18 (interview)		
Berg et al 1981	6–13	41	NW	29.3% (26.8%)		
				CBCL total >90th percentile		
Baeyens et al 2001	6–12	100	NW/DW	26%	10.0%	2.6
von Gontard et al 1999a	5–11	167	NW/DW	28.2%	10%	2.8
Hirasing et al 2002	6–15	91	NW	21%	10%	2.1
Van Hoecke et al 2004	9–12	84	NW/DW	20.4%	6.1%	3.3

Using the same instrument, the longitudinal study from Christchurch (New Zealand) reported similar rates for the children with primary nocturnal enuresis, while the children with secondary nocturnal enuresis showed a much higher rate of 52 per cent (McGee et al 1984). As the controls also showed high rates, the relative risk was 1.4 to 2.4 times higher. The same study was the only one to assess rates of DSM-III diagnoses at a later age – with marked differences between the children with primary and secondary nocturnal enuresis (Feehan et al 1990).

In the Dutch study by Hirasing et al (1997b) 23 per cent of children with enuresis scored in the clinical range of the CBCL total problem scale. In the cross-sectional Chinese study by Liu et al (2000) one-third of all wetting children were in the clinical range – 4.3 times the rate among controls. The US study by Byrd et al (1996) used the 32-item BPI (Behavior Problem Index), which is modelled on the CBCL. The rates are lower than in the other studies, but they include infrequent wetters (as low as one wetting episode per year).

In summary, the epidemiological studies show clearly that, depending on the definitions and instruments used, 20 to 30 per cent of all nocturnal enuretic children show clinically relevant behavioural problems – two to four times higher than the rate for non-wetting children. This is a substantial number of children, considering that the comorbidity of behavioural disorders among chronically ill children, some with severely incapacitating illnesses, is two to three times higher than that among healthy children (Cadman et al 1988, Eiser 1990).

The epidemiological studies report general prevalence in the population without selection biases. On the other hand, they usually rely on broad questionnaires as their only source of information. Clinical studies with smaller groups of children can address these questions in greater detail – but can reflect possible recruitment biases.

In an early study by Berg et al (1981) nearly 30 per cent of children who presented with enuresis in a paediatric clinic were deemed 'clinically disturbed' by non-standardized interviews and by the Rutter questionnaire (using a different cut-off from that in Rutter et al 1973 and McGee et al 1984). In another study in a paediatric setting, 20 years later, similar rates of 26 per cent were found (Baeyens et al 2001). These rates are almost identical to those in our own studies in a child psychiatric setting using the same instruments (von Gontard et al 1999a). The rates of a selected group of treatment-resistant children with nocturnal enuresis undergoing Dry Bed Training were 2.2 times higher (Hirasing et al 2002). In the study by Van Hoecke et al (2004), internalizing symptoms predominated in a mixed group of day- and night-wetting children, with significantly higher scores for withdrawal, physical complaints, anxious/depressed, social problems and internalizing behaviour scales compared to controls.

SPECIFIC COMORBIDITY

Regarding the subtypes of nocturnal enuresis, children with primary nocturnal enuresis showed lower rates of behavioural problems than those with the secondary type (von Gontard et al 1999a). The group with the lowest comorbidity – no higher than in the normative population – were those with monosymptomatic nocturnal enuresis without any daytime symptoms such as urge, postponement or dysfunctional voiding (see Table 6.3).

The difference between primary and secondary nocturnal enuresis has also been studied in epidemiological investigations. Children with primary nocturnal enuresis were not more deviant than controls in epidemiological studies (Feehan et al 1990). While developmental and genetic factors were associated with primary nocturnal enuresis, a variety of psychosocial factors were not (Fergusson et al 1986). On the other hand, secondary nocturnal enuresis was preceded by a higher rate of weighted life events (Järvelin et al 1990a) and was significantly associated with a higher rate of DSM-III psychiatric disorders, which can

TABLE 6.3
Subtypes of nocturnal enuresis: specific comorbidities of clinically relevant behavioural problems according to ICD-10 and CBCL in comparison to normative values, for different types of nocturnal enuresis (von Gontard et al 1999a; n=167, 5–11 years)

Measure (relative risk)	Enuretic children	Normative values	Higher risk
All children			
CBCL total >90th p.	28.2%	10.0%	2.8
ICD-10	40.1%	12.0%	3.3
Primary nocturnal enuresis			
CBCL total >90th p.	20.0%	10.0%	2.0
ICD-10	19.5%	12.0%	1.6
Primary monosymptomatic nocturnal enuresis			
CBCL total >90th p.	14.3%	10.0%	1.4
ICD-10	10.0%	12.0%	0.8
Primary non-monosymptomatic nocturnal enuresis			
CBCL total >90th p.	29.0%	10.0%	2.9
ICD-10	34.4%	12.0%	2.9
Secondary nocturnal enuresis			
CBCL total >90th p.	39.3%	10.0%	3.9
ICD-10	75.0%	12.0%	6.3

persist into adolescence (Feehan et al 1990). In a large longitudinal epidemiological study in New Zealand, 42 per cent of 11-year-old children with secondary, but none with primary nocturnal enuresis had a DSM-III diagnosis – a highly significant difference (Feehan et al 1990). These psychiatric disorders often preceded the relapse and were thus not a mere consequence of the enuresis.

There are two main age peaks for relapse: in infancy (2 to 3 years of age), and at preschool age (5 to 6 years). The most important life events were separation and divorce of parents (Järvelin et al 1990a). Other life events associated with relapse were birth of a sibling, entering kindergarten and school problems (von Gontard et al 1997). By adolescence, the attainment of dryness after the age of 10 years increased the risk for behavioural problems – independently of the primary or secondary status (Fergusson and Horwood 1994).

In contrast to marked differences regarding psychological factors, primary and secondary nocturnal enuresis do not differ regarding genetic (von Gontard et al 1997, 1998b) or other somatic factors – with the exception of constipation (Robson et al 2005) and late attainment of dryness (Fergusson et al 1990, Fergusson and Horwood 1994). Both are more pronounced in children with secondary nocturnal enuresis. The associations of genetic and psychological factors are summarized in Fig. 6.6. Primary and secondary enuresis are not distinct entities, but represent disorders on a spectrum.

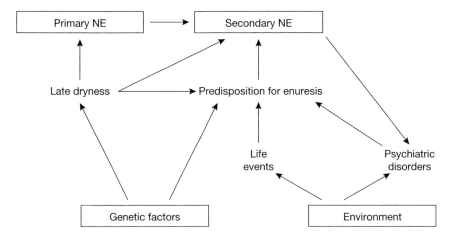

Fig. 6.6 Spectrum of primary and secondary nocturnal enuresis: genetic factors lead to late dryness and to a predisposition towards a relapse, which can be precipitated by stressful life events and behavioural disorders; these, in turn, reduce self-esteem and aggravate the psychiatric comorbidity.

TYPES OF DISORDERS

As regards the types of behavioural and emotional disorders, externalizing disorders predominate (von Gontard et al 1999a). Specifically, primary nocturnal enuresis has a low overall comorbidity with externalizing disorders predominating, while secondary nocturnal enuresis has a much higher comorbidity with both internalizing (emotional) and externalizing disorders occurring (see Table 6.4).

ATTENTION DEFICIT HYPERACTIVITY DISORDER (ADHD)

The most specific comorbid disorders with enuresis are ADHD (according to DSM IV) or hyperkinetic syndrome (according to ICD-10). In our own studies, the rates ranged from 9.3 per cent (HKS) to 13.5 per cent (HKS and ADHD) (von Gontard et al 1999a, Freitag et al 2006) – in children with primary and secondary enuresis (see Table 6.3). ADHD is not associated with any specific type of nocturnal enuresis (Baeyens et al 2004).

TABLE 6.4
Children with ICD-10 diagnoses – comparison between primary
and secondary nocturnal enuresis (von Gontard et al 1999a)

ICD-10 diagnostic groups	Primary nocturnal enuresis (n=82)	Secondary nocturnal enuresis (n=28)	p (chi²)
Externalizing disorders	12.2%	32.1%	*
Hyperkinetic syndrome	6.1%	17.9%	n.s.
Conduct disorder	6.1%	14.3%	n.s.
Internalizing (emotional) disorders	2.4%	25.0%	***
At least one diagnosis	19.5%	75.0%	***

In a retrospective study of patients with ADHD, 20.9 per cent wetted at night and 6.5 per cent during the day. The odds ratios were 2.7 and 4.5 times higher, respectively, which means that there is unspecific association of ADHD with both night- and daytime wetting (Robson et al 1997). In a study of 140 children with ADHD 25 per cent were affected by nocturnal enuresis, compared to 10.8 per cent of the 120 controls (Biederman et al 1995). The highest comorbidity rate for ADHD and nocturnal enuresis – 40 per cent – was reported by Baeyens et al (2004), possibly due to selection effects. Fifteen per cent had a combined type, 22.5 per cent an inattentive type and only 2.5 per cent a hyperactive type of ADHD. In a community-based sample, the prevalence rate was much lower (Baeyens 2005). In a two-year follow-up the disorder continued to be present in 72.5 per cent of children, indicating a high stability (Baeyens 2005). Also, nocturnal enuresis and ADHD are not transmitted together according to formal genetic findings (Bailey et al 1999). Molecular genetic studies have not been performed regarding this comorbidity, but the association is most likely to be based on common neurobiological factors.

In clinical practice, children with ADHD are more difficult to treat. In a retrospective study, 113 children with ADHD and nocturnal enuresis had a far worse outcome on alarm treatment than controls (with nocturnal enuresis only): 43 per cent (vs. 69 per cent) were dry at 6 months and 19 per cent (vs. 66 per cent) at 12 months. There was no difference in outcome if they were treated with medication, which does not require active cooperation. Non-compliance was reported in 38 per cent of children with ADHD, but in only 22 per cent of the controls (Crimmins et al 2003). Therefore, the comorbid diagnoses of both enuresis and ADHD require special attention – and each needs to be treated separately.

SUBCLINICAL PSYCHOLOGICAL SYMPTOMS
Subclinical behavioural signs and symptoms are common, understandable, appropriate reactions to the wetting problem and not disorders. Many studies have addressed the impact of wetting on children.

Self-esteem
One construct of special importance is that of self-esteem – or 'self-regard' or 'self-concept', which can be used synonymously. It has been defined as: '[a] relatively stable set of self-attitudes reflecting both a description and an evaluation of one's own behaviour and attitudes' (Piers 1984), and is an important attribute thought to be associated with mental health. In one study, lower self-esteem in children with enuresis disappeared upon attaining dryness (Hägglöf et al 1997). In another study, global self-esteem was significantly lower in children with nocturnal enuresis than in controls (Theunis et al 2002); but in yet another study, the self-esteem total score was higher among enuretic children than norms (Moffat et al 1987). It was thus concluded that there is no clear evidence that bedwetting leads to lower self-esteem (Redsell and Collier 2000) – but there can be no doubt that self-esteem can improve upon attaining dryness.

In a randomized study, 66 children were assigned to alarm treatment, and 55 to a three-month waiting list (Moffat et al 1987). The scores on the Piers–Harris self-esteem questionnaire increased significantly in the treatment group in those children who achieved total success and those who achieved partial improvement, but showed no increase in children with treatment failure. This implies that self-esteem improves even in children who achieve partial success.

The effects of 'good doctoring' can be seen even more clearly in another randomized study of 182 children treated by alarm, placebo or DDAVP (Longstaffe et al 2000). The scores on the Piers–Harris questionnaire increased after six months – regardless of any improvement. They increased significantly for the alarm and the DDAVP, but not for the placebo group. The authors conclude that 'frequent follow-up and emotional support and encouragement appear to be important components of an efficacious intervention for children with nocturnal enuresis' (Longstaffe et al 2000: 935). Caring for wetting children and their parents is an important factor – even if, or especially when, the treatment is not as successful as everyone (including doctors and nurses) would wish.

IMPACT ON PARENTS
Accompanying psychological problems may be just as distressing for parents and children as the wetting problem itself. Generally, parents are very concerned about the welfare of their child. In a population-based study, 17 per cent worried a great deal and 46 per cent 'some' or a little (Foxman et al 1986). In one study, the greatest maternal concerns were: emotional impact, social relationships, smell, extra washing, and financial aspects (Butler 1986).

Parents also believe that their child should be dry at night at a very early age: the mean anticipated age of dryness was 3.18 years in one study (Haque et al 1981) and 2.75 years in another (Shelov et al 1981). Parents believed that the causes responsible for their child's wetting were: developmental problem 33 per cent, emotional problem 29 per cent, heavy sleeping 20 per cent, physical or anatomical problem 13 per cent, small bladder 5 per cent (Shelov et al 1981); and emotional problem 35.5 per cent, heavy sleeping 38.2 per cent, physical problem 21.4 per cent, familial problem 28.9 per cent, small bladder 10.7 per cent (Haque et al 1981).

A minority of parents show an attitude that was described as 'maternal intolerance' by Butler (1986). These mothers are convinced that their child is wetting on purpose. They believe enuresis is controllable, and get angry at their child, do not invest energy in treatment, and withdraw and even punish their child. The reported rates of punishment ranged from 37 per cent (Butler 1987), 35.8 per cent (Haque et al 1981) and 23 per cent (Shelov et al 1981) to 5.6 per cent (von Gontard 1995). In other cultures, punishment is even more common: 42 per cent of Turkish children were spanked and 13 per cent beaten (Can et al 2004). Chinese parents show a high level of parenting stress associated with externalizing behavioural problems in their child (Chang et al 2002). These parental attributions and experiences have to be taken into account in all treatment plans for enuresis, as they can have a decisive influence on the outcome.

TOILET TRAINING

One issue parents often enquire about is the effect of toilet training on later wetting problems. Fortunately, it is easy to alleviate their fears. The best studies addressing this question are the two Swiss longitudinal studies conducted with an identical design in the 1950s and the 1970s. Due to the changes in toilet training practices the studies turned out to be a unique historical experiment.

In the 1950s, 96 per cent of mothers started toilet training within the first year of life – some at the age of 6 weeks, long before continence is physiologically possible. In the 1970s, due to more liberal attitudes and the advent of disposable diapers, toilet training started at 19–21 months, on average. Despite these different practices, there was no difference whatsoever regarding the age of continence at night. The authors therefore concluded that biological factors are mainly responsible for the attainment of night-time dryness. Environmental factors have little influence on this maturational process (Largo and Stützle 1977, Largo et al 1978, 1996). Also, early initiation of intensive toilet training means that it will take longer to complete – so that there is little benefit starting before the age of 27 months, as a recent study suggests (Blum et al 2003).

Assessment

PRIMARY EVALUATION

The primary evaluation of the enuretic child is simple and straightforward. History and a thorough physical examination will usually suffice to exclude those organic disorders that may present with bedwetting as a symptom – UTI, diabetes and kidney disease. Frequency-volume charts, urinalysis and sonography (in some centres) are sufficient for diagnosing most cases of nocturnal enuresis (Table 6.5). Most of the details regarding history and physical examination are given in Chapter 4 and in Appendix 1. Uncomplicated cases of

TABLE 6.5
Standard and extended assessment of nocturnal enuresis

Standard assessment
(sufficient for monosymptomatic nocturnal enuresis and for most other forms)
History
Frequency-volume chart
Questionnaires (in some centres)
Physical examination
Sonography (in some centres)
Urinalysis

Extended assessment
(only if indicated)
Urine bacteriology
Uroflowmetry
Laboratory tests
Child psychiatric assessment
Paediatric and urological assessment: radiology, cystoscopy, urodynamic investigations, etc.

enuresis do not need the attention of a specialist such as a paediatrician, urologist, urotherapist or paediatric psychiatrist, but can safely be evaluated by a general practitioner and followed up by a nurse.

The history should include questions regarding the type of enuresis (primary or secondary enuresis, monosymptomatic or non-monosymptomatic enuresis), frequency of wetting accidents, and daytime voiding habits. Urgency symptoms and signs of urinary tract infection should be enquired after, as well as symptoms suggesting constipation, such as encopresis. If the child is difficult to arouse from sleep at night – as the vast majority of bedwetters are – it is important to know whether the child, when awoken, is at all possible to communicate with, since this will have an impact on the feasibility of alarm treatment. It is of course also interesting to know whether the disorder runs in the family, although this will not affect treatment. Some brief questions should also be asked about the general health and well-being of the child, and about whether he or she experiences excessive thirst, especially in cases of secondary enuresis. A short list of the most important questions to ask appears in Table 4.3. It is important to find out whether the *child* regards the enuresis as a serious problem and how much it affects his or her life. Possible concomitant behavioural issues need to be addressed, but a detailed psychiatric evaluation is only needed if the child exhibits overt behavioural or emotional symptoms.

The physical examination should include height, weight, head circumference, inspection of the genitalia and a standard neurological examination. A rectal examination may be indicated if constipation is suspected. Even at this early stage a simple voiding chart completed by the patient is an invaluable aid when looking for signs of bladder dysfunction or excessive or reduced fluid intake. Blood samples or other invasive investigations are not usually needed. We recommend that a simple urine test for leukocytes, erythrocytes, glucose and bacteria is performed at the first visit in all children. This is particularly important in children with secondary enuresis, in whom excessive thirst, general malaise or weight loss may indicate diabetes (mellitus or insipidus) or kidney disease.

EVALUATION OF THERAPY-RESISTANT CHILDREN

Children with enuresis who do not respond to the alarm and to desmopressin in ordinary dosage, and non-responders to desmopressin in whom the alarm is considered unsuitable, should receive the attention of a specialist, usually a paediatrician with a specific interest in voiding problems, or a paediatric urologist. The help of a child psychologist or psychiatrist can be invaluable at this stage, as treatment outcome is poorer in children with comorbid disturbances. Symptoms and signs of constipation should be actively sought in all therapy-resistant children, and this may require a rectal examination.

The urodynamic and renal status of such children should be evaluated with extra care. These children should all complete a home voiding chart, so that voided volumes, micturition frequency and drinking habits can be documented and cases of excessive urine production detected. Uroflow and residual urine measurements are performed to detect signs of outlet obstruction and possible detrusor overactivity. In rare cases, a thirst provocation test (see Chapter 4), to assess renal concentrating capacity, is indicated if the child exhibits excessive urine production or fluid intake, but before this is considered the simple measurement of morning urine osmolality should be undertaken. It is our opinion that cystometry is still not necessary, provided that the above-mentioned examinations do not reveal signs of neurological disturbance, renal damage or bladder outlet obstruction. Nor will blood tests give much useful information.

Treatment

NON-PHARMACOTHERAPY

Preliminary steps

Before starting a specific treatment for nocturnal enuresis, several preliminary steps have to be considered. These are summarized in Chart 6.1. As always, treatment should only begin after a detailed assessment to rule out organic causes of the wetting and to identify psychiatric comorbid disorders and problems. Children should be at least 5 years old before treatment is initiated. It is important to remember that many parents believe that children should become dry at the age of 2 to 3 years (Haque et al 1981, Shelov et al 1981). These parents need to be counselled and advised to wait until their child reaches the age of 5 years (the definitional age of enuresis). Even some 5-year-olds will not be motivated enough for specific treatment, and in some countries waiting until the age of 6 to 7 years is recommended. If the family chooses to wait, then the child should be told that the bedwetting is not his or her fault and that effective treatment can be offered if the problem persists. Any constipation, encopresis and day-wetting problems should be addressed, in this order, first. Any other daytime symptoms (without wetting) should be treated before tackling the night-time wetting (in non-monosymptomatic nocturnal enuresis) (Kruse et al 1999). This is of great practical importance as some children will no longer wet at night once the daytime problems have been tackled.

One should also give advice about sound drinking and voiding habits, as described in Chapter 5. Thus, the child should know that instead of drinking large fluid volumes before bedtime extra fluid should be drunk during the day, that the bladder should be emptied regularly, about six times per day, etc. As has also been previously mentioned, it is part of good therapy to *explain*, *motivate* and provide *follow-up* to the patient, to reduce stress and alleviate possible guilt feelings. These unspecific, though effective principles are outlined in Chapter 5.

Non-effective forms of treatment

Many children who are referred have undergone or are receiving treatments or interventions that are not indicated. Some of them are harmless but have no effect in enabling the child to become dry. Other non-effective medications do have side effects. Many treatment recommendations have been shown to be clearly non-effective in reviews and meta-analyses (Butler 1987, 1994, Houts et al 1994, Lister-Sharp et al 1997). The methods that should be discontinued include:

- *Punishment*: up to 30 per cent of all enuretic children are still being punished and humiliated because of their enuresis (Butler 1987). In our own studies, 5.6 per cent of parents admitted they had punished their children (von Gontard 1995). In countries such as Turkey the rate of punishment is even higher – up to 40 per cent (Can et al 2004).

- *Inadequate rewards*: in our own studies, 24 per cent of parents used rewards in their endeavour to help their children. One pitfall is to reward dryness (which is not under the child's voluntary control) rather than cooperation and motivation (which are). Another pitfall is to promise large rewards (such as a bicycle) for dryness, instead of small positive reinforcements for intermediate successes. This can be extremely frustrating for those children who fail to reach the goal. Finally, non-material rewards (a trip to the cinema or to the swimming pool) can be a far greater incentive for children than material rewards.

- *Fluid restriction*: many doctors recommend that children should not drink in the evening, some suggest from afternoon onwards. In our own studies, 53 per cent of parents admitted that they tried to restrict fluids (von Gontard 1995). Considering the pathophysiology of nocturnal enuresis, this is, of course, not appropriate. It is unpleasant for children to be thirsty and fluid restriction has no influence on treatment success (Butler 1987, Lister-Sharp et al 1997). On the contrary, many children do not drink sufficient amounts of fluids – and should be encouraged to do so.

- *Waking*: many parents are convinced that they will help their child to become dry if they wake them during the night. In our own studies, 69 per cent of parents woke their children. Some woke them before they went to bed themselves; others even admitted setting the alarm clock several times during the night to wake the child. Empirical studies have shown that the likelihood that the child will remain dry that individual night will increase, but that the child will not remain dry if parents stop waking them (Butler 1987, Lister-Sharp et al 1997).

- *Lifting*: some parents do not even wake up their child, but lift them out of bed, carrying them to the toilet and back to bed without the child ever waking up. This popular method is equally ineffective (Lister-Sharp et al 1997). In some parents, this can be interpreted as a positive coping mechanism. By waking and lifting the child, parents have the feeling that they can do something actively for their child. This positive energy should, of course, be channelled into more effective forms of treatment.

- *Bladder training*: in the past, bladder retention control was recommended even for nocturnal enuresis. During the day, children were asked to postpone going to the toilet when they felt the urge to pass urine. The time interval between urge and going to the toilet was increased systematically. Studies have shown that this is not effective (Lister-Sharp et al 1997). From clinical observation, bladder retention can lead to excessive contraction of pelvic floor muscles and even induce dysfunctional voiding.

- *Cognitive-behavioural therapy without alarm*: as shown in Table 6.7, cognitive-behavioural therapy alone is not effective. Only one-third of all children achieve dryness, which is only half the success rate that alarm treatment can achieve.

- *Psychodynamic psychotherapy*: verbal and play psychotherapies are not effective for nocturnal enuresis, enabling only 21 per cent of the children to become dry (see Table 6.7). This is not very much higher than the 13 to 15 per cent of all children who achieve dryness spontaneously without any treatment at all. Psychodynamic, child-centred or analytical psychotherapy can be highly effective in comorbid emotional disorders. Enuresis, however, should always be treated in a symptom-oriented way, even in the case of coexisting psychological disorders.

- *Hypnotherapy* or *chiropractics* are not effective (Moffat 1997); *acupuncture* in contrast could have an effect but well-designed studies are still necessary (Hjälmås et al 2004); if these therapies have been implemented but have shown no success, it might be wise to discontinue them at this point in view of the treatment options with proven efficacy such as alarm treatment.
- *Anticholinergics* may be indicated if an urge syndrome or overactive bladder is present, even without daytime wetting. Anticholinergics can also be very helpful in combination with alarm treatment. If the alarm goes off several times every night, this could be an indication of bladder overactivity. Also, in treatment-resistant cases of nocturnal enuresis, anticholinergics have been recommended as a last resort, after a minimum of six months of unsuccessful treatment (Hjälmås et al 2004). In pure monosymptomatic nocturnal enuresis, however, anticholinergics have no place and should be discontinued (Homsy et al 1985).
- *Other medication*: only desmopressin and tricyclic antidepressants have a clear antienuretic effect. Neuroleptics, stimulants, tranquillizers, diuretics, alpha-blocking agents and other substances used in neurogenic urinary incontinence, such as phenoxybenzamine, are contraindicated and should be discontinued.
- *Other methods*: parents sometimes revert to recommendations outside of mainline medicine. Herbal teas, massages, creams, eucalyptus oil, dietary changes and diverse homeopathic mixtures are used but there is no evidence of their efficacy (Schönau et al 2005).

BASELINE TREATMENT

Baseline treatment can be considered to be a type of cognitive technique, consisting of counselling, provision of information, positive reinforcement, and increasing motivation. Children are asked to fill out a calendar or chart depicting wet and dry nights symbolically (for example with a 'sun' for a dry night and a 'cloud' for a wet night; or 'stars' for dry nights). In our experience, a baseline of four weeks is optimal, although two weeks is recommended by the American guidelines (AACAP 2004).

This four-week period should be modified in two situations. If all nights are consistently wet, baseline charts should be discontinued after 14 days. It would be extremely frustrating for a child to continue the process confronted with a calendar full of clouds. On the other hand, if the wet nights are markedly reduced after four weeks, continuing with these charts for a longer period – up to 8 or 12 weeks – may be beneficial. For some children, observation and recording, combined with praise and feelings of success, will accelerate the spontaneous rate of improvement and no other interventions will be needed.

These non-specific measures have been shown to be successful and are associated with fewer wet nights (Lister-Sharp et al 1997, Glazener and Evans 2002a). In one clinical trial, for example, 18 per cent of children became dry after an eight-week baseline (Devlin and

O'Cathain 1990). The authors of the recent Cochrane Review conclude that 'simple methods could be tried as first line therapy before considering alarms or drugs, because these alternative treatments may be more demanding and may have adverse effects' (Glazener et al 2004). For the 85 per cent of children for whom the baseline treatment is not sufficient, specific treatment such as alarm treatment is needed.

SPECIFIC MEASURES

The first-line treatment alternatives in uncomplicated nocturnal enuresis are the enuresis alarm or desmopressin. Our recommendation is that the advantages and disadvantages of these treatment modalities – summarized in Table 6.6 – be presented to the family and that they then choose which to start with. The indications for each are presented in the relevant sub-sections.

Since the most important determinant of success with the alarm is motivation, the families who choose the alarm will probably be those who are most likely to respond, and vice versa. The others should start with desmopressin. If the one does not work, the other should usually be tried (see Chart 6.2). Given the curative potential of the alarm, many families will opt for that treatment as their first choice. In the long run, the alarm is more effective than desmopressin (see Tables 6.6 and 6.7) (Wille 1986, Houts et al 1994, Schulman et al 2000, Glazener and Evans 2002b).

A combination of alarm and desmopressin can have synergistic positive effects, although the evidence regarding this is conflicting (see below). Only if one has exhausted these two possibilities should other treatment options be considered (see below).

ALARM TREATMENT

Alarm treatment is the most effective form of treatment of nocturnal enuresis, with the best long-term results (grade I level of evidence according to reviews and meta-analyses). Houts et al (1994) compiled a systematic review and meta-analysis of 78 randomized studies on nocturnal enuresis. As shown in Table 6.7, 62 per cent of children were dry at the end of treatment and 47 per cent at follow-up. The authors concluded that 'urine alarm treatments should not only be considered the treatment of choice, but the evidence from this review suggests that cure rather than management is a realistic goal for the majority of children suffering from nocturnal enuresis' (Houts et al 1994: 743).

Lister-Sharp et al (1997) provided a systematic review, including only randomized, controlled trials, on nocturnal enuresis (including 16 trials on alarms, 8 on DBT (dry bed training) and 2 on combined behavioural and drug approaches). The relative risk of attaining 14 consecutive dry nights was calculated. The likelihood of achieving 14 consecutive dry nights was 13.3 times higher with the alarm than without treatment (see Table 6.8). The authors concluded that 'in the long term, alarm treatment would appear to be the most clinically effective and, because of the cost of drug therapy recurring, also the most cost effective intervention' (Lister-Sharp et al 1997: 6).

Mellon and McGrath (2000) compiled a systematic review of 70 well-controlled outcome studies on psychological and behavioural interventions, which were categorized into 'efficacious', 'probably efficacious' and 'promising' treatments (Chambless criteria

Table 6.6
Advantages and drawbacks, and indications and possible contraindications
of the alarm and desmopressin as first-line enuresis treatment modalities

	Alarm	Desmopressin
Advantages	50–90% success (long-term after treatment)	50–90% success (only under medication)
	Harmless	Relatively harmless
	Curative potential	Easy to use
		Immediate effect
Drawbacks	Requires hard work	Low curative potential
	Takes time	Expensive
		Small risk of water intoxication
Indications	Whenever possible	Temporary, quick dryness (school outings, holidays, etc.)
		Treatment resistance and contraindications to alarm
		Lack of motivation
		Infrequent wetting
Contraindications	Lack of motivation in child and parents	
	Overt bladder dysfunction (overactive bladder, postponement, etc.), constipation, encopresis, behavioural disorders (ADHD) (treat these first)	
	Crowded living conditions	
	Familial stress and conflicts	
	'Parental intolerance'	
	Parental need for sleep (psychiatric disease such as depression, stressful working situation, having to care for infant)	

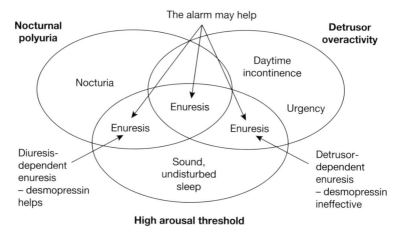

Fig. 6.7 Therapeutic response in relation to major pathogenetic factors in nocturnal enuresis.

TABLE 6.7
Effectiveness of different forms of treatment for nocturnal enuresis (percentage
dry at the end of treatment and at follow-up) (meta-analysis of Houts et al 1994)

Method	Percentage dry at the end of treatment	Percentage dry at follow-up (1–122 weeks; mean 21.2 weeks)
Non-pharmacotherapy		
Alarm alone	62%	47%
Alarm with behavioural therapy	72%	56%
Behavioural therapy alone	33%	30%
Verbal psychotherapy	21%	11%
Pharmacotherapy		
Tricyclic antidepressants	40%	17%
Desmopressin	46%	22%
Sedatives	27%	10%
Stimulants	18%	16%

TABLE 6.8
Relative risk of attaining 14 consecutive dry nights compared
to controls (meta-analysis of Lister-Sharp et al 1997)

Method	Relative risk of attaining 14 consecutive dry nights
Non-pharmacotherapy	
Alarm	13.3
Dry bed training (DBT)	10.0
DBT without alarm	2.5
Psychotherapy	No difference
Bladder training (retention control)	No difference
Pharmacotherapy	
Desmopressin	4.5 (no difference after discontinuation)
Imipramine	4.2

– Chambless and Hollon 1998). With a dryness rate of 77.9 per cent, alarm treatment was deemed clearly efficacious. A comprehensive narrative review was written by Moffat (1997), concluding that 'all the current evidence suggests that conditioning gives the best long-term outcomes for bed wetters'.

In 2002, a Cochrane Review of 22 randomized, controlled trials involving 1125 children concluded: 'Alarm interventions are an effective treatment for nocturnal enuresis. Desmopressin and tricyclics appeared as effective while on treatment, but this effect was not sustained after treatment stopped and alarms may be more effective in the long run' (Glazener and Evans 2002b). Therefore, when indicated, the alarm has been endorsed as a first-line treatment by multidisciplinary European (Läckgren et al 1999), world-wide (Hjälmås et al 2004), German (von Gontard 2006a) and American child psychiatric guidelines (AACAP 2004), as well as various individual authors (Butler et al 2004a).

What is an alarm?

An alarm consists of a pad or a metal sensor, which is connected to a bell by a wire. Once the sensor becomes wet, an electric circuit is closed and the alarm is set off. The mechanism is very simple and has been around for nearly 70 years (Mowrer and Mowrer 1938). Nowadays, the bell is powered by a small battery.

Two different types of alarms exist: body-worn and bedside alarms. In the case of body-worn alarms, the bell is strapped over the shoulder or pinched into a fold of the pyjamas, while the sensor is attached to the underpants. If desired, body-worn alarms can even be used with diapers. In the case of bedside alarms, a metal foil or a cloth pad (with integrated wires) is placed under the top sheet of the bed and is connected to an alarm next to the bed. Both alarms are equally effective (Fordham and Meadow 1989, Butler 1994, Lister-Sharp et al 1997, Butler 1998). Therefore, children should decide which alarm they would prefer. From our own clinical observations, younger children nearly always prefer the body-worn alarm, while older children and adolescents will choose the bedside alarm. Also, bedside alarms tend to be louder than the body-worn ones.

Indications for alarm treatment

For alarm treatment to be effective, both parents and children have to be motivated. In certain situations, it will not be advisable to start alarm treatment. These include sleeping disorders, stressful job obligations, and sometimes if there are other infants and siblings to look after. Another contraindication is when parents regard their child's enuresis as voluntary, a situation that Butler (1994) identified as 'parental intolerance'. In these cases, the alarm might be used in a negative way by the parents. Also, marked parent–child interaction problems can be a clear contraindication. If a child has an oppositional defiant disorder (ODD) he or she is likely to oppose alarm treatment and not cooperate sufficiently. Also, alarm treatment may be difficult if the child wets infrequently – simply because the alarm does not sound often enough to induce a sufficient training effect. In these cases, desmopressin might be the better choice. If the alarm sounds several times every night, this is often a sign of detrusor overactivity requiring additional anticholinergics. The alarm by itself will not be effective.

The child's goals, wishes and anxieties should be explored. Sometimes, children will only mention these if asked directly. Some children are worried that they will get an electric shock through the alarm. These fears are easily alleviated by showing them the small battery. Also, the child's motivation should be explored in detail. Some children may say quite frankly that they would like to be dry, but find alarm treatment too bothersome. Again, this would be a clear contraindication for alarm treatment. Instead, pharmacotherapy might be more advisable in these cases.

P.M., 7-year-old boy
Diagnosis: Monosymptomatic nocturnal enuresis

P. suffers from primary, monosymptomatic nocturnal enuresis, just like his father did as a child. There are no daytime bladder complaints or symptoms suggesting constipation.

Cognitive and physical development has been normal and P. is not excessively thirsty. He sleeps very soundly. P. tried the enuresis alarm a year ago with no effect, and desmopressin with partial effect. His parents are worried that their divorce, when P. was 3 years old, may have caused him to become a bedwetter.

Physical examination is normal. A frequency-volume chart also gives normal values for his age. P.'s mother recalls that the previous alarm treatment was conducted for three months, except for every second weekend when P. lives with his father, and there was never really any effect since P. sleeps so deeply. When the signal rang his mother stood by P.'s bed and waited – mostly in vain – for him to wake up. Now P. uses desmopressin and is dry approximately 50 per cent of nights, but is always wet without the drug. The mother is concerned about giving 'hormones' to her child.

First, the family were advised that the enuresis had nothing to do with their divorce. Second, proper instructions about how to use the alarm were given: P. must be helped to awaken to the signal, and the alarm must be used even when staying with his father. After six weeks of properly conducted alarm treatment P. became reliably dry.

Goals of treatment
The goal of alarm (as well as all other) treatment is complete dryness and not just a reduction of wetting frequency. Therefore, the following types of outcome have been defined (Butler 1991, Butler et al 2004b):

- Initial success: a minimum of 14 consecutive dry nights within 16 weeks of alarm treatment.
- Relapse: two wet nights in two weeks.
- Continued success: no relapse within six months after initial success.
- Complete success: no relapse within two years after initial success.
- Drop-out: two consecutive appointments missed or treatment discontinued.

For research purposes, Butler et al (2004b) suggested a simple 'dryness scale' (from 4 down to 0), again based on the percentage of dry nights: 4 = >90 per cent, 3 = 50–90 per cent, 2 = 25–49 per cent, 1 = 1–24 per cent and 0 = 0 per cent. The actual percentage and not the reduction from a baseline level is of greatest practical relevance.

The newer ICCS (Nevéus et al 2006) recommendations for treatment of all types of enuresis and incontinence are shown in Table 2.5.

How is alarm treatment conducted?
The alarm should not just be prescribed, but its functions shown and demonstrated. Children should feel responsible for their treatment. The instructions are extremely important and should be gone through in detail with parents and child.

Children are asked to go to the toilet before going to bed, something most of them do anyway. The alarm is attached and switched on. If the child has a dry night, nothing happens and the child can turn off the alarm the next morning. In case of wetting, the alarm is triggered and the child should wake up completely, either by him- or herself or with parental help. In some cases, parents will have to be quite imaginative in finding an optimal waking routine. Afterwards, the child goes to the toilet and is asked to urinate. Then, the pyjamas and the bedding are changed, and the alarm is reset. The child should be actively involved in this process. If the child wets a second time during the night, the whole routine is followed again. Parents are asked to mark all relevant data on a chart, which is depicted in Appendix 9 (adapted from Butler 1987).

To be successful, the alarm must be used every night for a maximum of 16 weeks. Some children become dry in only a few weeks; most will require 8 to 10 weeks and some a bit longer. After 14 consecutive dry nights, the alarm is discontinued and the child is considered to be dry. Parents are advised not to throw away their alarm but to keep it in case a relapse occurs, which happens in 30 per cent of cases within the first six months after treatment.

The rate of relapse has been underreported in some studies on alarm treatment (Kristensen and Jensen 2003). If a child wets only once for a single night, he or she should not despair but should be consoled – as this can happen to many children. A relapse is defined by Butler (1991) as two wet nights in two weeks, and in the ICCS terminology (Nevéus et al 2006) as more than one symptom recurrence per month. If a relapse occurs, alarm treatment should be restarted immediately, and most children will become dry again.

M.K., 7-year-old boy
Diagnosis: Primary non-monosymptomatic nocturnal enuresis

M. was referred because of nocturnal wetting. He had never been dry before, was wetting every night and wore diapers, which were completely wet. During the day, he used to wet quite often and had the tendency to postpone going to the toilet with holding manoeuvres. At the time of presentation he was wetting every three months during the daytime. The micturition frequency was four to five times a day. He used to soil his pants, but this had resolved spontaneously. There had been no previous therapies. The developmental history and family history were normal, and there were no major

112

behavioural problems. Physical examination, cognitive state and questionnaires were also normal.

M. was asked to increase his micturition frequency by going to the toilet seven times a day and noting this on a chart. Alarm treatment was also instituted, and M. became dry after eight weeks.

In this case, there were signs of voiding postponement, which was treated by asking M. to go to the toilet more often. The nocturnal enuresis was tackled successfully with alarm treatment.

Several factors influencing the outcome of the alarm treatment have been identified. These include: distance to the clinic, lack of treatment supervision, familial stressors, parental cooperation, cramped living conditions, maternal intolerance and anger, low self-esteem of the child, behavioural problems, previous treatment failure, daytime symptoms and secondary nocturnal enuresis (Butler 1994, Butler and Robinson 2002). The success rates in children with additional daytime wetting were lower than those in children with nocturnal enuresis alone (van Leerdam et al 2004), which means that any daytime wetting or other symptoms should be addressed first.

How does alarm treatment work?
As mentioned previously, alarm treatment is an operant type of behavioural treatment, which includes positive reinforcement such as praise and success, as well as aversive consequences such as getting up, going to the toilet and redoing the bed (Butler 1994). A classical conditioning paradigm using an ultrasound bladder-volume-controlled alarm has been described by Pretlow (1999).

Dryness can be achieved by two basic mechanisms: either the children learn to wake up and go to the toilet, or they sleep through the night.

1   Between 35 and 42 per cent of children choose the first route to success by waking up and developing nocturia (Bonde et al 1994, Hvistendahl et al 2004). This rate is much higher than the rate of nocturia in healthy school children (Mattsson 1994a). Those achieving dryness by developing nocturia through alarm treatment have a higher night-time urine production (Hvistendahl et al 2004). Nocturia can also be a persisting symptom of childhood enuresis in adults (Djurhuus et al 1999). On a neurophysiological basis, one could speculate that in these cases the nucleus coeruleus, which is responsible for arousal, might be stimulated in its activity by alarm treatment (Nevéus et al 2000).
2   Sixty-five per cent of dry children do not wake up but sleep through the night (Bonde et al 1994). In another study, 72 per cent did not wake up (Butler and Robinson 2002). The success is not mediated by reduced urine production or changes in the vaso-pressin secretion (Hansen and Jorgensen 1997). Instead, the bladder capacity increases through alarm treatment in dry, as well as wet, children (Oredson and Jorgensen 1998, Hvistendahl et al 2004). Neurophysiologically, one could hypothesize that the

113

micturition reflex is inhibited more completely by the pontine micturition centre in the brainstem (Ornitz et al 1999, Nevéus et al 2000, Freitag et al 2006).

K.W., 6-year-old girl
Diagnosis: Primary monosymptomatic nocturnal enuresis

K. was referred because of nocturnal wetting of large volumes. She had never been dry before and was a 'deep sleeper'. She became dry during the day at the age of 2½ years. There were no micturition problems and development was normal. Both parents had wetted as children. The paediatric examination and ultrasound were normal, the uroflow curve bell-shaped. Intelligence was in the normal range (IQ 105). There were no signs of behavioural or emotional symptoms. K. was treated with an alarm and became dry within a few weeks without nocturia.

This is a typical scenario for primary monosymptomatic nocturnal enuresis without any behavioural disorder. Genetic factors predominate. K.'s response to the alarm treatment was optimal.

Alarm treatment and behavioural treatment
The effect of alarm treatment can be enhanced by adding behavioural components to the treatment. Programmes that included the alarm in addition to other behavioural components showed the following general effects: 72 per cent of children became dry at the end of treatment, and 56 per cent remained so at follow-up (meta-analysis: Houts et al 1994 – see Table 6.7). Thus, combinations were considered as 'probably effective' (Mellon and McGrath 2000).

Specific programmes with the alarm include:

1   **Arousal training**: a simple, easily performed variation on the alarm treatment is the so-called 'arousal training' by van Londen et al (1993, 1995). When the alarm is triggered by wetting, children are instructed to turn off the alarm within three minutes, go to the toilet and reset the alarm. This goal is reinforced positively with two tokens, such as stickers, in case of success. If the goal is not reached, one token has to be returned.

In younger children, we found it advisable to modify this training: children receive one token if they are successful but do not have to pay back a token if they are not, which would be too frustrating for young children. The initial success rate (89 per cent) and the rate of dryness after 2.5 years (92 per cent) were higher than with alarm treatment alone (73 per cent and 72 per cent respectively) (van Londen et al 1993). Because of the high success rate and simplicity, arousal training has become the standard cognitive-behavioural therapy in our clinics if alarm treatment alone does not suffice.

2   **Dry bed training**: the best-known, and still widely used, training programme is the dry bed training (DBT) programme by Azrin et al (1974). It is an extremely complicated and difficult to perform programme, starting with an 'intensive night', followed by 'maintenance treatment':

- Intensive night: before going to bed, children receive detailed instructions on a so-called 'positive practice', clearly a euphemism. They are asked to lie on their bed, count to 50, go to the toilet and repeat this 20 times.

  They are woken every hour, fluids are offered and children are asked if they want to go to the toilet or not but are encouraged to retain the urine.

  After wetting, children have to take care of the dry bed-clothes (so-called 'cleanliness training') and must repeat the 'positive practice'.

- Maintenance treatment: on the following nights, children are woken only once per night, when the parents go to bed. If the child remains dry, they are woken half an hour earlier the following night. If, however, they wet the bed, they are woken at the same time as the night before. After dry nights, the child is praised. On wet nights, 'cleanliness training' and 'positive practice' are followed as previously described.

  After seven consecutive dry nights, the alarm is discontinued but 'positive practice' and 'cleanliness training' are still performed on dry nights.

  In case of a relapse (two wet nights per week), the alarm is reinstituted.

Despite high success rates reported in early studies (Azrin et al 1974), recent meta-analyses have shown that DBT is no more effective than alarm treatment alone (Lister-Sharp et al 1997 – see Table 6.8). The likelihood of attaining 14 consecutive dry nights was 10 times higher than in controls without treatment – but not different from alarm treatment alone. Also, the alarm is the most important component of DBT. DBT without the alarm showed only a 2.5 times higher likelihood of attaining dryness than the rate for controls. The relapse rates were not improved by DBT compared to alarm treatment alone (Lister-Sharp et al 1997).

As it is a cumbersome treatment, it is nowadays reserved for some children and especially adolescents with therapy-resistant nocturnal enuresis, as it 'may augment the effect of an alarm' (Glazener et al 2004). Thus, Hirasing et al (2002) could show that behavioural problems were reduced in children with persistent nocturnal enuresis treated with DBT.

Two other combinations should be mentioned. Although shown to be effective, they are more difficult to perform. In view of the good results of arousal training, they are not part of the therapeutical programme of our clinics:

3   **'Full spectrum home treatment'** is a combination package including a written contract, full arousal, 'overlearning' and bladder retention exercises (Houts et al 1994);

78.5 per cent of children became dry in two studies (Mellon and McGrath 2000), but the alarm exerts the main effect (Glazner et al 2004).

4   **'Overlearning'** is a relapse prevention programme: after attaining dryness, increasing amounts of fluids are given before sleep to stabilize the achieved effects (Morgan 1978). The relapse rate can be reduced from 20–40 per cent to 10 per cent through this 'provocation method'.

5   **Pharmacotherapy**: finally, alarm treatment can be combined with pharmacotherapy, although the evidence for combination treatment is conflicting.

   The combination of the alarm with six weeks of 40 µg desmopressin intranasally was better than alarm treatment alone, especially with high micturition frequency and comorbid behavioural symptoms (Bradbury and Meadow 1995). In a Chinese study comparing alarm treatment, desmopressin and a combined therapy, the combined therapy had the highest rate of sustained response (40.6 per cent). However, there was a high relapse rate after discontinuing medication (Ng et al 2005).

   In another randomized, controlled, double-blind study, three weeks of 40 µg and three weeks of 20 µg desmopressin in addition to the alarm led to a temporary, short-term reduction of wet nights compared to controls on alarm treatment and placebo (Leebeek-Groenewegen et al 2001). However, the long-term success rates were low and did not differ between the two groups (36 per cent and 37 per cent, respectively). In the subgroup of desmopressin non-responders, the combination of alarm plus desmopressin was less successful (51.5 per cent remission) than alarm plus placebo (48.1 per cent remission), so this cannot be recommended as a routine strategy (Gibb et al 2004).

   The combination of alarm and anticholinergics should be considered if an overactive bladder is suspected. If the alarm is set off several times per night, which is indicative of an overactive bladder, this combination has been proven to be successful. For example, 5 mg of oxybutynin in the evening combined with alarm treatment could be tried in these cases. If higher levels of anticholinergics are required, several doses should be given over the day. Even anticholinergics alone can be successful in treating non-monosymptomatic nocturnal enuresis. Predictive factors are age, frequency, small voids, small or variable wet patches and waking after wetting (Butler et al 2004b).

In conclusion, based on current evidence, alarm treatment alone should be started first. As an adjunct, arousal treatment is easy to perform and effective. Also, the combination of alarm and desmopressin or oxybutynin can be indicated. DBT and other programmes remain forms of treatment reserved for some therapy-resistant cases. In certain cases, alarm treatment will not be possible – such cases are prime indications for desmopressin.

Pharmacotherapy

DESMOPRESSIN

As stated above, desmopressin is one of the two first-line antienuretic therapies. Pharmacological details and safety aspects are discussed in Chapter 5.

Efficacy
Since the late 1970s many studies have shown that desmopressin is a useful treatment for enuresis (Dimson 1977, Birkasova et al 1978, Tuvemo 1978, Fjellestad-Paulsen et al 1987a, Terho 1991, Shu et al 1993, Matthiesen et al 1994, Stenberg and Läckgren 1994, Monda and Husmann 1995, Skoog et al 1997, Yeung 1997, Hjälmås et al 1998). In a recent meta-analysis it was concluded that desmopressin is better than placebo (Glazener and Evans 2002c). Reported success rates have varied between 40 and 80 per cent. A problem is that although the proportion of children with a moderate response to treatment is high, only a minority – perhaps as low as 25 per cent – achieve total dryness (Hjälmås et al 1998), and for many of those children the occasional wet nights still affect their self-esteem and lifestyle.

The group of enuretic children with the greatest chance of benefiting from desmopressin treatment are children with no daytime incontinence or urgency symptoms and normal voided volumes, i.e. those in whom nocturnal polyuria can be suspected to be the central pathogenetic factor (Nevéus 2001, Nevéus et al 2001b).

Most children successfully treated with desmopressin relapse after treatment, so the curative effect is low (Fjellestad-Paulsen et al 1987a, Stenberg and Läckgren 1994, Glazener and Evans 2002c). The curative rate amounted to a maximum of 18–38 per cent after discontinuing treatment in most studies (van Kerrebroeck 2002). Compared with the alarm, desmopressin has a distinctly lower curative effect in the long run (Moffatt et al 1993, Houts et al 1994).

How to start treatment
Pills and nasal spray have similar therapeutic efficacy (Fjellestad-Paulsen et al 1987a, Janknegt et al 1997), though with a possible bias towards higher intranasal efficacy (Matthiesen et al 1994). Since the tablets do not have to be swallowed whole and the efficacy of nasal spray is diminished in the presence of rhinitis, oral administration is often recommended, but that is a matter of preference.

Desmopressin should be taken in the evening, not earlier than one hour before going to bed. The usual dose is 0.2–0.4 mg orally (120–240 µg with the quick-melt formulation) or 20–40 µg intranasally. Some experts recommend medication to be started at the lower dosage and then increased in the absence of full therapeutic effect. Charts for documenting this strategy are shown in Appendices 7 and 8. Others prefer the opposite strategy – i.e. starting with a full dose and then diminishing it in case of full response – arguing that it is simpler and that it is a good strategy to 'let the first try be the best try', but that is also a matter of preference. As mentioned above, there is probably also a small group of therapy-resistant patients who may cautiously be given a dose as high as 0.8 mg orally (Nevéus et al 1999c), provided they adhere to strict fluid restriction (see below) during the evening and night.

One of the advantages of desmopressin is that one sees the effect – if there is any effect – immediately. We use a test period of two to four weeks; if there is no effect within this time, the family should discontinue treatment, and alternative treatments should be considered.

Whenever this drug is prescribed it is imperative that the family and child are informed about the small but significant risk of *water intoxication*. The typical nightmare scenario

117

is that the child goes to a party and consumes a litre or more of soft drinks and then takes his or her bedtime desmopressin. Ordinary fluid intake, say one or two glasses with the evening meal and one glass before going to bed, is acceptable, and extra water after strenuous physical activity is also allowable, provided the child only drinks *because he or she is thirsty.*

The sensation of thirst means that the CNS receptors have reacted to an increased serum osmolality, which means that it is safe and even desirable for the child to drink. But at an occasion like a school party children tend to drink not because they are thirsty but because it is fun. So, the important message is this: if the child is thirsty, they should drink (preferably water) to quench thirst only, and they can then safely take the medication; but if the child for other reasons drinks large amounts of fluid one evening, then the medication should be skipped that particular evening.

More exact fluid intake recommendations have been published for those who need an exact figure for how much can safely be consumed when taking desmopressin. Beach et al consider 30 ml fluid per kg body weight during the time span two hours pre-intake to eight hours post-intake to be the safety limit (Beach et al 1992), whereas Robson and co-workers give an allowance of a maximum of 240 ml during desmopressin nights (Robson et al 1996a). We prefer the more general recommendation stated above.

How to continue treatment

If desmopressin treatment is successful and the child and family are satisfied with the effect, the question often arises whether the drug should be taken every evening or only before 'important nights'. We strongly believe that this decision should be left to the family (and especially the child). There is no evidence that continuous desmopressin treatment hastens the spontaneous resolution of the disorder, and families who choose to only use the pills intermittently should not be given the impression that they are disobeying the doctor's orders. Usually, in the case of infrequent enuresis the family will choose intermittent treatment, and the child who wets almost every night will want to take the medication every night.

Families who choose to give desmopressin every night should be asked to discontinue treatment for one week every third month or so, in order to check whether the disorder has disappeared or not.

There are some data indicating that gradual tapering of desmopressin over one or several months may increase the chance of cure (Akbal et al 2004). In the well-motivated family this might be a recommended strategy to use after 6 to 12 months of treatment.

Sooner or later, in cases where the child does not manage to come off the medication without relapse, the parents will want to know how long it is safe to use desmopressin. This is a difficult question to answer with total confidence, but the studies performed so far indicate that the drug is safe to use for at least a few years (Knudsen et al 1991, Fjellestad-Paulsen et al 1993b, Sukhai 1993, Hjälmås 1995b), and we suspect that it may be used for even longer than that. If a relapse does occur after discontinuing medication, desmopressin can be reconsidered or alarm treatment tried (again).

What to do if it does not work

The child who does not respond to desmopressin should be encouraged to try the alarm, if it has not already been tried or judged unsuitable.

As stated above, the child who experiences no beneficial effect of desmopressin treatment within a few weeks should *not* be asked to continue medication. The case is not so clear-cut when the child shows a partial response. If there are additional symptoms suggesting detrusor overactivity, anticholinergic medication may be added; if not, the cautious use of high-dose desmopressin treatment may be tried (see above). Before trying this last treatment alternative, children on oral desmopressin should try switching to intranasal administration to see if it improves the situation. Otherwise, one test week of treatment with 0.8 mg orally or 80 µg intranasally will show if the child belongs to the small group of children requiring higher than normal dosage. The evidence base for the efficacy of supra-normal desmopressin dosage is, however, slim: just one open study and one placebo-controlled study (Skoog et al 1997, Nevéus et al 1999c). It is especially important that these children do not consume extra fluids during the evening and night, and it is the authors' recommendation that this treatment be used 'for important nights only' and not continuously.

Therapy-resistant cases

If primary treatment was tried two years ago or more, it should be tried again before anticholinergics are considered. Non-responders to desmopressin may, for obscure reasons (in the authors' unpublished experience), become responders, and – more importantly – the child may become easier to arouse from sleep or more motivated for alarm treatment as he or she grows older.

Children with 'diuresis-dependent enuresis' (i.e. with suspected nocturnal polyuria) usually respond to desmopressin (or alarm) treatment. However, in a minority of therapy-resistant children, diuresis dependency can still be suspected: for instance, children with a partial desmopressin response, children with normal voided volumes, and children with low renal concentrating capacity. In these children treatment with desmopressin 0.8 mg orally at bedtime could be tried, since it has been shown that there are some enuretic children who need such high desmopressin doses to achieve dryness (Nevéus et al 1999c). As already mentioned, during high-dose desmopressin treatment it is imperative that the child does not consume large amounts of fluids during the evening and night.

Many children who do not respond to either desmopressin or alarm treatment can be suspected to suffer from detrusor-dependent enuresis, since they have been found to have smaller bladders (functionally, not anatomically) (Rushton et al 1996, Eller et al 1997, 1998, Nevéus et al 1999b, Kamperis et al 2001, Nevéus 2001) and lower nocturnal urine production (Hunsballe et al 1995, Rittig et al 1997, Hunsballe et al 1998) than the responders, and cystometric studies have confirmed that detrusor overactivity is common in this group (Yeung et al 1999). Many of these children experience urgency symptoms, have small voided volumes, go to the toilet often and/or have current or previous daytime incontinence as well, and they are often constipated. Micturition chart data will often confirm that these children have enuresis of the non-monosymptomatic variety.

The first thing to do in the case of these children is to enquire if the alarm treatment was properly conducted. Many families fail with the alarm because they did not receive proper instructions (i.e. they were not told that most children need help to awake at the signal, that treatment needs to be continuous, etc.). If this is the case, then the family should be encouraged to try again, this time with proper follow-up. As previously mentioned, if the alarm sounds several times per night, this could be indicative of an overactive bladder requiring additional anticholinergics (although this clinical experience has not yet been confirmed by randomized trials).

The second step is to exclude or treat constipation. The strategies for this are discussed in Chapter 9.

If this has been done and the child is still not dry it is our clinical experience that anticholinergic treatment is effective in approximately 50 per cent of children, and in still more if desmopressin is added. Note, however, that these recommendations are not, as yet, grounded on a sufficient number of randomized, controlled trials.

If response to anticholinergics is partial, desmopressin should be added in standard dosage. Some doctors choose to start with combined treatment instead of anticholinergic monotherapy. Again, this is experience-based, not evidence-based, treatment.

ANTICHOLINERGICS
Since anticholinergic drugs are much more firmly established as a treatment of incontinence due to detrusor overacticity, the reader is referred to Chapter 7 for information about how to use these drugs and what precautions to take. Pharmacology, pharmacokinetics and side effects are covered in Chapter 5.) Here only the aspects specific to nocturnal enuresis are discussed.

Efficacy
The efficacy of anticholinergics as a treatment of enuresis without daytime incontinence is not scientifically proven. A moderately large number of studies on oxybutynin have been performed in children with enuresis (Buttarazzi 1977, Laurenti et al 1987, Lovering et al 1988, Persson-Jünemann et al 1993, Caione et al 1997, Kosar et al 1999, Nevéus et al 1999c), but the results are difficult to interpret because in most of these studies children with daytime incontinence have been included as well, and the efficacy in monosymptomatic enuresis is difficult to disentangle. In the one randomized, placebo-controlled study on enuresis without daytime incontinence published so far, oxybutynin was not found to be superior to placebo (Lovering et al 1988).

That said, the clear experience of the current authors is that there are enuretic children without daytime incontinence who become dry on anticholinergic medication. Our impression is that approximately 40 per cent of enuretic children resistant to first-line therapy respond to anticholinergics as monotherapy, and perhaps an extra 20 per cent or so if desmopressin is added. This is also logical, given the role of detrusor overactivity in nocturnal enuresis. In a well-designed Turkish study (Kosar et al 1999) in enuretic and/or incontinent children it was shown that oxybutynin was effective if the children were found to have detrusor overactivity, and ineffective if they were not, regardless of whether the presenting symptom was enuresis or daytime incontinence. Not surprisingly, the enuretic children who respond to anticholinergics usually have daytime symptoms such as frequency and/or urgency, detectable with a voiding chart, even in the cases without daytime incontinence. Their enuresis is of the non-monosymptomatic type.

Thus, we recommend that anticholinergics be used in enuretic children resistant to first-line therapy, provided that constipation has been treated or excluded and that the precautions regarding residual urine, UTIs, side effects, etc. (see Chapter 7) have been taken into account.

Strategy

Our practice is to give 5–10 mg oxybutynin, 5–10 mg propiverine or 1–2 mg tolterodine (though the last drug is still off-label in children and thus cannot be generally recommended) in the evening, starting with half that dosage during the first week. Medication is judged not necessary in the morning if there is no concomitant daytime incontinence. It may also be argued that if we administer the drug in the evening only, we lessen the risk of residual urine/UTI or constipation. Treatment success is estimated after approximately six weeks. If response is partial, the addition of desmopressin in standard dosage may be beneficial. It is our clinical impression that spreading the doses during the day (two or three doses) can be beneficial in severe cases.

Our experience is that enuretic children responding to anticholinergic therapy usually need to continue this medication for 4 to 12 months. During this treatment the child should try to develop sound, regular voiding habits and the family should watch out for signs of constipation or urinary tract infection. Tapering should be gradual.

If anticholinergics are used in the morning as well, residual urine should be measured regularly and, if present, the drug should promptly be temporarily withdrawn. In boys with no history of UTI, no voiding postponement behaviour and no daytime incontinence, follow-up of residual urine during treatment may be omitted.

If desmopressin, alarm and anticholinergic treatments have all been tried without success or have been judged unsuitable, the cautious use of imipramine might be warranted. This is a matter for specialist clinics, however, and not for the general paediatrician.

TRICYCLIC ANTIDEPRESSANTS

Tricyclic antidepressants – mainly imipramine – have for several decades now been used for nocturnal enuresis. Their usage has recently diminished considerably, since safer and/or simpler therapies have been developed. This changed attitude is laudable, but we do not agree with those authors who advocate the drug's complete abolishment from the antienuretic arsenal, since we believe that it still has a necessary role to play as a third-line treatment alternative in the hands of specialists.

The reason for this more permissive attitude is, first, that fatal side effects have only been reported when using doses *higher* (in antidepressive therapy) than those that are relevant in the treatment of enuresis, and second, because of the documented efficacy of the drug in children resistant to standard therapy.

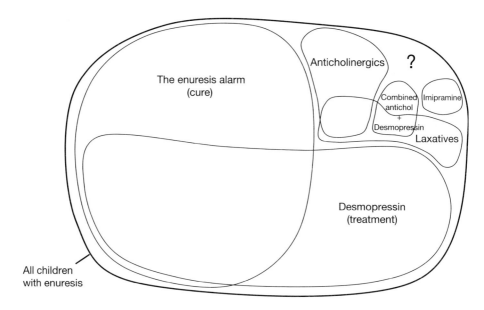

Fig. 6.8 How many enuretic children can we treat or cure? A graphic representation of evidence and clinical experience.

Efficacy

The efficacy of imipramine in nocturnal enuresis has been proven in several randomized, controlled studies (Poussaint and Ditman 1965, Kardash et al 1968, Miller et al 1968, Martin 1971, Rapoport et al 1980, Smellie et al 1996), and it is one of the two drugs that can be considered evidence-based as therapies for nocturnal enuresis (the other being desmopressin) (Glazener and Evans 2000). The proportion of unselected enuretic children responding to imipramine is approximately 40 per cent (Houts et al 1994; see Table 6.7). We have recently demonstrated that this holds true even in the group of children who are presently the only candidates for imipramine treatment, i.e. children who have not responded to the alarm, desmopressin or anticholinergics (Gepertz and Nevéus 2004). There are no clear clinical signs that indicate if a child will respond to treatment or not.

Tolerance may, however, be a problem. In our group it affected approximately 20 per cent of children with good initial therapeutic response (Gepertz and Nevéus 2004). And, as with all pharmacological therapies of enuresis, relapse after discontinuation is the rule rather than the exception.

Starting treatment

When imipramine treatment is considered, it is mandatory to (1) inform the family about the risks associated with overdosage and ensure that they keep the pills locked away; (2) inform the family that side effects can occur even in low doses; and (3) make sure that the child does not suffer from any heart condition. The child should be asked if they have ever fainted, if they tire easily, and if they have ever had attacks of palpitations. If the answer to any of these questions is affirmative, or there is any doubt, a long-time ECG recording with measurement of corrected QT time should be obtained before starting treatment. The same procedure should be used if anyone in the child's family has cardiac arrhythmias or other heart problems that are not attributable to hypertension, congenital malformations, arteriosclerosis or advanced age.

Being more cautious and conservative than paediatricians, child psychiatrists advise doing an ECG and blood test in every child treated with antidepressants (von Gontard and Lehmkuhl 1996, 2002, Gerlach et al 2004).

Also, every child on antidepressants should be followed up regularly (at closer intervals than with desmopressin) for somatic and psychological side effects. Changes in mood, motor activity and even suicidal ideation are rare, but possible, side effects even on low doses of tricyclics.

The ordinary antienuretic dose of imipramine is 10–25 mg given in the evening – the lower dosage is recommended for children below 9 years of age – which can then be increased to 25–50 mg. The effect should be seen within one month. If doses above 25 mg are reached, these should be divided into twice or three times daily. The antienuretic effects do increase by approaching antidepressive doses of a maximum of 3 mg/kg body weight/day in three doses – but this should only be done with special indication and under close clinical surveillance (Fritz et al 1994).

Continuing treatment
If the child responds to treatment, without significant side effects, the dosage can – and should – often be lowered without diminishing efficacy.

In our practice the development of tolerance – i.e. diminishing response during continuous treatment – has become less common since families have been routinely asked to discontinue treatment for at least two weeks every three months. In the small subgroup of children who experience side effects – palpitations, nausea – upon withdrawal of the drug, it should be withdrawn gradually the next time. Needless to say, the exclusive hardcore group of enuretic children receiving imipramine treatment should be followed up regularly by a specialist. We have no way of predicting how long the duration of imipramine treatment will need to be in the cases that respond. The decision to continue or discontinue long-term treatment must be made after balancing benefit, side effects and safety concerns on an individual basis.

What to do if it does not work
Some children with partial or no response to monotherapy with imipramine may become dry if desmopressin is added (Gepertz and Nevéus 2004). The nature of this synergism is unclear, but one explanation may be that desmopressin, by delaying bladder filling to a time of night when the child is more easily awakened, makes the job easier for the other drug. It may also be due to the possible CNS effects of desmopressin mentioned in Chapter 5.

**Diagnoses: Primary non-monosymptomatic nocturnal enuresis
(therapy-resistant); hyperkinetic syndrome with conduct disorder (F90.1)**

From the age of 9 years, P. had had contact with the child psychiatric team because of hyperactivity, distractability and impulsive behaviour. Regular contacts with a psychologist and adaptations of his school environment had diminished these problems considerably. The psychiatrist had concluded that stimulants were not necessary.

His nocturnal enuresis had, however, proven more difficult to treat. The bed-wetting frequency was irregular, but there were never more than seven dry nights in a row. Until a few years ago, he had occasionally also wetted his clothes during the daytime, but this had disappeared after contacts with a school nurse who provided basic urotherapeutic advice. He had 'restless' sleep and was difficult to arouse. P's father had become dry at the age of 8.

P. had no UTIs, was seldom ill, had a normal growth curve and was not described as excessively thirsty. There were no bowel-related complaints. There were no heart conditions in the family and P. himself had not suffered syncope, palpitations or other symptoms of cardiac disease.

P. had previously undergone several treatment attempts: desmopressin and the alarm were both unsuccessful. He was also given advice about regular voidings, fluid intake and sleep habits, but this had not improved his bedwetting situation. He was now becoming more and more concerned about this problem, and it was affecting his mood and behaviour negatively.

Physical examination revealed he was slightly overweight but nothing else. Ultrasound of the kidneys and urinary tract, as well as uroflow, were normal and there was no residual urine. A frequency-volume chart showed four to eight voidings per day with a voided volume between 50 and 250 ml. He was drinking about 1 litre of fluid daily, mostly at breakfast and lunchtime. Bowel movements occurred daily.

On the assumption that P. had nocturnal detrusor overactivity, anticholinergic treatment was given with oxybutynin 5 mg at bedtime. Due to lack of success, the dosage was increased to 10 mg after one month and 0.4 mg of desmopressin orally was added. This gave no extra benefit, but the parents noted that their son's temper was becoming difficult to control, with frequent outbursts of anger or sadness.

Given the severe therapy-resistance of his enuresis and the absence of cardiac risk factors, a trial of imipramine 50 mg orally at bedtime was deemed appropriate. The parents were instructed to keep the pills securely locked. After one week of treatment P. became dry. He had no subjective side effects and stayed dry for two consecutive months. All seemed well but then occasional wet nights started to reappear. The family were then instructed to provide regular medication-free periods of at least two weeks. This strategy alleviated the situation and made it possible to decrease dosage to 25 mg per night.

Other medication

Although there are presently only two drugs with proven antienuretic effect – i.e. desmo-pressin and imipramine – several other drugs have been claimed to be effective in a very limited number of studies. This is the case with amphetamine (Kapoor and Saksena 1969), sympathicomimetics (Penders et al 1984), androgens (El-Sadr et al 1990), carbamazepine (Al-Waili 2000), diuretics (given in the afternoon, not evening) (Dobson 1968, Moltke and Verder 1979, Scott and Morrison 1980, Nevéus et al 2004) and non-steroid anti-inflammatory drugs such as indomethacin or diclofenac (Batislam et al 1995, Sener et al 1998, Natochin and Kuznetsova 2000). Although it cannot be ruled out that one or several of these drugs will in the future prove to be useful in nocturnal enuresis we certainly do not have enough data to recommend their use in clinical practice.

ENT operations

In a bedwetting child who is reported to snore heavily and/or experience nocturnal apnoeas, tonsillectomy and/or adenoidectomy should be considered as a possible treatment, at least if ordinary antienuretic treatment fails.

Acupuncture

There are reasons to be cautiously optimistic about the possibility that acupuncture may be a useful therapy in a subgroup of children with nocturnal enuresis, since studies supporting its effectiveness are now accumulating (Song and Wang 1985, Zhong 1986, Tuzuner et al 1989, Björkström et al 2000, Serel et al 2001). The problem here is that many of the studies are of doubtful scientific quality and placebo-controlled trials are not feasible.

Diets

The proponents of the hypercalciuria hypothesis (see under pathophysiology, above) promote a low-calcium diet as a first-line treatment of nocturnal enuresis (Valenti et al 2002). The results of proper controlled studies of this treatment are needed before we can judge if this is a sensible strategy. A low-allergen diet is useful in the few cases of enuresis due to allergies (see Chapter 8).

Other methods

The orthodontic technique of 'rapid maxillary expansion', which entails the gradual widen-ing of the maxilla over a few weeks, and is used with the purpose of correcting malocclusion, has surprisingly shown positive results in reducing enuresis in two studies in the 1990s (Timms 1990, Kurol et al 1998), and a more recent report also gave moderate reasons for optimism (Usumez et al 2003). However, all of these studies have been uncontrolled, and the numbers have been small, so the procedure cannot, as yet, be generally recommended. Further studies may, of course, change the situation. The mechanism behind its possible efficacy may be related to the alleviation of subclinical upper respiratory tract obstruction. In the infrequent cases where such an obstruction is causing enuresis, specific and effective non-pharmacological therapies are available (see Chapter 8).

Biofeedback has shown some promise in the treatment of children with enuresis due to detrusor overactivity (Hoekx et al 1998, Yamanishi et al 2000).

Course and prognosis

NATURAL COURSE

As should be clear from the prevalence data, enuresis is a disorder that tends to disappear with increasing age. An annual spontaneous cure rate of 13 to 15 per cent is often quoted, but this figure should be treated cautiously. First, it is based on just one study (Forsythe and Redmond 1974), and second, it is now becoming increasingly clear that the chance of spontaneous resolution is much lower in enuretic teenagers and adults, than it is in younger children (Yeung et al 2004). Teenagers and adults with enuresis seem to represent a selected group of chronic enuresis, associated with a high wetting frequency, a lower educational level and more serious psychological and social effects (Yeung et al 2004).

Although there are no physical risks or adverse somatic consequences entailed in bedwetting *per se*, the psychological consequences of untreated or unsuccessfully treated nocturnal enuresis should not be underestimated. We can only speculate about the long-term social effects of this, but the impact of chronic low self-esteem in a growing individual may be considerable.

LONG-TERM OUTCOME WITH TREATMENT

The only antienuretic therapy with a clear curative potential is the alarm. Although the rate of relapse after successful treatment is about 20 per cent, a new session of treatment will usually solve the problem.

Whether pharmacological treatment shortens the natural course of the disorder is less clear. There may be some substance behind the claim that long-term desmopressin treatment hastens natural cure (Stenberg and Läckgren 1994), especially if it is tapered gradually, but the lack of an untreated control group in long-term studies makes these assumptions impossible to prove (Miller et al 1989, Knudsen et al 1991, Stenberg and Läckgren 1994, Hjälmås et al 1998). Even less can be said about the possible curative effects of imipramine or anticholinergics.

PERSISTENCE INTO ADULTHOOD

If children wet during the night, the risk for nocturnal enuresis as adults is increased eightfold. In a population-based study, the general prevalence of nocturnal enuresis in adults aged 32 to 60 years was 0.4 per cent in women and 0.3 per cent in men, for an occurrence at least once per month (and 1.7 per cent for both sexes, for less than once per month). With previous childhood enuresis, these rates increase to 3.0 per cent in women and 2.5 per cent in men (at least once per month) and 7.8 per cent for both sexes (less than once per month) (Hublin et al 1998).

In a longitudinal population-based study (the British National Birth Cohort of 1946) the effects of nocturnal enuresis at age 6 were analysed for 48-year-old women. These women had a 1.3 times higher rate of stress incontinence (66.7 per cent vs. 49.8 per cent) and urge symptoms (33.3 per cent vs. 22.3 per cent), and a three times higher rate of severe incontinence (22.2 per cent vs. 7.6 per cent) than women who did not wet at the age of 6 years (Kuh et al 1999). In other words, the genetic risk for nocturnal enuresis persists throughout life, can be reactivated by external stressors and predisposes not only to nocturnal enuresis, but unspecifically to other types of incontinence as well (Foldspang and Mommsen 1994).

In the same birth cohort of 1946, women who had wetted several times a week as children had a significantly higher rate of psychiatric disorders (31 per cent) at the age of 36 years than controls. There was no association if the nocturnal wetting occurred from time to time or at a later age, and there was no association in men (Rodgers 1990). In other words, childhood nocturnal enuresis, if severe enough, can be associated with an increased risk for psychological problems at a later age.

Summary and clinical guidelines

Before starting treatment of nocturnal enuresis, a few preliminary steps have to be considered (Chart 6.1). Organic causes, UTIs, encopresis, constipation and marked comorbid behavioural disorders need to be addressed first. If any daytime wetting is present, this also requires treatment first (see Chart 7.1 on page 181). If nocturnal wetting is the only problem, Chart 6.2 can be followed.

Nocturnal enuresis is usually caused by excessively deep sleep (difficulty in waking up) and lack of inhibition of the micturition reflex, combined in some cases with nocturnal polyuria and/or nocturnal detrusor overactivity. Primary assessment of a child with enuresis consists of history, physical examination, urine dipstick test for glucose and leukocytes/ bacteria, a voiding chart and sonography (in some countries). Blood tests and other invasive procedures are only very rarely needed. History should focus on daytime micturition and bowel habits, growth, general health and development, previous micturition problems, sleep and behaviour.

Treatment is indicated when the bedwetting threatens to become a social or psychological problem for the child, starting at the age of 5 years. In non-monosymptomatic nocturnal enuresis, daytime symptoms (without daytime wetting) should be treated first. Provision of information includes advice regarding fluid intake (extra fluid in the morning and at lunch) and regular voiding habits (approximately six micturitions per day). Ineffective treatment is discontinued and simple charts are filled out, registering wet and dry nights, usually for four weeks, but for longer if effects are seen.

The first-line antienuretic treatment is either the enuresis alarm or desmopressin medication. The alarm is potentially curative but demands motivation and commitment, whereas desmopressin is easy to administer but has a low or no curative potential. If the alarm is chosen, treatment should be consistent (no weekend interruptions), follow-up and encouragement should be provided and the parents should be instructed to help the child to wake up at the alarm signal. Treatment should continue until 14 consecutive dry nights have been achieved within a maximum of 16 weeks. Alarm treatment can be combined with other behavioural techniques such as 'arousal training'.

If desmopressin is chosen, parents need to be informed about the risk of water intoxication if the drug is combined with excessive fluid intake. Desmopressin is given orally (0.2–0.4 mg) or intranasally (20–40 µg) at bedtime; the doses should be titrated individually. Effects should be evident within a maximum of four weeks. If the child is a desmopressin non-responder, medication should be discontinued. If it is effective, it can be given at the lowest dose necessary in 12-week blocks, followed by a withdrawal for a week. In case of a relapse, new 'blocks' of up to 12 weeks can be started again. If the first first-line treatment is not effective, one should switch to the other.

If both first-line therapies are ineffective, then anticholinergic medication, possibly combined with desmopressin, may be considered. There is still a place for imipramine treatment of severely therapy-resistant enuresis, but only by specialists in the field and after proper evaluation. Finally, in therapy-resistant cases, detailed urological and child psychiatric assessment, inpatient and day-care treatment may be considered. Subgroups such as those with secondary nocturnal enuresis have a higher rate of comorbid psychiatric disorders which need to be addressed if present.

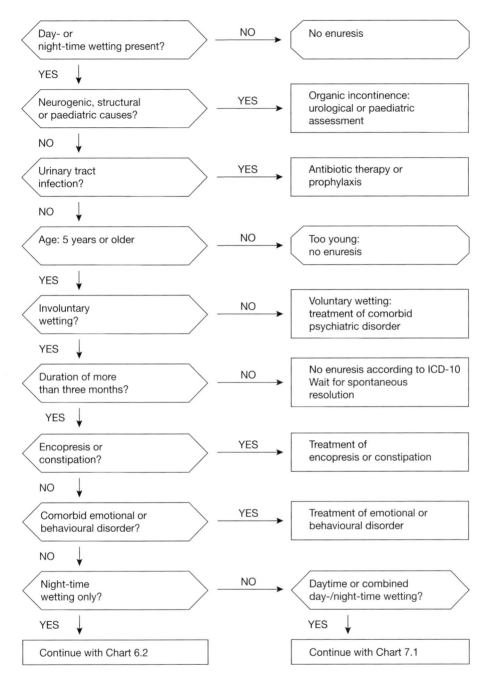

Chart 6.1 Diagnostic steps: enuresis and functional urinary incontinence

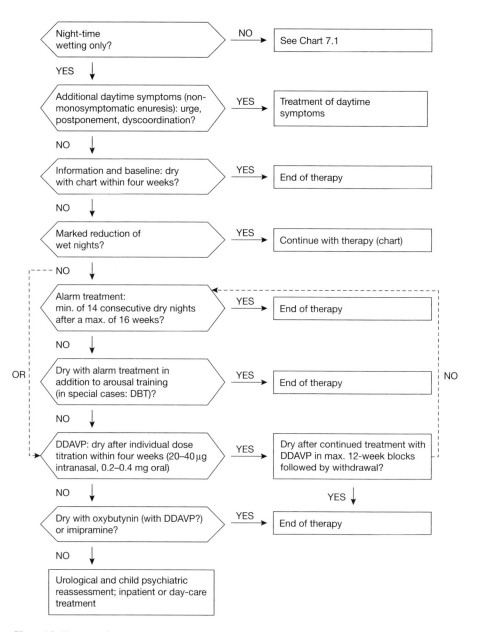

Chart 6.2 Therapy of nocturnal enuresis

7
FUNCTIONAL URINARY INCONTINENCE

Definitions and classification

As mentioned before, urinary incontinence denotes any involuntary passing of urine at an inappropriate time and place in a child past the age of usual bladder control. In this chapter all types of functional urinary incontinence except nocturnal enuresis will be discussed. Incontinence can occur in the context of the following conditions.

The *urge syndrome* or *overactive bladder*, caused by detrusor overactivity, is urinary incontinence in a child who experiences urgency symptoms but does not regularly postpone micturition or exhibit holding manoeuvres. The micturition frequency is often high and the voided volumes small.

Voiding postponement is the term used in those children who habitually postpone micturition, using various holding manoeuvres, often until it is too late and incontinence is the result.

Dysfunctional voiding denotes the tendency towards intermittent or continuous sphincter contractions during bladder emptying, commonly resulting in residual urine and UTIs. Since incontinence is common in these children it is included in this chapter even though the term dysfunctional voiding *per se* says nothing about the continence of the child.

Stress incontinence – a very rare condition in the neurologically intact child – occurs on exertion and is caused by an underactive or damaged sphincter. *Giggle incontinence* is the peculiar and uncommon condition where laughter, specifically, triggers apparently complete bladder emptying. *Detrusor underactivity* (or 'lazy bladder' in older terminology) is defined as the non-neurogenic inability of the detrusor to completely empty the bladder, forcing the child to strain with the abdominal musculature or apply manual suprapubic pressure during micturition, and often resulting in incontinence due to bladder overfilling. Table 7.1 summarizes the characteristics of overactive bladder, voiding postponement and dysfunctional voiding.

Epidemiology

Approximately 5 per cent of 7-year-olds suffer from daytime urinary incontinence of one type or another (Nevéus et al 1999a). The decreasing prevalence with increasing age of the child, so typical for nocturnal enuresis, is less clear here, and in adulthood the prevalence rises again, especially among women (Foldspang and Mommsen 1994, Kuh et al 1999, Andersson et al 2004). The estimated prevalence of daytime urinary incontinence among children in various age groups is shown in Table 7.2. Little is known as regards the prevalence of the various subtypes of daytime urinary incontinence, but bladder overactivity

TABLE 7.1

TABLE 7.1
Characteristics of overactive bladder, dysfunctional voiding and voiding postponement

	Overactive bladder	Dysfunctional voiding	Voiding postponement
Frequency	Usually >7 per day	Varying	<5 per day
Urgency	Yes	Varying, decreasing with age	Yes
Incontinence	With or without urge incontinence	Varying, decreasing when severity increases	Incontinence, varying amounts
Uroflow shape	May be tower-shaped	Staccato	Normal bell-shaped or staccato
Residual urine	Mostly <20 ml	Significant (>20 ml)	Varying
Main presenting symptoms	Frequency, urgency, incontinence	Recurrent UTIs, incontinence	Typical holding manoeuvres, incontinence

is probably the most common, especially among girls, and incontinence with voiding postponement the second most common; stress incontinence is rare.

Comorbid paediatric conditions

URINARY TRACT INFECTION (UTI) AND ASYMPTOMATIC BACTERIURIA (ABU)
UTI and ABU are overrepresented in children suffering from daytime incontinence (Berg et al 1977), and UTI is often suspected, rightly or wrongly, by the doctor attending to the incontinent child. This state of affairs has caused a tremendous amount of confusion and many unnecessary antibiotic prescriptions. The facts are as follows:

1 Residual urine entails a risk for UTI. Residual urine is often present in incontinent children with voiding postponement, dysfunctional voiding or detrusor underactivity.
2 Detrusor overactivity, such as is present in most children with urge incontinence, seems to be a risk factor *per se* for the development of UTI (Moore et al 2000), regardless

TABLE 7.2
Prevalence of daytime incontinence (symptom frequency at least once per month, when stated) among different age groups

Reference	N	<7 years	7–10 years	10–15 years
Bakker et al 2002	4332			6%
Bower et al 1996	2292		5.5%	
Hansen et al 1997	1557		*c.* 2%	
Hellström et al 1990	3556		*c.* 5%	
Järvelin et al 1988	3206		3.4%	
Kajiwara et al 2004	6917		9%	2%
Nevéus et al 2001a	1300		4%	
Söderström et al 2004	1478		6.3%	4.3%
Sureshkumar et al 2000	2020	<19.2%		
Weighted summary		**10%?**	**2–9%**	**2–6%**

of residual urine. The suggested mechanism is that the intermittent funnelling of the bladder neck during uninhibited detrusor contractions leads to bacteria being brought into the bladder from the lower urethra.

3   UTI may give rise to incontinence *de novo*, or worsening of a previously present incontinence, due to bacterial irritation of the urothelium.

4   Children with ABU often have an underlying disturbance of bladder function which does not improve with the eradication of the bacteria (Hansson et al 1990).

5   Falsely positive bacterial cultures due to contamination are common in children.

The practicalities of these complex associations of UTI and wetting are discussed later in this chapter (see page 138).

VESICO-URETERIC REFLUX (VUR)
VUR is an intermittent backflow of urine in the wrong direction through the ureterovesical junction. It is detected radiologically using a micturating cystourethrogram (MCU) and subdivided into grades I to V, with grades III and above assigned to cases with varying degrees of upper urinary tract dilatation (see Figs 7.1 and 7.2 and Table 7.3). Only dilated

TABLE 7.3
Grades of reflux according to the International Reflux Study Committee classification

I	Reflux into ureter only
II	Reflux into renal pelvis and calyces but no dilatation
III	Mild to moderate dilatation but minimal blunting of calyces
IV	Moderate dilatation, loss of angles of fornices, papillary impressions in calyces still present
V	Gross dilatation and tortuosity, papillary impressions no longer visible

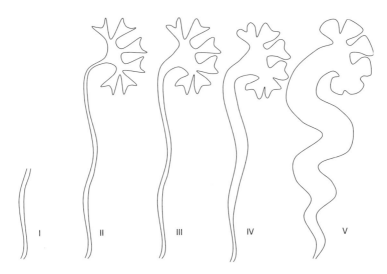

Fig. 7.1 Grades of vesico-ureteric reflux according to the International Reflux Study Committee classification.

133

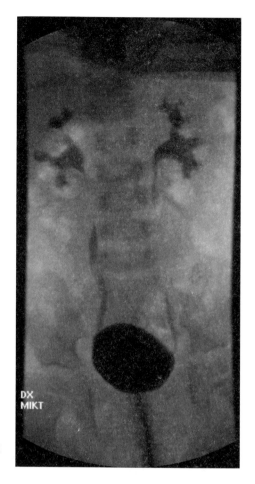

Fig. 7.2 Vesico-ureteric reflux, grade II left and grade III right.

VUR is significantly associated with kidney damage and/or risk for pyelonephritis (Goldman et al 2000a, 2000b).

It is now increasingly clear that VUR is associated with conditions that have in common a tendency towards high intravesical pressure, such as posterior urethral valves, neurogenic bladder disturbance, detrusor hyperactivity and dysfunctional voiding (van Gool et al 1992a). It is, however, not the pressure *per se* that is the cause of the reflux (Griffiths and Scholtmeijer 1987), but rather alterations of the anatomy (bladder wall thickening, changes in the ureterovesical junctions) which are induced by the chronic effects of sustained high pressure (Sillén 1999). The fact that the spontaneous resolution of VUR is slower in children with concomitant voiding disorders (van Gool et al 1992c, Koff et al 1998) also supports the hypothesis that the bladder disturbance is causing the reflux and not the other way round (Hjälmås 1992).

Approximately 50 per cent of children with VUR have detrusor overactivity and/or dysfunctional voiding, the former being the most common and the latter being more

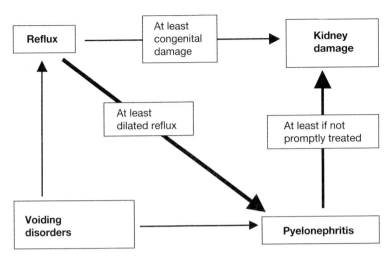

Fig. 7.3 The relationships between reflux, bladder/bowel malfunction, pyelonephritis and kidney damage.

associated with kidney damage (Koff 1983, Griffiths and Scholtmeijer 1987, Scholtmeijer and Nijman 1994, Sillén 1999). And, among children with dysfunctional voiding, as many as 50 per cent may have VUR (Allen 1977, Mayo and Burns 1990).

From the above it should be clear that incontinent children can be suspected to have a higher prevalence of VUR than the general population. This, emphatically, does *not* mean that every incontinent child should be submitted to an MCU. VUR should be sought not because the child is incontinent but because he or she has febrile UTIs.

The MCU is an examination that is often painful or at least uncomfortable for the child, especially after the first few years of life. The reason for looking for VUR is to find out why an infant or small child has had pyelonephritis. In older children, VUR is much less likely to be the cause of pyelonephritis. Thus, an MCU is only seldom indicated in these children. However, even in these children reflux will have to be excluded if febrile UTIs are recurrent or if ultrasound reveals upper tract dilatation. One way of circumventing the need for urethral catheterization may be to perform an indirect cystourethrogram via MAG3 scintigraphy.

Recent preliminary findings (Läckgren, personal communication) suggest that girls with relapsing cystitis often have VUR and that endoscopic treatment of this VUR may have positive effects on bladder function. If this should prove true, then the future indication for cystography (standard MCU or MAG3 scintigraphy) may widen.

If reflux, of grade III or higher, is found in a child, two things need to be done: (1) look for kidney damage, preferably via DMSA scintigraphy; and (2) reach a careful decision regarding treatment (or non-treatment) of the reflux. Since VUR has a spontaneous tendency towards resolution, albeit mostly in infants and toddlers, and kidney damage in the setting of VUR may be congenital, as well as caused by pyelonephritic episodes, there is no clear consensus regarding how – or, indeed, *if* – to treat it (Jodal et al 1992, Smellie et al 1992). There are presently four alternatives:

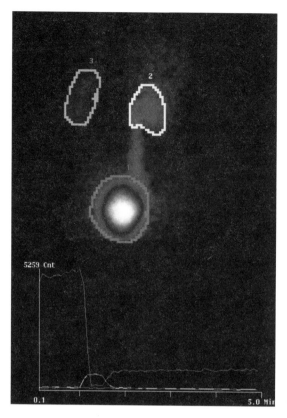

Fig. 7.4 Left-sided vesico-ureteric reflux, as detected by MAG3-renography. Radionuclide detection curves for the left renal pelvis and for the bladder.

1   Long-term antibiotic prophylaxis, while waiting for the VUR to resolve.
2   Watchful waiting, with prompt treatment of febrile UTIs, while waiting for the VUR to resolve.
3   Surgical correction with reimplantation of the refluxing ureter.
4   Endoscopic correction of the VUR via the injection of a suitable material adjacent to the ureteric orifice (Läckgren et al 2001).

The choice of correct treatment is not completely clear, and falls outside the scope of this text, but suffice it to say that the introduction of the injection technique (alternative 4 above) has greatly decreased the need for open surgery (alternative 3 above), and the important point is not to treat the reflux but to prevent (further) kidney damage. It also has to be kept in mind that long-term antibiotic prophylaxis entails risk for the evolution of bacterial resistance.

The key point is this: although refluxing ureters are often associated with disturbed bladders, this does not mean that bladder malfunction *per se* is an indication for looking for VUR.

136

PELVIC PAIN SYNDROMES

The term *interstitial cystitis* has been used in adults with chronic severe suprapubic pain and disturbances of bladder function (urgency, frequency, incontinence, terminal haematuria). Cystoscopy typically reveals so-called 'diffuse glomerulations' of the mucosa upon water distension of the bladder. The condition probably exists in children as well, although it is very rare (Close et al 1996, Kusek and Nyberg 2001). These children are reported to suffer from urgency, frequency and – specifically – pain, but do not show clear detrusor overactivity on cystometry. Instead they have a low-volume threshold for the sensation of bladder filling. Repeated water distension during cystometry is the treatment of choice (Close et al 1996), although the tricyclic antidepressant amitriptyline has shown effect in adults (van Ophoven et al 2004).

So-called *pelvic floor spasms* have also been found and urodynamically described in a group of children. These children (mostly girls) have mainly nocturnal attacks of severe pelvic floor pain with increased pelvic floor muscular activity and high urethral pressure. Concomitant daytime incontinence due to detrusor overactivity is often present, and pelvic floor relaxation is helpful in the majority of cases (Hoebeke et al 2004).

FUNCTIONAL FAECAL INCONTINENCE (ENCOPRESIS)

The high comorbidity of functional faecal incontinence with daytime wetting has been described in many studies. Between 12 and 29 per cent of children with functional faecal incontinence and constipation also wet during the day (Benninga et al 1994, Loening-Baucke 1997). Among daytime wetting children, 25 per cent also have functional faecal incontinence (Berg et al 1977). In our own study, 18.2 per cent of children with urge incontinence, 25 per cent with voiding postponement and 42.9 per cent with dysfunctional voiding also had functional faecal incontinence – rates that were much higher than the 5.5 per cent of children with nocturnal enuresis (von Gontard and Hollmann 2004). Children with combined urinary incontinence and functional faecal incontinence seem to have especially high rates of behavioural problems.

In a large sample of 1000 children with wetting problems who underwent videourodynamic investigations, 17 per cent were constipated. Boys with detrusor underactivity had the highest rate of constipation (25 per cent) (Hoebeke et al 2001). The close association of wetting and soiling can be explained by local factors associated with the accumulated faecal masses. Other, central nervous factors will be involved in children with functional faecal incontinence without constipation. Regarding treatment, functional faecal incontinence with or without constipation should be treated first, as this alone will lead to a marked reduction of day- and night-time wetting (Loening-Baucke 1997).

Behavioural disorders

No population-based studies have yet addressed the comorbidity of behavioural problems and daytime wetting. Only clinical studies with possible selection biases exist so far. In an early study, which does not fulfil current child psychiatric standards, 30 per cent of day-wetting children had behavioural disturbances (Fielding 1980). In another study, 25 per cent of children had definite and another 14 per cent possible emotional disorders (Halliday

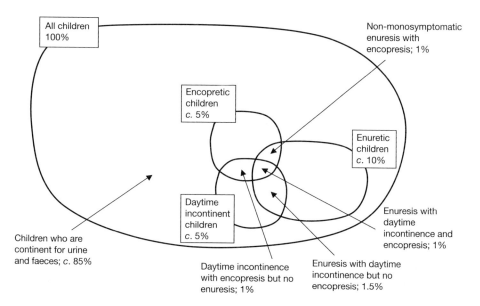

All children
100%

Non-monosymptomatic
enuresis with
encopresis; 1%

Encopretic
children
c. 5%

Enuretic
children
c. 10%

Daytime
incontinent
children
c. 5%

Enuresis with
daytime
incontinence and
encopresis; 1%

Children who are
continent for urine
and faeces; *c.* 85%

Daytime incontinence
with encopresis but no
enuresis; 1%

Enuresis with daytime
incontinence but no
encopresis; 1.5%

Fig. 7.5 Graphic representation of the approximate prevalences of enuresis, daytime incontinence and encopresis, and their overlap, among 7-year-olds. The areas and their overlap are proportionate to the percentages they represent.

et al 1987). In our own study, 53 per cent of day-wetting children fulfilled the criteria for at least one diagnosis according to ICD-10 (von Gontard et al 1999a).

In a study in a paediatric setting of 418 children aged 5–17 years, day-wetting children were described as being more stubborn, oppositional and secretive than nocturnal enuretic children (Kodman-Jones et al 2001). In a subgroup of 58 children, those with and without urinary tract infections were compared: 11 per cent of day-wetting children with UTIs had a CBCL total score in the clinical range, 35 per cent of day-wetting children without UTIs, and 16 per cent of nocturnal wetters. In other words, the subgroup with the highest risk for behavioural problems was day-wetting children without UTIs (Kodman-Jones et al 2001). In another study, 90 girls with recurrent UTIs had significantly more behavioural abnormalities than controls (Stauffer et al 2004). The issue of behavioural problems in children with and without UTIs therefore remains unresolved.

Compared to children with nocturnal enuresis, more children with daytime wetting had at least one ICD-10 diagnosis (52.6 vs. 33.6 per cent); 34.5 per cent of day-wetting children had a total problem score on a CBCL questionnaire, compared to 25 per cent with night-time wetting (von Gontard et al 1999a; Table 4.10). There is, therefore, a difference between the scores of day- and night-time wetting children, but it is not highly significant. This is due to the fact that among both the day- and night-wetting children there are subgroups with higher and lower comorbidity. Some subgroups of day-wetting children definitely have higher risks than others. Thus, children with voiding postponement had significantly higher rates of any ICD-10 diagnosis (53.8 per cent vs. 28.6 per cent) than children with urge incontinence. Also, 37.3 per cent had a total problem score on the CBCL questionnaire, compared to only 13.5 per cent of children with urge incontinence (von Gontard et al 1998a, Lettgen et al 2002).

ADHD is also a common problem among day-wetting children. Compared to controls, children with ADHD had more symptoms of incontinence, constipation, infrequent voiding and dysuria (Duel et al 2003). With ADHD, treatment outcome is worse. In a retrospective analysis, 68 per cent of day-wetting children with ADHD became dry, compared to 91 per cent of controls. Non-compliance was much higher for children with ADHD when they were treated by timed voiding (Crimmins et al 2003).

In adults, depression and incontinence are closely associated – possibly due to a common neurochemical (mainly serotonergic) pathogenesis (Steers and Kyu-Sung 2001). This association is not typical in children.

Toilet training
Two Swiss longitudinal studies by Largo et al (1978, 1996) (described in Chapter 6 – see page 102) – reported that, in the 1950s, Swiss mothers began toilet training early, before the age of 12 months. Later, in the 1970s, toilet training began around 20 months. While a greater proportion of the children trained earlier became dry during the second year of life, from the age of 3 years onwards the more liberally trained children of the 1970s were more often dry. By the age of 5 years (the definitional age), there was no difference at all between the groups.

The authors recommended that parents should positively reinforce their child's signal of wanting to become dry. The process of gaining continence entails two aspects: the voluntary initiation and the stopping of a micturition – a developmental task most children are proud of. Both a *laissez-faire* and a coercive attitude are unfavourable. Fortunately, most parents by the 1970s were able to provide this support intuitively, as there was a great congruence between the child's asking for the potty and parental prompting (Largo et al 1996).

General approaches to day-wetting children
The general approaches outlined for the assessment of nocturnal enuresis (Table 6.4) apply to day-wetting children – except that the somatic and psychological assessments need to be conducted in much greater detail and with more scrutiny due to the higher rate of associated conditions such as UTIs, residual urine, VUR and behavioural problems (see above).

History
Obviously, the central issue in the case history of a child with daytime incontinence is the wetting. One needs to get a detailed description of *when, how often, how much* (damp, wet or soaking) and *in which circumstances* the wetting accidents occur. Other micturition symptoms such as urgency, holding manoeuvres and straining need to be specifically asked about, as well as encopresis and other symptoms of constipation. The general neurological development of the child should be superficially assessed and, importantly, previous UTIs should be enquired after.

The guidelines given in Table 4.4 are useful to bear in mind when evaluating the answers to the questions regarding micturition and incontinence.

Voiding Charts

The value of a voiding chart in the assessment of a child with daytime incontinence is hard to overestimate. As described in Chapter 4, it is our opinion that it should be part of the standard diagnostic work-up in all these children.

Physical Examination

All these children should undergo a standard physical examination at least once. Genital inspection should be part of that examination, as should inspection of the spine and a simple neurological examination (leg reflexes, Babinski's sign). Rectal examination is indicated if the history suggests that constipation may be present.

Urine Analysis and Culture

A standard urine test for red and white blood cells and bacteria is obligatory at the first assessment of these children, especially those who have previously been dry. When evaluating the results of this test, however, it is important to consider the caveats mentioned in Chapter 4 (see page 35).

If the child has cystitis and is treated with antibiotics to which the bacteria are sensitive (or intermediately sensitive), symptoms should disappear *promptly* – i.e. within one to two days. If this does not happen, then the bacteria were probably not responsible for the condition, and treatment should be directed at the bladder, not the bacteria.

Flowmetry and Residual Urine Measurements

Flowmetry (always combined with residual urine measurements), if available, is very useful in the evaluation of children suffering from daytime incontinence. In wards provided with the equipment it should be used in every incontinent child. Children with therapy-resistant incontinence, repeated UTIs or in whom treatment with anticholinergic drugs is being considered should always be referred for such an examination.

Cystometry

Cystometry is not indicated in incontinent children as often as was previously thought. The only place for this procedure in incontinent children is when history, physical examination or repeated flowmetries give rise to the suspicion of neurogenic bladder disturbance. It may also sometimes be used in extremely therapy-resistant cases of urge incontinence/voiding postponement.

Ultrasound

As already mentioned, the routine use of ultrasound in incontinent or enuretic children varies greatly between different cultures and countries. Ultrasound should at least be carried out in all children who have a history of UTIs.

Urography is mandatory in children with suspected ectopic ureter. Otherwise, X-ray is of little benefit in incontinent children. Urography is also an alternative, albeit inferior, to scintigraphy when looking for kidney scars in children with past febrile UTIs.

BLOOD TESTS
Blood tests have no place in the evaluation of daytime incontinence, unless the child has suffered from repeated febrile UTIs, in which case serum creatinine should be measured (and the presence of kidney scars also needs to be determined).

Overactive bladder

DEFINITION
Overactive bladder is defined in this text as the presence of incontinence in association with urgency symptoms in a child who has a normal or increased micturition frequency and who does not habitually postpone voidings. If involuntary detrusor contractions are observed via cystometry, this is termed detrusor overactivity. Other terms used for the same condition are: bladder instability, unstable bladder, urge incontinence, and, in older terminology, spastic/automatic/uninhibited bladder.

EPIDEMIOLOGY
Although overactive bladder is the most common daytime micturition disturbance in children, its true prevalence is difficult to assess, since most epidemiological studies do not differentiate between different kinds of daytime incontinence. The vast majority of children suffering from daytime incontinence also suffer from urgency symptoms (Kajiwara et al 2004) – the hallmark of detrusor overactivity – and can be assumed to belong to either the overactive bladder group or the voiding postponers.

The prevalence of daytime incontinence in 7-year-olds is approximately 6 per cent for girls and 4 per cent for boys (Hellström et al 1990, Söderström et al 2004); the majority of these children can be presumed to suffer from overactive bladder, and most of the remainder probably belong to the voiding postponement group (see below). The prevalence of *severe* incontinence in the same age group is lower – about 2 per cent wet every week and 0.5 per cent every day – and more evenly distributed between the sexes (Hansen et al 1997).

Urge incontinence, and presumably overactive bladder, often coexists with other voiding disorders in the same child, reflecting common or interrelated pathogenetic mechanisms, or in some cases just coincidence. Thus 15–30 per cent of enuretic children (Forsythe and Redmond 1974, Järvelin et al 1988, Hellström et al 1990, Hirasing et al 1997b, Gümüs et al 1999, Nevéus et al 2001a, Yeung et al 2004) and 12–30 per cent of children suffering from encopresis or constipation also experience daytime accidents (Loening-Baucke 1997).

Bladder overactivity is caused by detrusor overactivity, but the pathogenesis of detrusor overactivity itself is not clear. What was regarded as one clinical entity is found to be several. A jumble of different subentities has thus emerged, such as motor and sensory detrusor instability, central and peripheral, myogenic and psychogenic variants and so on.

It is clear that the pathogenesis of detrusor overactivity is multifactorial (Bulmer and Abrams 2004). The situation in children is further complicated by the fact that most studies have been performed in adult women or elderly males (and some in animals), and we obviously cannot assume that these results can be carried over to boys without prostate hypertrophy or girls who have not borne any children. An additional source of confusion is that the correspondence between bladder and detrusor overactivity may not be so clear-cut after all, since it has been shown that not all patients with the urge syndrome exhibit detrusor overactivity on conventional cystometry (Powell et al 1980) and that many patients without such symptoms may have involuntary detrusor contractions when examined with ambulatory cystometry (Heslington and Hilton 1996). The following section is an attempt to sort out the confusion, roughly following the outline provided in Table 7.4 below.

Micturition reflex

In many, but not all, patients, the involuntary detrusor contractions are preceded by an involuntary sphincter relaxation – more or less as in the normal micturition – indicating that in these cases it is the micturition reflex that is pathologically easy to elicit (type A in the table below), not the detrusor contractions *per se* (Low 1977, Bergman et al 1989, Koonings and Bergman 1991, Wise et al 1993, Artibani 1997, Marinkovic and Bedlani 2001). This phenomenon has been labelled 'type II detrusor instability' and is associated with CNS pathogenesis (Blaivas 1982), low cystometric bladder capacity (McLennan et al 2001) and a poor response to anticholinergic treatment (Bergman et al 1989). How common it is in

TABLE 7.4
Hypotheses of detrusor overactivity pathogenesis (adapted from Bosch 1990)

Underlying disturbance	Pathogenetic mechanism
A Micturition reflex	1 Increased peripheral afferent activity 2 Decreased suprasacral inhibition 3 Decreased peripheral (sphincter, pelvic floor) inhibition
B Neurotransmission	1 Changed type of neurotransmitter 2 Changed quality of neurotransmitter 3 Increased detrusor receptor density 4 Increased detrusor receptor affinity
C Myogenic	1 Abnormal synchronization of spontaneous activity 2 Biochemical detrusor muscle disturbance 3 Membrane instability (denervation supersensitivity)
D Psychogenic	

incontinent children is not known, but there is no reason to suspect that it is rare, since in adults it has been found to be exclusively associated with urge incontinence as opposed to stress incontinence (McLennan et al 2001).

The hypothesis of detrusor overactivity secondary to increased peripheral efferent activity, with resultant increased peripheral afferent activity to the bladder (case A1 above), is supported by the finding that adult women with detrusor overactivity have more dense subepithelial sensory nerves than controls (Moore et al 1992a). Animal studies on the nociceptive C-fibre bladder afferents are relevant here in the paediatric setting (de Groat et al 1999). These unmyelinated afferents are involved in foetal and neonatal micturition, but also when the micturition reflex is disturbed, as in UTI and spinal cord injury.

It is common knowledge that cerebral damage of various kinds – cerebrovascular insults, neurodegenerative disorders, multiple sclerosis, etc. – often gives rise to incontinence and neurogenic detrusor overactivity, cystometrically similar to idiopathic detrusor overactivity (Awad et al 1984, Van Arsdalen and Wein 1991, Sakakibara et al 1996, Dmochowski 1999, Marinkovic and Bedlani 2001). Type II detrusor instability, as described above, is the disturbance most commonly seen (Marinkovic and Bedlani 2001), and loss of suprabulbar inhibition of the micturition reflex is the suspected mechanism.

Although children with idiopathic detrusor overactivity are of course not suspected of having significant congenital brain damage, it cannot be excluded that lack of central inhibition of the detrusor reflex is the pathogenetic mechanism in some of these children (case A2 above). An indication that central neuropathology may be operative in children with urge incontinence comes from studies that have shown that the bladder cooling reflex (see Chapter 4) may be positive in up to 50 per cent of these children (Gladh et al 2004).

Neuroanatomically, the anteromedial aspect of the frontal lobes, their descending pontine connections and the basal ganglia are thought to be especially crucial (Van Arsdalen and Wein 1991, Sakakibara et al 1996, Dmochowski 1999), whereas neurochemically, loss of GABA-mediated inhibition (Kanie et al 2000) and increased dopamine D2-receptor-mediated excitation of the micturition reflex are implicated (Yokoyama et al 1999, Pehrson and Andersson 2003). The enkephalins, acting on endogeneous opioid receptors in the CNS, have also been implicated, since IV morphine and its antagonist naloxone have detrusor-relaxant and micturition-inducing properties, respectively (Murray and Feneley 1982, Malinovsky et al 1998). The enkephalins inhibit the detrusor presynaptically, except in the trigonum and bladder neck (Klarskov 1987). It is thus speculated that a lack of endogenous opioids could cause detrusor overactivity.

The well-documented association between constipation (Loening-Baucke 1997) and incontinence also fits well with the idea of the uninhibited micturition reflex, since the stimulus of the distended bowel compressing the bladder may lead to an interruption of the normal peripheral inhibition of micturition provided by the sphincter and pelvic floor (case A3 above).

Neurotransmission
If the micturition reflex as such is not disturbed but detrusor contractions appear without warning, the explanation could be that neurotransmission to the detrusor is disturbed (B in

Table 7.4). Given the confusing number of transmitters, besides norepinephrine and acetyl-choline (Hoyle 1994), involved in bladder control, it should come as no surprise that several neurotransmitters have been postulated to play causative roles in detrusor overactivity and incontinence (Andersson and Hedlund 2002). Dopamine has already been mentioned (Andersson 2003), as have the enkephalins. Serotonin and norepinephrine may also be implicated, as antidepressant drugs with noradrenergic and/or serotonin reuptake inhibitor properties possess some detrusor-relaxant effects (Rabey et al 1979). For norepinephrine this is easy enough to explain, since this input to the sphincter is tonically active during urine storage. The effects of serotonin and of serotonin receptor-subtype-specific agonists and antagonists are, however, forbiddingly complicated and incompletely understood (de Groat 2002).

Somewhat surprisingly, the overactive detrusor has been found to possess a *decreased* density of cholinergic nerve endings, but with hypersensitivity of those nerve endings (case B3 or B4, above) (Harrison et al 1987, Speakman et al 1987). The proposed mechanism behind this *denervation hypersensitivity* is detrusor damage secondary to raised intravesical pressure due to intrauterine vesical obstruction, a hypothesis that has gained support in animal experiments (Sibley 1985, Brading and Turner 1994) and has a clinical analogue in the extreme case of the highly disturbed bladder function of boys with congenital urethral valves.

The *purinergic* contribution to detrusor activity and its possible role in detrusor overactivity has recently come into focus, and is probably a fruitful path to follow (Andersson 2003). As mentioned in Chapter 3, the purine ATP is a parasympathetic co-transmitter in the detrusor and plays a role in the initiation of the detrusor contraction (Theobald 1995). ATP is released by the distended urothelium and leads to contraction via stimulation of the cholinergic nerve endings (Fry et al 2004a). This purinergic contribution has been shown to be exaggerated in overactive detrusors (O'Reilly et al 2002, Kumar et al 2003). Support for this idea comes partly from well-designed studies which have shown that patients with urge incontinence show more purinergic activity upon nerve stimulation than controls (Bayliss et al 1999, O'Reilly et al 2002), and that the pattern of ATP-specific receptors in the detrusor of patients both differs from that of controls and has similarities with that of small children (Moore et al 2001).

Myogenic
The smooth muscle cells of the detrusor are continuously electrically active, but the fact that every cell is just linked to a few of its immediate neighbours indicates that this activity is asynchronous and does not result in detrusor contractions. A disturbance of this coupling has been proposed as a mechanism leading to detrusor overactivity (Fry et al 2004b). The detrusors of elderly patients with detrusor overactivity, when examined with electron microscopy, have shown cell junction patterns that would permit rapid propagation and possibly synchronization of impulses (El-Badawi et al 1993, Brading 1997). Doubt has, however, been thrown on this explanation by the findings of a recent investigation in adult women with detrusor overactivity and controls, in which no differences in cell junction patterns could be found (Carey et al 2000).

Smooth muscle hypertrophy and connective tissue infiltration are associated with detrusor overactivity in men with benign prostatic hypertrophy (Andersson 2003). Also, detrusor biopsies in adults with detrusor overactivity resistant to anticholinergic treatment have been shown to contain exaggerated numbers of mast cells (Moore et al 1992b). The relevance of these findings to the paediatric population remains to be shown, but is probably not great.

Psychogenic
Detrusor overactivity is sometimes claimed to be psychogenic in origin, and perceived differences in behaviour or psychological profile between women with and without urge incontinence have been put forward as support for this view (Freeman et al 1985). It may be that hypotheses about psychogenicity just reflect our imperfect knowledge. Some support for theories of behavioural origin may be provided by the finding that children with urge incontinence have often been potty-trained by inadequate methods (Bakker et al 2001).

Although there are no formal genetic studies on overactive bladder, the concurrence in families is high – often with several other family members affected. In view of newer molecular genetic findings with positive linkage to chromosome 17 (Eiberg et al 2001), associated psychological signs and symptoms are more likely to be a consequence and not a causative factor of overactive bladder.

To conclude, the pathogenesis of detrusor overactivity – which causes bladder overactivity and the urge syndrome – is multifactorial, sometimes involving overactivity of only the detrusor and sometimes of the entire micturition reflex. The lack of central supraspinal inhibition may be causative in some cases, whereas peripheral myogenic or neurogenic factors are crucial in others. Whatever the cause, this detrusor contraction leads *either* to the sensation of urgency and the more or less successful attempt by the child to inhibit the contraction by forcefully contracting the sphincter, *and/or* the sudden wetting of the pants.

PSYCHOLOGICAL ASPECTS
Children with urge incontinence were previously considered to have few behavioural problems. If these did occur they were considered to be secondary effects of the wetting (van Gool and de Jonge 1989, Olbing 1993). Thus, only 13 per cent of girls were described as having 'behavioural problems', assessed in a non-standardized manner and interpreted as 'related to acceptance and understanding of their incontinence problem by peers and parents' (van Gool and de Jonge 1989). According to a two-centre paediatric and child psychiatric study, however, the comorbidity rate does seem to be higher than this (Lettgen et al 2002): 29 per cent of children with urge incontinence had an ICD-10 diagnosis and 14 per cent had an internalizing disorder. In another study 13.5 per cent had a clinical total problem score on the CBCL – again mainly internalizing problems (von Gontard et al 1998a). Subjectively, nearly 80 per cent of children saw a disadvantage in their wetting and were distressed (von Gontard et al 1998a).

In summary, children with urge incontinence have a low rate of comorbid psychiatric disorders. If they are affected, emotional, introversive symptoms predominate. The children

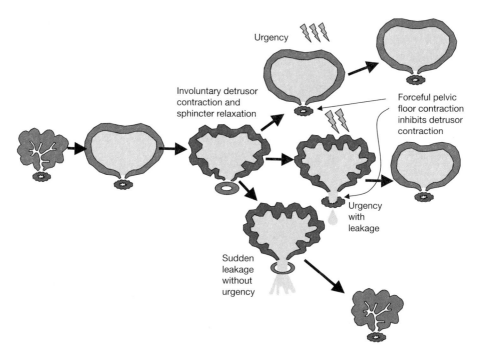

Fig. 7.6 Detrusor overactivity.

are distressed by their wetting, and family functioning is intact (Lettgen et al 2002). One could therefore speculate that urge incontinence is, indeed, very unlikely to be a syndrome of psychogenic aetiology. Other factors, such as genetics, maturation and urinary tract infections, are far more important.

CLINICAL SIGNS AND SYMPTOMS
Due to the pathogenetic considerations above, the symptoms of most children with overactive bladder vary between two extremes:

1 Sudden, intense urgency but no wetting or just a small wet spot – this means that the child managed to interrupt the detrusor contraction on this occasion.
2 The child becomes soaking wet without any warning at all – this means that the child did not even have the time to experience urgency, let alone contract the sphincter.

Thus, the typical child with bladder overactivity wets varying amounts of urine, sometimes with and sometimes without urgency (Jabs and Stanton 2001). But they can all describe typical urgency symptoms and tend to go often (more than six times daily) to the toilet (Bauer et al 1980, van Gool and de Jonge 1989). Wetting can happen any time during the day, but usually more often in the afternoon when the child is becoming more tired, and it can happen during all sorts of activities.

146

UTIs do often occur in these children (van Gool and de Jonge 1989), but not as often as in children with voiding postponement or dysfunctional voiding. The *physical examination* of the child with overactive bladder is usually unremarkable, but perigenital eczema is not uncommon.

The *micturition chart* data in a child with overactive bladder supports the history data. Thus, in a typical case one finds that the child goes often to the toilet, voids small volumes, often experiences urgency and wets small or large amounts. Urgency and incontinence usually start at the end of the morning and become worse in the afternoon (van Gool and de Jonge 1989). For an example of this pattern, see Fig. 7.7.

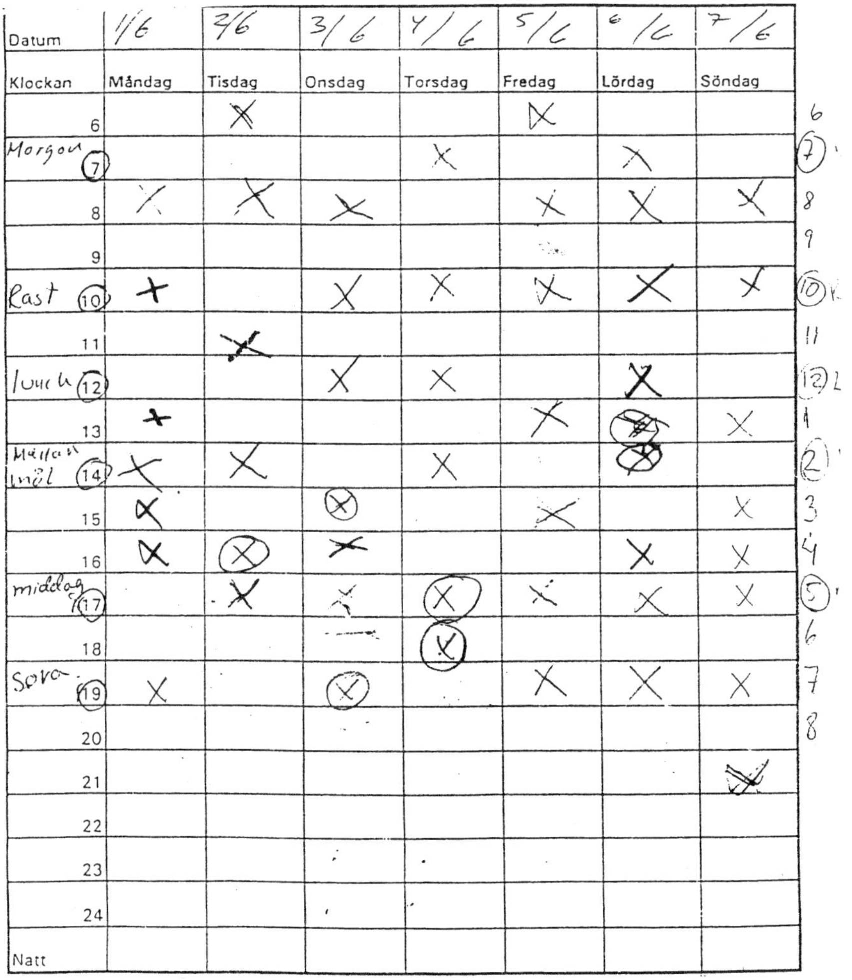

Fig. 7.7 Typical frequency-volume chart of a child with urge incontinence due to bladder overactivity (voidings marked with X, incontinence episodes marked with X and a ring).

147

Flowmetry typically reveals a bell-shaped curve with an early peak. It may also look entirely normal. If the child has managed to push him- or herself and postpone micturition longer than normal, he or she often produces a tower-shaped – i.e. short and high – curve. Residual urine is usually not present.

ASSESSMENT

A thorough clinical history, supported by a voiding chart and a urine test to rule out UTI, should be enough in most instances. Flowmetry with residual urine measurement is also very useful but can in clear-cut cases be omitted if the equipment is not readily available.

If the urine test is positive for leukocytes, erythrocytes or bacteria, a urine culture should be taken. If the culture turns out to be positive, a short antibiotic treatment is warranted – at least if the incontinence is secondary – but if this does not give clear and prompt symptom relief, then treatment of the bladder, as described below, should be started.

If the diagnosis is not clear, flowmetry and residual measurement should (if available) be performed, and if there is a suspicion of neurogenic bladder, cystometry should be considered.

TREATMENT

Although there is a general consensus that urotherapy (bladder control therapy) is the first-line treatment in the overactive bladder syndrome, opinions differ as to which kinds of urotherapy are to be used in which situation. Different strategies are used in different parts of the world, and comparisons between them are almost impossible. The problem here, as always, is the lack of good randomized, controlled studies. Consequently, there is as yet no truly evidence-based treatment of daytime urinary incontinence in children (Sureshkumar et al 2003). But treat them we must, and our suggestion is that one starts with a basic urotherapeutic approach which is simple and can be started, at least, by anyone. We suggest two different alternatives below, both of which make use of the therapeutic voiding chart.

Training

Alternative A is to focus on conscious bladder control. The child is instructed to go immediately to the toilet at the first sign of urge, without using any holding manoeuvres, and then mark on the voiding chart (with appropriate signs or symbols such as 'flags' and 'clouds') whether the underpants were dry or wet (van Gool et al 1984, 1992b, Olbing 1993, von Gontard 2001). This is in reality a simple kind of cognitive-behavioural therapy.

Alternative B is even simpler (for the caregiver, that is). The child is asked to go to the toilet regularly, approximately every two hours, regardless of whether there is a sensation of bladder fullness or not, and to record the effects on a voiding chart (Hellström et al 1987). Both alternatives should include instructions about the function of the bladder, voiding posture, adjustment of drinking habits and the liberal treatment of possible constipation. We suggest that this simple bladder training is used for a minimum of one to two months, with follow-up visits to the outpatient ward (nurse or doctor appointment), during which charts are reviewed and feedback is given.

Pharmacotherapy

If this fails and constipation has been excluded or eradicated, then *anticholinergic* treatment may be warranted (Soomro et al 2001). The drugs that have been used in this context are oxybutynin, propiverine and tolterodine. Most paediatric data are available for oxybutynin, but the newer drugs tolterodine and propiverine may also turn out to be useful alternatives. The choice about which drug to use will be dictated mostly by availability and personal experience, but oxybutynin may not be the drug of choice in children with ADHD or other neuropsychiatric problems, since psychic side effects (aggressiveness) seem to be more common with this drug (Jonville et al 1992, t'Veld et al 1998). Pharmacological and pharmacokinetic data for the anticholinergic drugs are provided in Chapter 5; practical advice about how to use them in this setting is given below. Please note that hard facts are lacking here and the advice given constitutes the authors' own views, not evidence-based medicine.

Before starting anticholinergic treatment a few precautions are mandatory:

1   *Exclude residual urine.* Anticholinergics may aggravate or cause the accumulation of residual urine, with a concomitant risk for UTI. Thus, all incontinent children in whom anticholinergic treatment is considered need to undergo flowmetry and ultrasound measurement of residual urine. If there is significant residual urine, this should be eliminated via bladder training – ideally with the help of a urotherapist – before treatment can start.
2   *Exclude or treat constipation.* Anticholinergics may aggravate or cause constipation, which may in its turn result in low treatment efficacy and bowel symptoms. If the child needs laxatives to get rid of constipation then this treatment should continue during anticholinergic treatment.
3   *Continue bladder training.* The family must be aware that the sound voiding and drinking habits described earlier must continue during anticholinergic treatment. The pills are no excuse for neglecting the bladder. Specifically, the child should not postpone voidings during medication, since this may result in residual urine and UTIs.
4   *Inform the family about risks and common side effects.* The family should watch out for signs of UTI (this is perhaps the most important message) or constipation and ensure that the dental hygiene of the child is good (since salivation is decreased during treatment).

Ordinary dosage, when giving anticholinergics for daytime incontinence is: oxybutynin 2.5–5.0 mg bid or tid (or 0.3 to max. 0.6mg/kg/day), propiverine 2.5–5.0 mg bid or tid (or 0.4 to max. 0.8mg/kg/day), or tolterodine 0.5–1.0 mg bid (off-label for children), with even larger doses sometimes necessary and tolerable in older children, if lower dosage did not result in significant side effects (Hjälmås et al 2001). Maximum daily dosage, however, is 15 mg oxybutynin/propiverine or 4 mg tolterodine – these dosages should not be exceeded. Treatment should start with a low dose and only slowly be increased every two to three days, to reduce side effects. If ineffective after one month, the dosage can be increased again.

There are various figures for how efficient anticholinergic drugs are in urge incontinence, but a rough estimate is that between one-half and two-thirds of these children show a clear benefit (Nagy et al 1990, Primus and Pummer 1990, Malone-Lee et al 1992, Mazur et al 1995, Rentzhog et al 1998, Larsson et al 1999, Ruscin and Morgenstern 1999). Extended release preparations (of oxybutynin or tolterodine) might have advantages in the future, but further studies are needed (Reinberg et al 2003). Treatment effect may take some time, but should be seen within one to two months. If the effect is then satisfactory, gradual tapering (over a few weeks) is advised after three to four months, and then at least twice per year as long as the drug is needed. And the child should always be reminded that the pills are only half the treatment – the bladder needs to be trained as well.

We recommend that residual urine be monitored after a few months of anticholinergic treatment, and then perhaps every six months as long as the drug is needed. If significant residual urine accumulates, the medication should be discontinued, at least temporarily, while the child again learns how to empty the bladder completely. The anticholinergic medication may then be cautiously reintroduced, if it was effective.

If the child develops a symptomatic UTI during anticholinergic treatment, residual urine accumulation should immediately be suspected and the drug discontinued. UTI should be suspected if there is dysuria, sudden aggravation of incontinence and/or unexplained fever. The UTI should, of course, be treated with antibiotics, and anticholinergic treatment should only be reintroduced if the child needs it, residual urine has been clearly eradicated and it is known that the child complies with the bladder regime, as described above. Routine urine cultures in asymptomatic children on anticholinergic treatment are *not* warranted: asymptomatic bacteriuria should not be treated with antibiotics. If, however, the child has recurrent symptomatic UTIs which are not associated with residual urine, then a combination of prophylactic antibiotics (see Chapter 8) and continued anticholinergic treatment may be needed, but only with persistent focus on bladder training.

Finally, a few more words about constipation in children taking anticholinergic medication. Symptoms may naturally be bowel-centred – i.e. stomach pains, encopresis, hard stools, etc. – but a very common way for this side effect to manifest itself is just by a gradually diminishing treatment efficacy. Thus, in the child who initially had a good reduction of wetting and urgency, but now experiences more and more accidents in spite of continuing drug treatment, constipation should be the prime suspect. In these children, and in those with more evident constipation, we suggest that anticholinergic treatment be discontinued and bowel treatment with enemas and bulk laxatives such as lactulose started. After two weeks or more of this treatment, anticholinergics may once again be added. If the bladder improves, then the suspicion of constipation was grounded and laxatives should be taken as long as the anticholinergics are needed.

L.K., 5-year-old girl
Diagnoses: Urge incontinence; primary nocturnal enuresis

L. was referred for day- and night-time wetting. She had been dry during the day at the age of 2½ years, but had experienced a relapse after the birth of her younger brother, and had wetted ever since then. She went to the toilet up to 20 times a day, sat on her heels and used other holding manoeuvres. At age 3 she had had several UTIs. She wet every night and had never been dry. The wetting volumes were large and it was difficult to wake her. Previously she had been treated with propiverine without success. Alarm treatment had been discontinued after three months, as the alarm sounded several times a night. The parents were very concerned and play psychotherapy had been conducted for a period of 18 months.

The frequency-volume chart showed a frequency of 11 times per day with volumes of 35 to 70 ml. The bladder wall was slightly thickened (3.9 mm); residual urine was only 2 ml. On the Child Behaviour Checklist (CBCL) the parents reported symptoms in the clinical range for the total score, externalizing and internalizing behaviours, especially anxious, depressive and thought problems. There were overt signs of interactional problems between parents and child.

L. was instructed to go to the toilet as soon as she sensed an urge and to refrain from using holding manoeuvres. This was documented on a chart. In addition, she received oxybutynin with a maximum dose of 15 mg per day in three doses. There was a marked reduction of wetting episodes as well as micturition frequency. Unfortunately, she developed residual urine of up to 100 ml and two urinary tract infections. Oxybutynin was discontinued, but the charts remained as the main line of treatment. Simple family counselling was conducted to reduce tension between L. and her parents. Also, behavioural therapy with a simple token system was instituted to increase motivation.

After several months, the daytime wetting episodes were reduced to a maximum of once a week. As soon as she becomes dry during the daytime, a new round of alarm treatment will be instituted.

This case is typical for a protracted course of urge incontinence. The tensions within the family were a consequence of the wetting problem. The play therapy was certainly not indicated and showed no effect. The alarm treatment was started too early, when the overactive bladder was still leading to several wetting episodes per night. Unfortunately L. did not respond to one anticholinergic (propiverine), and developed residual urine with the other (oxybutynin). With counselling and behavioural therapy alone a marked response could be achieved.

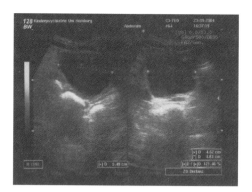

Fig. 7.8 L.K.: ultrasound: residual urine of 100 ml under oxybutinin, which had to be discontinued.

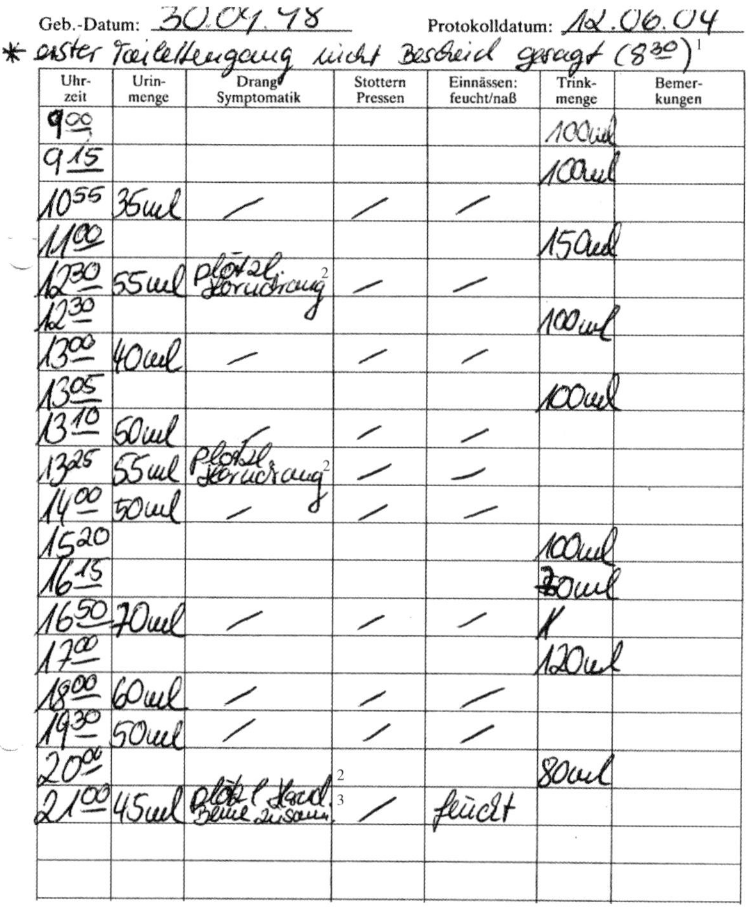

Geb.-Datum: _30.09.78_   Protokolldatum: _12.06.04_

✱ *erster Teiletengang nicht Bescheid gesagt (8³⁰)*[1]

Uhr-zeit	Urin-menge	Drang Symptomatik	Stottern Pressen	Einnässen: feucht/naß	Trink-menge	Bemer-kungen
9⁰⁰					100ml	
9¹⁵					100ml	
10⁵⁵	35ml	⟋	⟋	⟋		
11⁰⁰					150ml	
12³⁰	55ml	*plötzl. Harndrang*[2]	⟋	⟋		
12³⁰					100ml	
13⁰⁰	40ml	⟋	⟋	⟋		
13⁰⁵					100ml	
13¹⁰	60ml		⟋			
13²⁵	55ml	*plötzl. Harndrang*[2]	⟋	⟋		
14⁰⁰	50ml	⟋	⟋			
15²⁰					100ml	
16¹⁵					80ml	
16⁵⁰	70ml	⟋	⟋	⟋	⟋	
17⁰⁰					120ml	
18⁰⁰	60ml	⟋	⟋	⟋		
19³⁰	50ml	⟋	⟋	⟋		
20⁰⁰					80ml	
21⁰⁰	45ml	*plötzl. Harnd.²³ Beine zusam.*	⟋	feucht		

Fig. 7.9 L.K.: frequency-volume chart: 11 micturitions per day with volumes of 35 ml to 70 ml and urge symptoms; fluid intake of 920 ml. (Translations: 1 did not notify (mother) regarding first voiding; 2 sudden (imperative) urge; 3 legs together (a holding manoeuvre.)

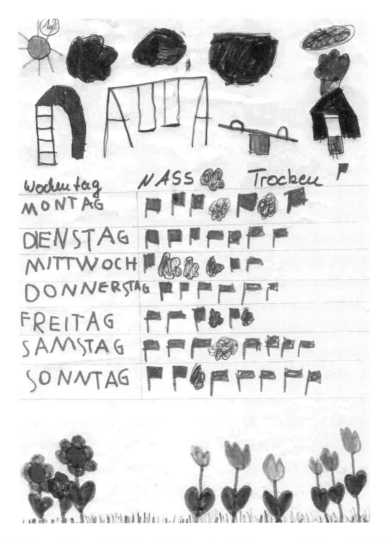

Fig. 7.10 Chart of 'flags and clouds', which L. drew herself (Nass = wet; Trocken = dry; the days of the week are on the left).

Therapy-resistant cases

So what about the child who is still wetting, in spite of standard urotherapy and anticholinergic treatment? One possibility might be that emotional and behavioural problems are decreasing motivation and compliance, in which case these problems need to be addressed. If no such problems are present, we recommend that in these cases ultrasound and a full urodynamic investigation with cystometry – ideally of the ambulatory natural-fill kind – be performed. This procedure will help clarify pathogenetic mechanisms and identify the few patients with previously undetected neurogenic bladder.

These therapy-resistant children can probably benefit from more advanced modes of urotherapy, although, as stated above, there is no firm evidence-base (yet) for this. Among the procedures that have been tried, with encouraging results, is transcutaneous electrical nerve stimulation (TENS) of various kinds (Bower et al 2001, Soomro et al 2001), using repetitive electrical stimulation of the tibial nerve (Amarenco et al 2003, de Gennaro et al 2004) or the anogenital area (Shepherd et al 1984, Trsinar and Kraij 1996, Gladh et al 2001), as a complement to ordinary urotherapy. There is now grade 4 evidence to support such therapy in children with detrusor overactivity (Bower et al 2004). Biofeedback may be useful in these children (Cardozo et al 2000, Yamanishi et al 2000), although its role in the treatment of voiding dysfunction is more established.

Acupuncture (Philip et al 1988) may also have a role to play in these children, although it is too early to recommend or discourage this treatment, with the very scant data available today. The use of botulinum toxin A, injected into the detrusor, will probably be a future treatment alternative for children with severe, therapy-resistant detrusor overactivity (Leippold et al 2003). Intensive, inpatient urotherapy, as practised during 'voiding schools' and similar arrangements, is time-consuming and costly but probably very useful.

COURSE AND PROGNOSIS

The natural course and long-term outcome of urge incontinence are considerably less studied than enuresis, and only very hazy figures can be given. Some caveats are needed: first, as mentioned above, urge incontinence is not uncommon among adult women and elderly men, and there are some indications that childhood bladder malfunction is a predisposing factor, at least in the former group (Kuh et al 1999). Second, children who present with urge incontinence may later change their voiding pattern and be found among the dysfunctional voiders or voiding postponers instead.

Hellström and her collaborators reexamined a group of children in their late teens who had first been evaluated at age 7 (Hellström et al 1995). From this study a spontaneous yearly resolution tendency of 20 per cent for girls and 25 per cent for boys can be calculated. The shorter follow-up study by Swithinbank indicated that the prevalence shrank from 15 per cent at age 11 to 3 per cent at 16 (Swithinbank et al 1998). A retrospective evaluation of the outcome of conservative management indicated that 70 per cent became symptom-free and 17 per cent had a partial response within a few years (Curran et al 2000).

To summarize, it seems that the prognosis for boys is generally better than for girls, and that a general resolution tendency of around 15 per cent per year can be surmised, while awaiting further studies.

SUMMARY AND CLINICAL GUIDELINES

Chart 7.1 presents an overview of the most important subgroups of daytime wetting. If overactive bladder/urge incontinence is present, Chart 7.2 shows the recommended sequence of therapeutic steps.

Overactive bladder is caused by uninhibited, involuntary detrusor contractions in the absence of (known) neuropathy. The symptoms present as varying degrees of intermittent incontinence and urgency. Voiding frequency may be increased but dysuria is usually absent. Concomitant constipation is very common and may be an aggravating or causative factor.

The condition needs to be distinguished from cystitis, by a urine dipstick test (and culture if this test turns out positive), and from neuropathic bladder disturbance, by history and physical examination. A voiding chart should also be completed. Ultrasound examination of the urinary tract should be performed, at least if there is a history of urinary tract infection or if the condition proves resistant to standard treatment. Uroflow/residual urine measurement should also be performed, at least in therapy-resistant cases.

Continuous, dribbling incontinence, leakage on exertion, and physical signs such as leg asymmetry, increased tendon jerks and lower lumbar hair tufts or dimples should prompt cystometric evaluation. Signs or symptoms of constipation (infrequent defecations, hard stools, encopresis, stomach-ache) should be actively sought. Blood tests are not indicated but uroflow measurement (with assessment of residual urine) is very useful, if the equipment is at hand. Otherwise it can be reserved for therapy-resistant cases. Behavioural problems and possible signs of reduced self-esteem should be looked for.

The first-line treatment is non-pharmacological and consists of the institution of regular voiding habits (approximately six times per day) and adequate fluid intake. Specifically, children are asked to register any signs of urge and go to the toilet immediately and to refrain from using holding manoeuvres. Charts are filled out. Each voiding is registered, with different signs for wet (e.g. 'clouds') or dry (e.g. 'flags') underpants. This can be considered to be a type of cognitive-behavioural treatment. Relaxation techniques can also be included. Regular follow-up and encouragement are recommended.

The second-line treatment of bladder overactivity is anticholinergic medication (oxybutynin, propiverine, tolterodine), provided that there is no residual urine, or advanced or intensified urotherapy. Switching from one anticholinergic to another in case of treatment resistance is recommended. The bladder training should continue under medication. Long-term antibiotic prophylaxis may be needed in children with overactive bladder and concomitant urinary tract infections, as an interim measure while the bladder disturbance is treated. If comorbid behavioural and emotional symptoms are present, counselling and psychotherapy might be indicated.

Voiding postponement

DEFINITION
Voiding postponement (also known as micturition deferral or psychogenic urinary retention) is defined as daytime wetting following the postponement of micturition in characteristic situations (such as play, watching TV, and school). The child postpones the imminent micturition until overwhelmed by urgency, uses holding manoeuvres such as crossing the legs and moving back and forth in a restless fashion, holding the abdomen and genitalia, sitting on the heels, etc. When about to burst, the child rushes to the toilet. As they are often too late, they wet their clothes.

This syndrome was first described by Olbing (1993) and later by Beetz (1993). As in all functional syndromes, neurogenic and other organic causes need to be ruled out. Of the functional syndromes, dysfunctional voiding has to be excluded explicitly.

Robson et al produced a similar description of a condition called 'micturition deferral':

> The most common cause of daytime wetting in a preschool child is holding the urine to the last minute, or micturition deferral. Children commonly become absorbed in play activities and ignore the need to void. After several signals are ignored, a detrusor contraction occurs that the child cannot suppress, and an incontinent episode results.
>
> (Robson et al 1996b: 91)

EPIDEMIOLOGY

Voiding postponement is one of the most common disorders of daytime wetting. Due to inconsistent definitions, reliable epidemiological data are lacking. In children referred to a paediatric setting for wetting disorders, it was just as common (23.5 per cent) as urge incontinence (22.5 per cent) (Olbing 1993). In our own studies of consecutively presented children in a child psychiatric setting, voiding postponement was even more common (16.8 per cent) than urge incontinence (13.2 per cent) (von Gontard et al 1999a). More boys are affected (65.4 per cent) compared to urge incontinence (38.1 per cent) (von Gontard et al 1999a).

AETIOLOGY

Voiding postponement is considered to be an acquired syndrome of behavioural origin (Olbing 1993). From clinical observations, dysfunctional family interactions, behavioural problems and lack of motivation were described (Olbing 1993). In some children without behavioural problems, voiding postponement can be a mere habit. Once learned, this habit is maintained despite obvious disadvantages. In other children, voiding postponement can develop out of urge incontinence by the excessive use of holding manoeuvres. The progression from urge incontinence to voiding postponement to dysfunctional voiding and underactive bladder has been observed in many children, but not the other way round.

CLINICAL SIGNS AND SYMPTOMS

A typical sign is the postponement of micturition in certain situations in which the children do not want to void. Typical situations are: on the way back home from school; or during play with friends – some children will even say they were afraid of being left out if they left the play situation and then went back. Some children are afraid to go to the school toilets, either because they think they are dirty or because they are afraid other children might disturb them. Many children avoid school toilets altogether, especially for defecation (Vernon et al 2003). Others are afraid to leave the classroom, or afraid to ask to go to the toilet. Another typical situation is while watching television or reading – they are so absorbed that they are afraid of missing something (Robson et al 1996b).

The urge to void is usually of normal intensity to begin with. The children do not react but try to postpone micturition voluntarily for as long as possible. The longer they postpone micturition, the stronger the urge becomes, so they use typical holding manoeuvres until, finally, incontinence occurs.

In voiding postponement exactly the same type of holding manoeuvres can be observed as in the overactive bladder syndrome. The children press their legs together, twitch back and forth, and even sit on their heels. The pathophysiology of the two disorders is completely different, however. In the overactive bladder there are sudden increases of intravesical pressure, which are counteracted by holding manoeuvres. In voiding postponement, there is no primary bladder overactivity; instead, the bladder storage capacity is pushed to its limits by voluntary contractions of the pelvic floor muscles.

In some children, the sequence of urge incontinence, voiding postponement, dysfunctional voiding and the end-stage of underactive bladder can be observed. This sequence does not necessarily occur, as each syndrome can arise in a primary form without precursors (Hoebeke et al 2001).

A very common symptom, in addition to the postponing behaviour, is a low micturition frequency of less than four to five times a day. In extreme cases, children go to the toilet only one to three times a day. This low micturition frequency is often not registered by children and parents and is only detected via micturition charts. Infrequent voiding can be associated with night-time wetting only. In one study, night-time wetting improved in 55 per cent of children by simply increasing the number of micturitions (Kruse et al 1999). In contrast, children with urge incontinence usually have a much higher micturition frequency – over seven times per day.

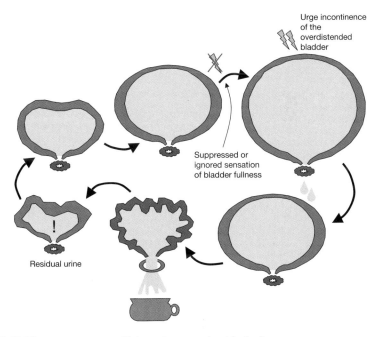

Fig. 7.11 Voiding postponement with incontinence and residual urine.

157

Because of this repetitive retention of urine, the mean voided volume is higher than in children with urge incontinence (Lettgen et al 2002). Urinary tract infections occur in 19.2 per cent of children, a significantly lower rate than in urge incontinence (50 per cent). Children also have increased rates of residual urine and bladder wall thickening (von Gontard 1995). Although most children had normal, bell-shaped uroflow curves, the rates of plateau-shaped curves (12.2 per cent) and staccato curves (18.4 per cent) were high.

In addition to the retention of urine, faecal retention is common: 23 per cent of children had encopresis (von Gontard et al 1998a). Faecal, scybalous masses can be palpated abdominally. Signs of retrovesical impressions can be seen on ultrasound. The coexisting retention of both urine and stools can be understood physiologically: the pelvic floor is one physiological unit, so its contraction will enhance retention in both systems. The association of infrequent voiding, behavioural abnormalities, poor fluid intake and functional stool retention was significantly more common in girls with recurrent UTIs than in controls (Stauffer et al 2004).

P.Q., 8-year-old girl
Diagnoses: Urinary incontinence; recurrent UTIs;
voiding postponement; encopresis with constipation;
oppositional defiant disorder (F 91.3)

P. became day- and night-dry at the age of 3 but started wetting again during the daytime from the age of 5 onwards. Wetting frequency varied from several times daily to once a week. Sometimes the urine came suddenly, without warning, and sometimes she sensed an urgent need to urinate but didn't make it to the toilet in time. Since P. started school two years ago, the incontinence episodes had become less frequent, but instead she had had several UTIs, with dysuria and dramatically increased voiding frequency as presenting symptoms. Antibiotic response had been prompt and there had been no febrile UTIs. The parents noted that she would some-times squat or stand on tiptoe in order to avoid going to the toilet. Also, there had been instances of encopresis more recently. Peer relations at school were problematic, since P. has a short temper, and school performance was hampered by the fact that she is easily distracted. She had no close friends. A school psychologist was involved and special education was considered.

Physical examination was normal except for moderate obesity. She was oppo-sitional and would not let the doctor inspect her genitalia or perform a rectal examination. Uroflow revealed a plateau-shaped curve and there was 35 ml of residual urine after voiding 145 ml. The urine dipstick test was negative so no culture was taken. A voiding chart revealed that P. voided irregularly, two to five times per day with volumes between 50 and 400 ml, that she drank little and that defecation occurred every other day. Incontinence episodes, with just dampness of the underwear, occurred twice during the recording week. An ultrasound showed no kidney or urinary tract abnormalities but confirmed residual urine.

It was concluded that P. had disturbed bladder function with urgency, voiding postponement and residual urine, that the UTIs were probably secondary to the bladder disturbance, and that there was probably constipation as well. Furthermore, it was suspected that she also needed psychological/psychiatric counselling.

With the aid of a urotherapist, bladder training was started, and laxatives and bowel advice were also given. Progress was slow and she had two more cystitis episodes, but after involving the child psychiatric department compliance with treatment increased.

PSYCHOLOGICAL ASPECTS

In adults, 'psychogenic urinary retention' was described in patients with a wide variety of severe psychiatric disturbances (Allen 1972, Montague and Jones 1979). It was hypothesized that 'the retention of urine was an active aggressive phenomenon rather than a passive one' (Allen 1972: 304); or that the retention could also have stimulating effects (Bass 1994), or be associated with guilt feelings (Bird 1980).

From clinical observation, two groups of children can be described. On the one hand, some children show a habitual postponement of micturition but no other behavioural symptoms. One has the impression that they get used to this habit and simply continue with it because it is convenient not to go to the toilet in certain situations. Although the postponement is voluntary initially, as time goes on, the habit is maintained without thinking much about it.

In other children, voiding postponement can be interpreted as one of many oppositional symptoms. Indeed, one of the most common coexisting disorders is oppositional defiant disorder (ODD). Parents describe how in addition to avoiding the toilet, children refuse to blow their nose and use a handkerchief, to tidy their room, brush their teeth and to obey instructions. They are often late because they dawdle and take too much time to get dressed before going to school or kindergarten. Food refusal, selective eating, selective mutism and even psychogenic vomiting have been observed. Other children refuse to drink sufficient amounts of fluids.

In a systematic study of children with voiding postponement in a paediatric and child psychiatric setting, 53.8 per cent fulfilled the criteria for at least one ICD-10 diagnosis (von Gontard et al 1998a). These were mainly externalizing disorders, in one-third of all children, supporting the hypothesis of oppositional defiant disorder (ODD). Also, 37.3 per cent of children had a CBCL total score in the clinical range, again with externalizing symptoms predominating. In this case, it is interesting to look at the single items of the CBCL. The children showed a wide variety of behavioural problems, including attention problems (including items such as 'acts too young', 'can't concentrate', 'can't sit still', 'impulsive', etc.) and delinquent behaviour ('lacks guilt', 'lies', 'bad companions', 'swearing, obscenity', 'steals at home', etc.). High rates were registered for withdrawn ('would rather be alone',

159

'refuses to talk', 'secretive', 'sulks', 'unhappy, sad, withdrawn', etc.) and aggressive behaviour ('argues', 'mean to others', 'demands attention', 'destroys own things', 'jealous', 'fights', 'stubborn', 'irritable', etc.). Compared to the normative population, the rates of behavioural problems were four to ten times higher (von Gontard et al 1998a). Subjectively, these children are just as distressed as children with urge incontinence: 64 per cent could state clearly that they saw and felt disadvantages as a result of their wetting problems.

In addition to individual problems, there were clear signs of dysfunction, as measured using a questionnaire on family adaptability and cohesion (FACES-III, Olson et al 1985). Most of the families had a rigid type of adaptability and a disengaged type of cohesion (Lettgen et al 2002).

Adaptability denotes the extent to which the family system is flexible and able to change: rigid families adjust too little to change, they continue to use the same ways of solving problems regardless of changes within the family or the surroundings (Dundas 1994). Family cohesion denotes the degree to which family members are separated from or connected to their family, including such dimensions as emotional bonding, boundaries, coalitions, time, space, friends, decision making, interests and recreation (Olson et al 1985). Families with voiding postponement tend to have a low level of cohesion and to be disengaged: high levels of autonomy are encouraged, members are independent and their commitment and attachment to the family are low (Dundas 1994, Olson et al 1995). The combination of 'rigid' adaptability and 'disengaged' cohesion is an especially problematic constellation: of the 16 possible family types, it ranked 14th regarding general contentment and 16th regarding marital satisfaction in a large analysis of 2440 families (Green et al 1991).

In summary, voiding postponement occurs in children either as a habit, or as part of an oppositional defiant disorder or other behavioural disorder. Also, families with voiding postponement have more extreme types of family dysfunction – much more so than families with urge incontinence.

ASSESSMENT

As a behavioural syndrome, close attention has to be paid to the voiding postponement behaviour, which cannot be separated from the holding manoeuvres. Therefore, an exact history, observation, questionnaires and micturition charts are essential. These will show a low micturition frequency, associated with a more or less voluntary postponement of micturition in certain situations. Also, large voided volumes, thick bladder walls, residual urine, abdominal masses and encopresis predominate. The uroflow curves do show slight abnormalities, but no typical pattern. Dysfunctional voiding, with consistent repeated staccato or interrupted uroflow curves, needs to be excluded. Because of the high comorbidity of behavioural disorders, a careful assessment of this comorbid disorder is necessary.

TREATMENT

Overall, the quality of treatment studies for day-wetting children is not based on a high level of evidence; thus only five randomized, controlled studies could be identified in total for all types of daytime wetting (Sureshkumar et al 2003). The recommendations for voiding postponement, as for most other forms of daytime wetting, are therefore based on clinical experience or non-randomized studies.

A symptom-oriented approach is indicated in all cases of voiding postponement. The first step is provision of information and psychoeducation. Often, parents and children are unaware of the association of voiding postponement, retention of urine and incontinence.

Children and parents are instructed to increase micturition frequency (Kruse et al 1999). The goal is to go to the toilet seven times a day, at regular intervals. The child should sit on the toilet in a relaxed way, and take plenty of time. If encopresis or constipation are also present, this also has to be treated. The micturitions on the toilet, as well as wetting episodes, are noted on a chart (see Appendix 12). Quite often, parents have to take an active role and send their child to the toilet. To increase motivation, a simple token system with positive reinforcement can be used. The cooperation of the child should be reinforced either by small material rewards (such as stickers, playing cards, etc.) or by social rewards (playing together, going to the swimming pool, etc.).

In older children, digital wrist alarm watches or countdown timers can be of help in reminding the child to go to the toilet: intervals of one and a half to three hours can be set (Meadow 1990). One advantage of this method is that the child takes on more responsibility for treatment success. In case of residual urine, ultrasound can be used therapeutically with success, by visualizing the bladder and enhancing the child's understanding of retention (MacKinnon et al 2000).

A.B., 9-year-old boy
Diagnoses: Voiding postponement; primary nocturnal enuresis

A. was referred for day- and night-time wetting. He wetted his bed three to four times per week with large urine volumes, was a deep sleeper and difficult to wake. He wetted small amounts every day. He very often used holding manoeuvres and postponed micturition, with a micturition frequency of only four times per day. No further behavioural problems were reported. Sonography was normal without residual urine. Uroflowmetry showed a bell-shaped curve.

Treatment consisted of increasing the micturition frequency to seven times per day and keeping the micturition intervals as short as possible. A. was asked to refrain from using holding manoeuvres and to fill out charts for documentation. Without any other intervention, nocturnal enuresis decreased to once every two weeks and ceased completely after eight weeks. Daytime wetting decreased slowly to two to four times a week after eight weeks, and stopped after 16 weeks.

In this case, typical voiding postponement was treated by regulating toilet habits, increasing the micturition frequency and refraining from holding manoeuvres. No other treatment was needed.

However, often these symptom-oriented approaches are not sufficient because of the high behavioural comorbidity. Other child psychiatric and psychotherapeutic interventions are often needed (Beetz 1993). These can consist of behavioural and cognitive techniques in conduct disorders, as well as stimulant therapy in ADHD. In those few children with emotional disorders, psychodynamic therapy may be indicated. In cases of family dysfunction, family counselling and even family therapy may be indicated. In severe cases, an outpatient setting will not suffice, and day clinic or even inpatient treatment may be necessary. This will lead to a reduction of interfamilial attention, so that the child's individual problem can be treated in a different context.

M.S., 8-year-old girl
Diagnoses: Hyperkinetic syndrome with conduct disorder (ICD-10: F 90.1); voiding postponement; recurrent UTIs; recurrent constipation

M. had become dry at 2½ years of age, had started wetting at 3 years, and had had recurrent UTIs requiring antibiotic prophylaxis since then. She had been operated on because of a bladder diverticulum at the age of 7 years. During play she habitually postponed going to the toilet and sat on her heels. She was verbally aggressive when asked to go to the toilet. Sometimes she had to strain to get the micturition going. The urine flow was only occasionally interrupted. She used to have recurrent constipation, which had resolved. She showed many problems in her social behaviour. She dawdled, did not tidy her room, refused certain types of food, did not do her school work, provoked her mother, was not accepted by peers and was often sad and depressed. M.'s development had been fairly normal; her mother was a single parent having to look after three children.

The paediatric examination was normal. Ultrasound revealed that the bladder wall was thickened (3.9 mm), there was residual urine of 5 ml and there were retrovesical impressions. The uroflow curve was bell-shaped, the EMG relaxed. In the mental state examination, M. was shy and socially withdrawn, uncooperative, demonstrative, oppositional and depressed. The IQ was in the normal range (K-ABC; Kaufman and Kaufman 1983). The family relations test (FRT) showed negative tendencies towards her mother and her younger siblings.

A child psychiatric day clinic treatment was initiated because of the severity of the behavioural disorder. M. was sent to the toilet regularly – no further treatment was needed for the constipation or her day wetting. Because of the hyperkinetic syndrome, stimulant therapy with methylphenidate (25 mg per day) was initiated, which led to a reduction of the hyperactivity and increased attention span. Individual play therapy, as well as mother–child interactional therapy, was also needed. After marked reduction of conduct and affective problems, counselling was continued on an outpatient basis.

In this case, the psychiatric disorder was the main problem and required day clinic treatment. The voiding problems were treated relatively easily in this setting.

COURSE AND PROGNOSIS
If the voiding postponement is a mere habit and children are motivated, the prognosis is favourable. Within a few weeks, an increase of micturition frequency and reduction of incontinence can be achieved. In case of comorbid disorders, especially oppositional defiant disorder, treatment can be very difficult indeed as compliance is low and children will not adhere to the treatment regimes. In some children, the postponement will persist; and in some, dysfunctional voiding and underactive bladder may follow.

SUMMARY AND CLINICAL GUIDELINES
The therapy of voiding postponement is purely non-pharmacological. As indicated generally, encopresis, constipation or UTIs should be treated. Information on regular voiding and drinking habits should be provided. Children should be encouraged to go to the toilet regularly seven times a day and to fill out charts (Chart 7.3). This can be encouraged with a simple token system (rewards). Digital wrist alarm watches can act as useful reminders in older children. As the comorbidity of behavioural and emotional disorders is high, additional counselling, psychotherapy and other child psychiatric interventions are often required.

Dysfunctional voiding

DEFINITION
In contrast to the previous syndromes, dysfunctional voiding is a disorder of the emptying phase of the bladder. It is defined urodynamically by a lack of relaxation and a dyscoordinated contraction of the external sphincter during micturition. An interrupted or staccato uroflow curve with marked EMG contractions is typical. Milder forms are called dysfunctional voiding; more severe forms are termed 'Hinman syndrome' after Hinman who first described the disorder. Other terms used are: detrusor–sphincter dyscoordination, non-neurogenic neurogenic bladder, and occult neurogenic bladder, etc., in earlier terminology.

One should note that the term dysfunctional voiding is often used indiscriminately in the United States for all sorts of urinary incontinence, even disorders of the filling phase. Strictly, it denotes a disorder of the emptying phase alone.

EPIDEMIOLOGY
Epidemiological data are not available. It is a rare, often overlooked syndrome. In a series of patients referred for wetting problems in a paediatric setting, only 3 per cent had dysfunctional voiding (Olbing 1993). In our own studies, 4.2 per cent of all wetting children fulfilled the criteria when uroflow and EMG were performed routinely (von Gontard 1995). Among children with UTIs, only 0.9 per cent were affected (Hellerstein and Linebarger

2003). In other clinical samples the rates were 16.8 per cent (Hoang-Böhm et al 1999) and 32 per cent (Hoebeke et al 2001). In a recent review, the prevalence was estimated at between 5 and 25 per cent (Hoang-Böhm et al 2004). Evidently, selection biases and accuracy of assessment play a decisive role and population-based studies are urgently needed.

While all other incontinence-related symptoms decrease as the child approaches adolescence, emptying difficulties (interrupted stream and prolonged voiding time) actually increased up to the age of 17 years in a population-based follow-up study (Hellström et al 1995).

AETIOLOGY

The syndrome was first described by Hinman and Baumann (1973, Hinman 1974, Hinman and Baumann 1976, Hinman 1986). Hinman described the syndrome as a behavioural, acquired reversible disorder which could be ameliorated by suggestive and behavioural techniques. He interpreted it as a 'bad habit in certain personalities in unfavourable family settings' (Hinman 1986). According to clinical observations, anxious, depressed, shy and timid behaviour are common, as well as oppositional tendencies. Allen (1977) saw hyper-activity as a typical sign and speculated that psychological factors would play a major aetiological role in at least 50 per cent of the 21 cases he studied. Family stressors such as parental alcoholism, divorce and dominant fathers were described (Allen 1977).

In contrast, other authors have postulated that there are no associations with emotional or psychosocial problems (van Gool et al 1984). Instead, a maturational delay of the CNS and a dysfunction of the urethral sphincter were hypothesized. A genetic component cannot be excluded in individual families but genetic factors play a lower role than in other syndromes, such as nocturnal enuresis and urge incontinence (Hjälmås 1995a). As Hinman (1986) pointed out, this syndrome has two prerequisites: a failure to inhibit the detrusor reflex and an over-compensation by the external sphincter.

In most cases, however, it is a learned behaviour. It can develop out of urge incontinence and voiding postponement, but it can also develop without these precursors. In some children, signs of urge incontinence and voiding dysfunction coexist (Vijverberg et al 1997).

CLINICAL SIGNS AND SYMPTOMS

Children are often referred because of the wetting problems and not because of their dysfunctional voiding. These specific symptoms are often not registered by the children or their families and have to be actively looked for. Typical signs are: straining to get the micturition started against the resistance of the contracted sphincter; and a staccato or interrupted uroflow curve. The urine stream is not very strong, as the pelvic floor does not relax completely. Residual urine and urinary tract infections are common. The bladder wall is thickened. The micturition frequency can vary. Not all symptoms are always present in every patient (Hoang-Böhm et al 2004).

For the diagnosis of voiding dysfunction, these uroflow abnormalities must persist in repeated measurements. A single abnormal finding is not sufficient for diagnosis, as 30 per cent of normal children show a staccato and 6 per cent an interrupted curve (Bower et al

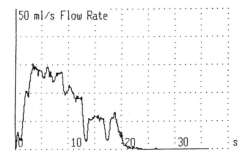

Fig. 7.12 Typical staccato uroflow curve of a child with voiding dysfunction (residual urine 19 ml, voided volume 340 ml).

2004). As a result of the repeated and habitual contraction of the pelvic floor, stool retention, constipation and encopresis can occur (Ab et al 2002).

As the intravesical pressure is increased, vesico-ureteric reflux and obstruction of the upper urinary tract can develop (Hinman 1986, van Gool et al 1992c). Even renal insufficiency has been described as a long-term consequence of this functional syndrome (Varlam and Dippel 1995). If the dysfunctional voiding is not treated, complications following surgery can occur (Hinman and Baumann 1976, Allen 1977).

PSYCHOLOGICAL ASPECTS
Systematic investigations of psychological aspects are rare. From our own observations and studies, dysfunctional voiding is clearly a heterogeneous disorder. Four typical constellations can be observed:

1   It can occur as a temporary symptom in day-wetting children or in non-monosymptomatic nocturnal enuresis. In these cases the habit is not yet fixed and can easily be changed by more regular, relaxed toilet habits or a short course of biofeedback.
2   Dysfunctional voiding can be present in children with no psychological disorder, and in these cases it represents a chronic, habitual behaviour.
3   In up to half of the children, severe, marked, psychiatric disorders such as severe depressive episodes and elective mutism can occur. Also, dysfunctional voiding following severe sexual abuse and deprivation as well as other familial stressors such as migration has been described in case reports (Varlam and Dippel 1995). Some of these children would be considered to have signs of posttraumatic stress disorder. In the first report by Hinman and Baumann (1973), most patients (13/14) were said to have 'neuropsychiatric defects' (hyperkinesis, neurosis or chronic anxiety) as well as 'failure personalities'.
4   In addition, dysfunctional voiding has been observed anecdotally in children with neurological disorders such as spastic diplegia. In chronic neurological diseases, such as spinal muscular atrophy, dysfunctional voiding can occur as a functional problem (von Gontard et al 2001b, van Gool 1997). Also, 60 per cent of children with severe mental and motor retardation showed voiding dysfunction (Van Laecke et al 2001).

Uroflowmetry with EMG should be performed, if available, in every case of dysfunctional voiding. Typically, staccato or interrupted uroflow curves with reduced maximal flow rate and prolonged micturition time occur. The EMG shows contraction either intermittently or continuously. Ultrasound should also be performed: typical signs are a thickened bladder wall, extreme residual urine (Hoang-Böhm et al 1999) and retrovesical impression from faecal masses. In ultrasound of the kidneys, fluids can sometimes be detected in the renal pelvis. Because of the high rate of urinary tract infections, urine analysis and, if indicated, bacteriology are often necessary. In chronic cases, further urodynamic and radiological investigations may be indicated.

TREATMENT

Because of the long-term organic consequences, dysfunctional voiding has to be treated actively. The treatment method of choice is biofeedback, which is defined as a variety of techniques by which physiological activity is made conscious through visual and acoustic signals (Kjolseth et al 1993).

The treatment of dysfunctional voiding includes cognitive-behavioural elements combined with general increase of motivation (van Gool et al 1992b, Olbing 1993). Information should be provided and the coordination of detrusor and sphincter explained. UTIs, constipation and encopresis should be treated. If necessary, voiding frequency and oral fluids should be increased. Toilet training should be initiated. It is recommended that children take a lot of time, sit in a relaxed manner on the toilet seat, spread their legs apart and have contact with the floor – either directly or with a foot stool. The children are asked to relax completely, initiate micturition without straining and simply let the urine flow until they have the feeling that the bladder is empty. General relaxation methods can be useful. In contrast, any type of physiotherapy aimed at strengthening the pelvic floor is contraindicated.

In addition to these general measures, specific uroflow biofeedback training should be initiated. Different techniques are available. Usually, visual uroflow and acoustic EMG biofeedback with perianal surface electrodes are combined. Only a few centres use anal-plug EMG biofeedback (de Paepe et al 2000).

Children are asked to look at the monitor and follow their uroflow curve. At the same time, they can listen to the biofeedback of the EMG and register if their pelvic floor is relaxed or not. Following the micturition, residual urine is measured. The results are discussed with the child and goals are defined. Obvious goals are a relaxed pelvic floor, a bell-shaped curve and no residual urine. If one or more of these goals are achieved, this can be reinforced with a reward or token. After micturition, children are encouraged to drink fluids, so that the training can be repeated several times in one session. From clinical experience, two to six sessions, each with three to four training units, are usually sufficient to achieve coordination. If this is not possible, children can be admitted to day clinic or inpatient treatment. Specific programmes, usually for small groups of two to four children, are offered in several hospitals.

In a recent review of eight different biofeedback studies, 90 per cent success rates for daytime incontinence and nocturnal enuresis were reported, and marked reductions of UTIs and vesico-ureteric reflux were achieved (Hoang-Böhm et al 2004). Most cases can be treated on an outpatient basis. A more intensive approach is inpatient treatment which should be reserved for severe cases. An excellent programme was described by Vijverberg et al (1997). The success rate for a mixed group of urge incontinence and dysfunctional voiding was good for 68.4 per cent, and average for 12.6 per cent, while 19 per cent did not improve – due to young age and psychological problems requiring more intensive mental health treatment. Other programmes start with inpatient therapy and instruction and then, as soon as possible, continue on an outpatient basis (Hoang-Böhm et al 1999). It is important to follow up the patients for a long time – the mean follow-up time was 18.6 months with a range of 3 to 39 months.

The effectiveness of uroflow biofeedback has been shown by Kjolseth et al (1993), who followed 32 children with voiding dysfunction over four years. The number of sessions varied between one and nine, with 47 per cent needing only four to five sessions. Half of the children were cured, eight showed a marked improvement, and only seven no effect. The uroflow was completely normalized in 55 per cent of the children. After four years, eight of the initially cured patients had completely normal curves, two had had relapses, and three had current urinary tract infections.

In another study of 16 children treated for dysfunctional voiding, 10 were free of symptoms after a six-month follow-up, and 13 after a five-year follow-up (Hanson et al 1987). Nocturnal enuresis also ceases: the success rate was 87 per cent after two years, and 80 per cent at the four-year follow-up (Porena et al 2000). Despite the effectiveness of biofeedback, it is not clear which components are the decisive therapeutic elements.

T.F., 10-year-old boy
Diagnoses: Dysfunctional voiding; primary nocturnal enuresis

T. was referred for day- and night-time wetting. He had never been dry at night, wetted large amounts of urine into his bed and was difficult to arouse. During the day, he wetted smaller amounts three to four times per week. He went to the toilet eight to ten times a day despite taking oxybutynin. Straining and an interrupted urine stream were also reported, but only when asked specifically. There were no other signs of behavioural problems. Sonography showed a thickened bladder wall, retrovesical impressions and large residual urine volume – between 40 and 70 ml. The initial uroflowmetry showed an interrupted curve. The micturition protocols showed that T. went to the toilet only five times a day and that his fluid intake was only 650 ml per day.

Treatment consisted of increasing fluid intake and micturition frequency. T. was asked to relax and initiate micturition without straining. In addition, biofeedback training was conducted on an outpatient basis. In only six training sessions, a coordinated micturition with a bell-shaped curve and a reduction of residual urine

167

to 2 ml was attained. In each session, T. was asked to drink plenty of fluids and, as soon as his bladder was filled, uroflowmetry and sonography were performed. Goals and results were discussed and successes reinforced by praise. Under this treatment, day wetting ceased almost completely. Nocturnal enuresis was treated with 20 µg of desmopressin. T. was a full responder but had a relapse as soon as medication was discontinued. Dryness was finally achieved with alarm treatment.

This is a classic case of dysfunctional voiding, which probably developed from initial urge incontinence. The symptoms of straining and interrupted urine stream are often overlooked by children and their parents, but can be detected by a careful history and uroflowmetry. Because of possible secondary effects, coordination has to be achieved first, before other treatments for daytime incontinence and nocturnal enuresis can follow.

Recently, EMG biofeedback systems for home use have been marketed. These are often attractive for children as they look like computer games. In one type, children can see a school of fish on the monitor. If their pelvic floor is relaxed, a whale swims up to sea level and squirts out water. If the pelvic muscles are contracted, the whale swims to the ocean floor. The disadvantage of these systems is that only the pelvic floor (by EMG), but not the actual emptying of the bladder (by uroflow), is controlled. On the other hand, the repeated training effect in the home environment is far less cost intensive than clinic treatment. In

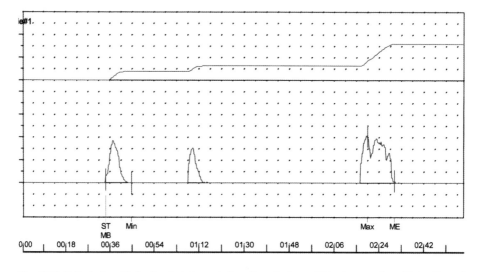

Fig. 7.13 T.F.: before biofeedback: interrupted uroflow (volume 161 ml, max. flow 10.4 ml/sec, 3 fractions) and residual urine of 40 ml.

168

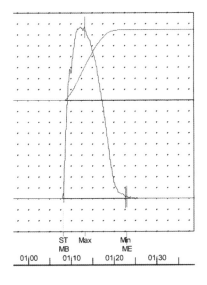

ST   Max   Min
      MB   ME
01¦00 | 01¦10 | 01¦20 | 01¦30 |

Fig. 7.14 T.F.: after biofeedback: bell-shaped curve (324 ml, max. flow 39.3 ml/sec) and residual urine of 2 ml (normal).

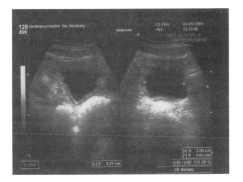

Fig. 7.15 T.F.: ultrasound before: residual volume of 40 ml at the beginning of biofeedback training (longitudinal view left, transversal view right).

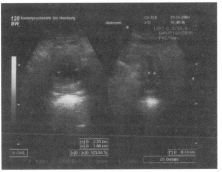

Fig. 7.16 T.F.: ultrasound after: residual volume of 2 ml at the end of training two months later (transversal view left, longitudinal view right).

home training, parents need close instruction and supervision. Frustrated families and interactional problems have been observed if families are not supervised properly.

Biofeedback should be conducted in every case of persisting dysfunctional voiding. Other modes of treatment might possibly have a place in the future. A recent review concluded that there were clear benefits from the use of electro-neuromodulation in different forms of incontinence – not just dysfunctional voiding (Bower and Yeung 2004). Based as it is on six studies and a low grade of evidence, this approach requires further studies before it can be recommended.

If comorbid behavioural disorders are present, these, of course, need separate treatment. Psychotherapy and other child psychiatric interventions may be indicated, as in the case

169

reports of Varlam and Dippel (1995). The first cases reported by Hinman and Baumann (1973) were treated by hypnosis, with suggestions regarding bladder control and anti-depressant medication. The technique was later outlined in greater detail by Baumann and Hinman (1974): patients were relaxed, asked to pretend they were doing an activity they liked and, when they entered a hypnotic state, positive suggestions were made, such as 'you can learn how good it feels to empty your bladder completely . . .', etc. Although they did show a good effect, these approaches have been dropped nowadays – not always to the advantage of the patients.

Summary and Clinical Guidelines
Dysfunctional voiding is associated with a high risk for UTIs, encopresis and constipation, requiring additional therapy. In addition to providing information and regulation of voiding and drinking habits, the specific and most effective form of treatment is biofeedback training (Chart 7.4). A visual biofeedback with uroflow and/or an acoustic biofeedback with pelvic floor EMG can be employed. Relaxation techniques can be added. Residual urine should be checked after each voiding. In most cases, coordination can be achieved on an outpatient basis. In severe cases, more intensive day-care or even inpatient training may be required. In subgroups of children with comorbid behavioural disorders, counselling, psychotherapy and other child psychiatric interventions are indicated. Wetting usually subsides once stable coordination is achieved. Any persistent wetting (with coordinated emptying of the bladder) is then treated as indicated in other cases.

Stress incontinence

Definition
Stress incontinence occurs on exertion (coughing, straining or any other cause of increased abdominal pressure) and is associated with an underactive or damaged sphincter.

Epidemiology
Although common among adult women, especially women who have borne children (Persson et al 2000), genuine idiopathic stress incontinence is exceedingly rare in childhood. When it occurs it uniformly affects adolescent girls. Girls with cystic fibrosis for some reason seem to have a higher prevalence of stress incontinence than other girls (Nixon et al 2002).

The condition is not uncommon, however, in children with sphincter underactivity due to neurogenic bladder dysfunction. In these cases, it is not a functional but a neurogenic type of incontinence. These children are discussed in Chapter 8.

Aetiology
Stress incontinence is incontinence due to urethral inability to overcome a raised intra-abdominal pressure that is transmitted into the bladder. The underlying cause in the few cases that present in childhood is unknown. As usual, aetiology may be partly hereditary (Ertunc et al 2004).

It should be noted that in some cases it may not be a low urethral resting tonus that is responsible, but an extreme intra-abdominal pressure; stress incontinence in the presence of a normal pelvic floor has been noted in 80 per cent of teenage elite trampolinists after a few years of training (Eliasson et al 2002).

The debated so-called 'congenital wide bladder neck anomaly' that has sometimes been found on video urodynamic evaluation of incontinent girls (Murray et al 1987) may in some cases be related to stress incontinence, but is more probably an incidental finding of low differential diagnostic value in children with detrusor overactivity. An attractive – albeit speculative – alternative explanation is that the wide bladder neck anomaly represents the sphincter relaxation of an overactive micturition reflex, as discussed in the earlier section on the aetiology of bladder overactivity (see pages 142–143).

CLINICAL SIGNS AND SYMPTOMS

The typical presentation of stress incontinence is the leakage of small amounts of urine during situations of raised intra-abdominal pressure, such as laughing, coughing or straining. Urgency is probably not part of the symptomatology (at least not in children), neither is an increased or diminished micturition frequency. This last point is important, since stress incontinence is often confused with the much more common situation where children with voiding postponement or detrusor underactivity experience 'pseudo-stress incontinence' due to bladder overfilling (see page 176). A high micturition frequency may be present, indicating the child's attempt to decrease the risk of leakage. The risk for UTIs is not increased in genuine idiopathic stress incontinence.

The symptomatology is unclear even in the adult population, since it has been shown that symptoms of stress incontinence and overactive bladder can overlap (Cardozo and Stanton 1980). Women with symptoms suggesting the one can by cystometry be found to have the other, and vice versa. The fact that the presence of urine in the proximal urethra may, in itself, elicit involuntary detrusor contractions may be an explanation for this phenomenon (Jung et al 1999). Whether these considerations have any bearing at all in children is an open question.

It should be kept in mind that stress incontinence is often confused with urge incontinence, i.e. an emptying reflex is elicited when the child with overactive bladder is exercising. As mentioned above, stress incontinence in childhood is very rare.

PSYCHOLOGICAL ASPECTS

Children may be highly distressed and may often be teased. Social withdrawal and emotional symptoms are common (Olbing 1993). Systematic studies are lacking.

ASSESSMENT

The first step in the evaluation of children with suspected stress incontinence is, apart from history and physical examination, the completion of a voiding chart. With the help of voiding chart data, the much more common conditions of voiding postponement, urge incontinence and detrusor underactivity can be excluded, and the specific situations in which incontinence episodes occur can be described. The leakage of large amounts of urine, the presence of

171

urgency, and abnormally low micturition frequency are all symptoms that speak against a diagnosis of stress incontinence.

The next step is uroflowmetry, which typically is unremarkable.

Every child with stress incontinence needs to see a urologist or a gynaecologist. The condition is so rare in childhood that paediatricians cannot be expected to have enough experience to handle it alone. The first task of the urologist will usually be to submit the child to cystometric evaluation, in order to confirm or exclude the suspected diagnosis and – importantly – to exclude or detect neurogenic bladder disturbance.

TREATMENT
Treatment of idiopathic stress incontinence is complicated. Mild forms, especially in younger women, can be treated by pelvic floor training alone (Moore 2000, Simpson 2000), while in moderately severe cases the addition of an alpha-adrenergic agonist such as phenylpropanolamine or ephedrine may be beneficial (Rees and Ransley 1980, Alhasso et al 2003). The modern antidepressant duloxetine, with noradrenergic and serotoninergic effects, has also been shown to be useful in randomized, controlled studies (Norton et al 2002). In severe or therapy-resistant cases, surgery often has to be resorted to. The large number of different surgical procedures available reflects the fact that, as in neurogenic bladder disturbance, there is no one procedure that is universally curative.

COURSE AND PROGNOSIS
Stress incontinence is usually a lifelong condition that will worsen as pelvic floor muscular support grows weaker.

SUMMARY AND CLINICAL GUIDELINES
Genuine stress incontinence is extremely rare in children and adolescents. Bladder overactivity and/or voiding postponement or detrusor underactivity are much more common. If genuine stress incontinence is suspected in a child it should be verified cystometrically and a urologist or a gynaecologist should be consulted.

Giggle incontinence

DEFINITION
Giggle incontinence (also known as giggle enuresis, enuresis risoria) is defined as a complete emptying of the bladder with large urine volumes which are elicited reflexively by laughing. In contrast to stress incontinence, micturition is induced by a neurological reflex and not by increased intra-abdominal pressure. Therefore, micturition does not stop immediately if laughing is interrupted.

EPIDEMIOLOGY
No population-based studies have been conducted so far. Although a rare condition, it is often overlooked in the clinical context.

Giggle incontinence is a genetic syndrome affecting both boys and girls, with a female preponderance (Sher and Reinberg 1996). It is probably transmitted only by females: 5/9 mothers and one grandmother (Elzinga-Plomp et al 1995), and 10 female relatives of 4/7 families were affected, respectively (Sher and Reinberg 1996). This is an unusual phenomenon known only in genetic imprinting or in mitochondrial inheritance. A receptor-mediated imbalance of the cholinergic and monoaminergic systems has been postulated (Sher and Reinberg 1996).

Giggle incontinence and its association with cataplexy were first described by MacKeith (1959). Sher and Reinberg (1996) showed that during giggle incontinence, a loss of control of other bodily functions develops; thus some children cannot remain seated or standing (Elzinga-Plomp et al 1995). Although the genetics and neurobiology of giggle incontinence have not yet been elucidated, it is interesting that an overlap exists with cataplexy, but not with narcolepsy or any other type of excessive sleepiness.

Cataplexy is characterized by a sudden loss of muscle control evoked by emotions, especially laughter – but not by coughing, sneezing or straining. In healthy controls, the emotional context of laughter (and not just the respiratory effects alone) had the greatest effect on suppressing motor neuron activity (Overdeem et al 2004). Narcolepsy, characterized by sleep attacks, hypnagogic hallucinations and sleep paralysis, is an abnormality of REM sleep often associated with cataplexy. Both have a clear genetic component.

In one study, narcolepsy–cataplexy was inherited in an autosomal dominant mode in a large French family. Positive linkage to a locus on chromosome 21q, with LOD score of 4.0, was found (Dauvilliers et al 2004). Also, patients with narcolepsy–cataplexy have a specific reduction of hypocretin-1 levels in their spinal fluid (Dauvilliers et al 2003). Although giggle incontinence was not reported in these series, these findings might point towards a common aetiology.

Typical for giggle incontinence is the apparently complete, reflectory emptying of the bladder during laughter. The frequency in one study varied between twice a week and four times a day (Elzinga-Plomp et al 1995). This means a marked restriction of social activities in these children. The urodynamics are normal. Therefore the name 'giggle enuresis' or 'enuresis risoria' was suggested by some authors (Elzinga-Plomp et al 1995).

The main differential diagnosis is stress incontinence, in which unspecific increases of intra-abdominal pressure will lead to small amounts of incontinence, but not to a complete emptying of the bladder. This was reported in an early questionnaire survey of student nurses, 25 per cent of whom experienced some 'bladder responses to laughter at some time in their life' (Glahn 1979). In cases of urine retention, small changes of intra-abdominal pressure can induce wetting of small amounts. Giggle incontinence can also be mistakenly diagnosed in children with overactive bladder, as incorrectly reported by Chandra et al (2002).

Psychological Aspects

There have been no systematic investigations of children with giggle incontinence. From clinical experience, they are highly distressed by the symptom and try to avoid situations in which they might be forced to laugh. Social withdrawal, not going to parties and not meeting with friends have been observed. It is not known if the rate of behavioural disorders is increased, however.

Assessment

The assessment of giggle incontinence does not differ from that in other syndromes of functional incontinence. As a disorder of the central nervous system, peripheral bladder function is usually not affected.

Treatment

Two different types of treatment have been suggested: pharmacotherapy and behavioural therapy. Due to the co-occurrence with narcolepsy, stimulant treatment is effective (see Chapter 5). The doses required are higher than those prescribed for ADHD. Thus, 0.3 to 0.5 mg of methylphenidate per kg bodyweight every four to five hours during the day should be prescribed. In addition, 5 to 20 mg of methylphenidate should be taken before engaging in social activities which might induce laughing. Despite these high doses, side effects are not typical and all children remain dry even one to five years later (Sher and Reinberg 1996).

In contrast, Elzinga-Plomp et al (1995) described a conditioning treatment with an aversive stimulant (a mild electrical current), which was employed by the children themselves when they had to laugh. Later, this was replaced by an 'imaginary shock'. It was hypothesized that this stimulus would inhibit the micturition reflex. After intense training with video films and role-play, the aversive stimulus was replaced by the imaginary stimulus. In approximately eight sessions, the incontinence frequency could be reduced by 90 per cent, even on a long-term basis.

According to anecdotal reports, some cases of giggle incontinence resolve within a few months with supportive treatment and anticholinergic medication only (Brocklebank and Meadow 1981), but these cases may not represent giggle incontinence in a strict sense, but misdiagnosed 'overactive bladder' (Chandra et al 2002). Most children will require a more intensive and specific treatment. Antidepressant medication used in narcolepsy has not been described in the treatment of children with giggle incontinence.

I.L., 13-year-old girl
Diagnosis: Giggle incontinence

I. had had no bladder complaints until the age of 9 when she started wetting with increasing frequency. Her family history was negative for incontinence and her medical history was normal. She had tried intense bladder training with voiding schedules and urotherapeutic advice several times, and she had had several antibiotic treatments for suspected UTI, since there had sometimes been bacteria in her urine, but this had not helped. She had also received anticholinergic treatment with tolterodine 2 mg bid, with only marginal benefit.

She had many friends and was a very good football player but her incontinence had had an increasingly negative impact on her social activities. Her previous doctor had told her that the problem would disappear by puberty, but she had passed menarche at the age of 12 and she was still wetting at least three to four times per week.

The incontinence appeared only when she laughed. Exercise, increased abdominal pressure or emotional distraction *per se* never caused incontinence. And when she wetted, it was not just a damp spot on her underwear but her trousers were soaking wet. To try to cope with this situation she had adopted the habit of tying a sweater around her waist so that her trousers were hidden if she had to laugh.

After verifying the history with a frequency-volume chart, methylphenidate treatment was started under the supervision of a child psychiatrist. With a dosage of 10 mg bid she is now wetting only once or twice per month, which is a great relief. She has medication-free intervals when the social situation permits, e.g. during the school holidays, but the main problem now is that nobody can tell her how long she will need to take this drug to stay dry.

SUMMARY AND CLINICAL GUIDELINES

In addition to the general provision of information and regulation of voiding and drinking habits, the main lines of treatment are either pharmacological or cognitive-behavioural. Due to the coexistence of cataplexy, stimulant medication is recommended. The doses required are higher than in the treatment of ADHD. Charts documenting the effects should be filled out.

The other mode of treatment is cognitive-behavioural, with a classical conditioning paradigm substituting an aversive stimulus by an imaginary stimulus in situations in which giggling and incontinence might occur. This type of treatment should be carried out only by therapists or physicians with training in CBT.

Underactive bladder

DEFINITION

Bladder underactivity replaces the older term 'lazy bladder' (or detrusor decompensation) as the paediatric term indicating non-neurogenic underactive or acontractile detrusor. Much semantic and pathogenetic confusion is attached to this condition. We are talking here about children without (known) neurological malfunction who, on urodynamic testing, are found to have large, hypocontractile bladders, and need to use raised intra-abdominal pressure to void.

The condition is distinguished from voiding postponement by the bladder's inability to empty without the help of abdominal pressure. Voiding postponement and detrusor underactivity may be said to represent two extreme points on a scale, although this does not imply that the one necessarily, if left untreated, leads to the other.

Detrusor underactivity is a term that can be applied when cystometry has revealed that the detrusor is hypocontractive, which is often the case in children with underactive bladders.

Epidemiology

Not much is known about the prevalence and incidence of bladder underactivity, due to changing and confusing terminology. The condition is more common among girls than among boys, and can be postulated to be less common than the syndrome of voiding postponement. Diagnosis is usually made by the age of 8 to 10 years.

Aetiology

Detrusor underactivity is often the result of long-standing voiding postponement, which in its turn can be suspected to have mainly behavioural or psychogenic causes. It may also have myogenic causes, and utrastructural cellular changes have been found in the detrusor of adults with detrusor underactivity (Brierly et al 2003).

Dysfunctional voiding may coexist with detrusor underactivity, as may, paradoxically, detrusor overactivity – that is, there may be involuntary detrusor contractions, but the detrusor is unable to build up and sustain enough pressure to attain normal bladder emptying. Sometimes a clinical progression may be seen, with urge incontinence starting in the preschool years, then evolving in the early school years into dysfunctional voiding and voiding postponement due to attempts to counteract the detrusor overactivity, and then progressing after a few more years into the 'end stage' of bladder underactivity.

Clinical Signs and Symptoms

The syndrome of bladder underactivity presents with incontinence, UTI, or a palpably distended bladder, which may be detected incidentally when the child is undergoing a physical examination for other reasons. The majority of UTIs in these children are lower urinary tract infections, since the condition is not usually associated with pathology of the upper urinary tract. Since residual urine is always present the risk for UTI is high.

The type of incontinence varies according to the child's micturition habits and the presence or absence of detrusor overactivity. Overflow incontinence or 'pseudo-stress incontinence' may occur due to bladder overfilling. The incontinent episodes may then coincide with giggling, straining or physical activity, and the volumes lost are typically not large. If detrusor overactivity is present, then varying degrees of urgency and/or urge incontinence are also present. And some children with underactive bladders may be continent.

Psychological Aspects

In the original article, the 'lazy bladder syndrome' was described as an acquired behaviour which has 'developed from the habitual neglect of the patient to empty the bladder on getting the urge to micturate' (de Luca et al 1962). Systematic studies on comorbid behavioural problems have not been performed, although from clinical impressions the rate of associated problems is high.

ASSESSMENT

The history taking should focus on micturition problems, UTIs and behavioural disturbances. A detailed history can in many, but certainly not all, cases reveal the disease progression delineated above, with previous urge incontinence and a more recent tendency towards postponement of micturitions, often coinciding with the advent of recurrent UTIs and amelioration of incontinence. As in children with voiding postponement, behavioural deviations are common and may be detected by careful questioning.

A distended bladder may be palpable on physical examination and is very suggestive of the syndrome. If, however, incontinence can be elicited by compression of the distended bladder then neurogenic bladder disturbance should be suspected.

In children with bladder underactivity the micturition chart again provides invaluable information. These children void spontaneously only once or twice a day, although they may sometimes experience incontinence more often than that. When incontinent, the children are more often damp than soaking wet. Urgency symptoms may or may not be present.

Uroflowmetry should also be performed. Typical cases will show an interrupted (fractioned) curve with low maximum urine flow, prolonged voiding time and large voided volumes. If myography is included, the presence of concomitant dysfunctional voiding may also be detected. Residual urine is almost invariably present. Ultrasound, which is strongly recommended in these children, will show no upper tract dilatation; if it does, then neurogenic bladder or urethral valves (in boys) should be suspected. The bladder wall may be of increased thickness but it should not be sacculated as is the neurogenic bladder. It is recommended that an MCU is seriously considered in all boys who on clinical history and uroflow appear to be suffering from detrusor underactivity, since it may instead be a case of posterior urethral valves (see Chapter 8).

Cystometry is indicated in the children in whom neurogenic bladder disturbance cannot be excluded, or in severely therapy-resistant cases (and in them too the main point of cystometry is to exclude neurogenic bladder disturbance).

TREATMENT

If the distended bladder is only discovered incidentally in a child with neither incontinence nor UTIs then specific treatment may not be absolutely necessary. These children should, however, be strongly advised to go to the toilet more often, since they run a high risk of getting UTIs, and they should be followed up – preferably by a urotherapist.

Otherwise, urotherapy – with the help of a skilled urotherapist – is the treatment of choice. The goal is for the child to learn to void more often and, importantly, to empty the bladder completely. This usually means that the child is instructed in double-micturition – that is, voiding two or three times in immediate succession at each toilet visit. The results are monitored with regular voiding charts.

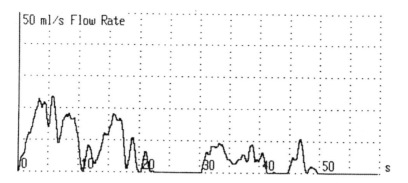

Fig. 7.17 Interrupted uroflow curve of a child with underactive bladder (residual urine 98 ml, voided volume 320 ml).

Anticholinergic medications are obviously not indicated in these children, unless they have successfully eliminated their residual urine and still have urge incontinence. Long-term antibiotic prophylaxis may, on the other hand, be indicated if UTIs occur and the residual urine has not (yet) disappeared. But, as always, the antibiotic should not be an isolated intervention but an interim measure while awaiting the effects of bladder training.

If residual urine proves impossible to eliminate, bladder drainage by CIC may have to be resorted to, especially if there are UTIs in spite of antibiotic prophylaxis. Surgical drainage, as in the neurogenic or valve bladder, is not indicated in these children, since the condition is expected to remit spontaneously.

COURSE AND PROGNOSIS

Despite the sometimes very troublesome nature of the condition the long-term prognosis is not known, as follow-up studies are lacking. In some patients, the course can be favourable; in others, chronic persistence of incontinence and recurrent UTIs have been observed. The prognosis is dependent on compliance with therapeutic measures such as CIC.

SUMMARY AND CLINICAL GUIDELINES

Bladder underactivity is the term used in children who seldom void and need to apply abdominal pressure in order to do so. The condition is commonly accompanied by incontinence, residual urine and/or urinary tract infections.

These children need to be evaluated with a voiding chart and with repeated uroflow measurements and assessment of residual urine. Ultrasound of the kidneys and urinary tracts should be performed.

Urotherapy is the treatment of choice. The children need to learn to go to the toilet regularly (approximately six times per day), to adopt a good voiding posture and to empty their bladders completely. Constipation, if present, should be treated, and some children may need antibiotic prophylaxis until residual urine has disappeared.

178

In severely therapy-resistant children who suffer from repeated urinary tract infections and cannot eliminate their residual urine, clean intermittent catheterization may be needed.

Other forms of functional urinary incontinence

VAGINAL REFLUX

Incontinence secondary to vaginal reflux is not uncommon in prepubertal girls, perhaps accounting for as much as 12 per cent of the daytime incontinence seen in this patient group (Mattsson et al 2003). During normal micturition some urine gets trapped between the labiae and leaks up into the vagina. Subsequently, when the girl rises and leaves the toilet, the refluxing urine leaks into the underwear.

This condition is very easy to distinguish by history alone, since the incontinence episodes exclusively occur within five to ten minutes of normal micturition. The urine volumes are not large, but may be enough to cause wetting of more than just the underwear. Treatment of vaginal reflux is usually straightforward. The child is instructed to adopt a good, relaxed voiding posture, with foot support and the bottom low on the toilet seat, and after each micturition to apply manual pressure, with a piece of toilet paper, to the perineum until the reflux urine is voided. Anatomical changes at puberty will eventually cause the problem to cease.

EXTRAORDINARY DAYTIME URINARY FREQUENCY

A subtype of overactive bladder with daytime urinary frequency (without incontinence) was described by Koff and Byard (1988). It is considered to be a benign, self-limiting condition lasting an average of 2.5 months. The aetiology is unknown, 'but it may be predominantly behavioural' (Koff and Byard 1988: 1280). In the authors' experience it is not uncommon and seems to be more common among boys.

Typical signs are that, during toddler or preschool years, children suddenly have to void very often for no obvious reason. They may need to go to the toilet every 15 minutes or even more frequently, but the disturbance is characteristically limited to the waking hours; enuresis or frequent nocturia are *not* an essential part of the condition. Daytime

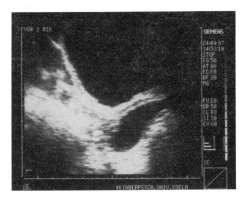

Fig. 7.18 Vaginal reflux: J.T., a 12-year-old girl with dysfunctional voiding, developed vaginal reflux. An ectopic ureter was excluded. The reflux ceased under urotherapy.

incontinence may be present but is of minor magnitude compared to the extreme urinary frequency. Urine production is not increased, so voided volumes are very small.

The important thing to remember in the evaluation of these children is to take a urine sample in order to exclude UTI and diabetes (glycosuria). If the history is typical, no other investigation (besides physical examination) is needed. A standard voiding chart would be scribbled full of ridiculously small urine volumes, and reliable uroflow measurements would be impossible to obtain due to the small voided volumes.

Treatment is notoriously unsatisfactory, although detrusor relaxant drugs such as oxybutynin have been tried. Prognosis, though, is excellent. The parents should be informed that the condition will remit spontaneously within a few months.

UROFACIAL SYNDROME

The urofacial syndrome, or Ochoa syndrome, is a peculiar disturbance of bladder function and of facial expression that is inherited recessively on chromosome 10q23–q24 (Ochoa and Gorlin 1987, Ochoa 2004). Approximately 100 cases world-wide have been reported to date, but the syndrome is probably more common than that. These patients were originally described as suffering from enuresis, but they can have any kind of bladder and bowel disturbance and are characterized by an inability to smile in a normal way. When trying to smile they displace the angles of the mouth laterally to produce a melancholy, bitter or even sad appearance (Ochoa 2004). Although this syndrome is providing interesting insights into the genetics of bladder function, there is, as yet, no reason to believe that the bladder/bowel problems of these people should be treated differently from others.

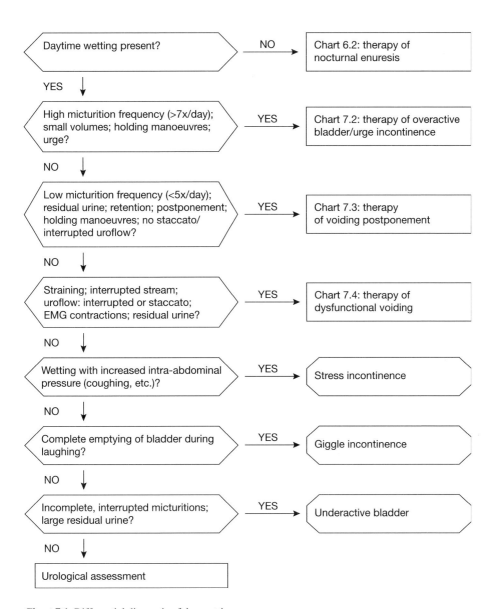

Chart 7.1 Differential diagnosis of day wetting

181

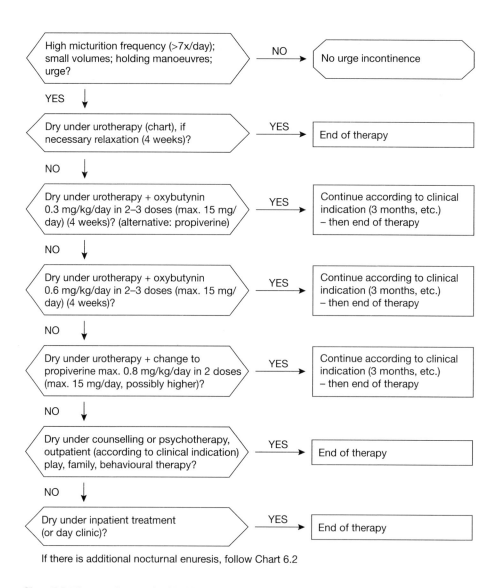

High micturition frequency (>7x/day); small volumes; holding manoeuvres; urge?	**NO** →	No urge incontinence

YES ↓

Dry under urotherapy (chart), if necessary relaxation (4 weeks)?	**YES** →	End of therapy

NO ↓

Dry under urotherapy + oxybutynin 0.3 mg/kg/day in 2–3 doses (max. 15 mg/day) (4 weeks)? (alternative: propiverine)	**YES** →	Continue according to clinical indication (3 months, etc.) – then end of therapy

NO ↓

Dry under urotherapy + oxybutynin 0.6 mg/kg/day in 2–3 doses (max. 15 mg/day) (4 weeks)?	**YES** →	Continue according to clinical indication (3 months, etc.) – then end of therapy

NO ↓

Dry under urotherapy + change to propiverine max. 0.8 mg/kg/day in 2 doses (max. 15 mg/day, possibly higher)?	**YES** →	Continue according to clinical indication (3 months, etc.) – then end of therapy

NO ↓

Dry under counselling or psychotherapy, outpatient (according to clinical indication) play, family, behavioural therapy?	**YES** →	End of therapy

NO ↓

Dry under inpatient treatment (or day clinic)?	**YES** →	End of therapy

If there is additional nocturnal enuresis, follow Chart 6.2

Chart 7.2 Therapy of overactive bladder/urge incontinence

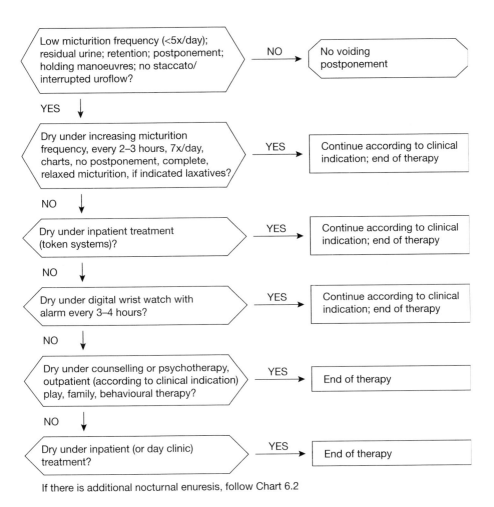

Low micturition frequency (<5x/day); residual urine; retention; postponement; holding manoeuvres; no staccato/ interrupted uroflow? — NO → No voiding postponement

YES ↓

Dry under increasing micturition frequency, every 2–3 hours, 7x/day, charts, no postponement, complete, relaxed micturition, if indicated laxatives? — YES → Continue according to clinical indication; end of therapy

NO ↓

Dry under inpatient treatment (token systems)? — YES → Continue according to clinical indication; end of therapy

NO ↓

Dry under digital wrist watch with alarm every 3–4 hours? — YES → Continue according to clinical indication; end of therapy

NO ↓

Dry under counselling or psychotherapy, outpatient (according to clinical indication) play, family, behavioural therapy? — YES → End of therapy

NO ↓

Dry under inpatient (or day clinic) treatment? — YES → End of therapy

If there is additional nocturnal enuresis, follow Chart 6.2

Chart 7.3 Therapy of voiding postponement

183

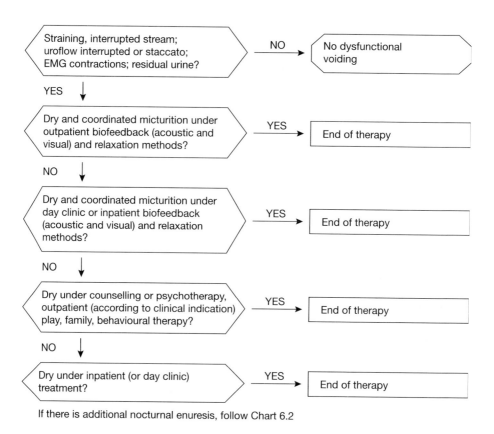

Straining, interrupted stream; uroflow interrupted or staccato; EMG contractions; residual urine? — NO → No dysfunctional voiding

YES ↓

Dry and coordinated micturition under outpatient biofeedback (acoustic and visual) and relaxation methods? — YES → End of therapy

NO ↓

Dry and coordinated micturition under day clinic or inpatient biofeedback (acoustic and visual) and relaxation methods? — YES → End of therapy

NO ↓

Dry under counselling or psychotherapy, outpatient (according to clinical indication) play, family, behavioural therapy? — YES → End of therapy

NO ↓

Dry under inpatient (or day clinic) treatment? — YES → End of therapy

If there is additional nocturnal enuresis, follow Chart 6.2

Chart 7.4 Therapy of dysfunctional voiding

8
ORGANIC URINARY INCONTINENCE

Structural urinary incontinence

A child may be incontinent for anatomical reasons. Children who have undergone surgical urinary diversion and are incontinent as a result are obvious such cases, but since these children constitute no differential diagnostic dilemma and are dealt with extensively in urological textbooks they will not be discussed here. The same can be said about children with bladder extrophy, cloacal malformations and other complex urogenital malformations which are evident from the start. We will therefore focus here on the few conditions that may go undetected throughout early childhood and present with incontinence/enuresis or UTI.

Urogenital sinus anomalies can be considered incomplete versions of the cloacal malformations mentioned above. Ureteric ectopy and ureterocoele belong to the spectrum of *duplication anomalies* of the upper urinary tract (Whitten and Wilcox 2001), which in one way or another affect approximately 1 per cent of the population and are inherited as an autosomal dominant trait with incomplete penetrance. The most common manifestation of duplication is when one or both kidneys are drained by two ureters that unite before entering the bladder. This anomaly is of no clinical consequence, except in cases with very low confluence of the ureters, where vesico-ureteric reflux (VUR) may be common. The risk for clinically relevant conditions such as VUR, ureterocoele, upper polar renal dysplasia or ectopy of the ureteric orifice only occurs when the duplication is complete, and it is then usually the ureter draining the upper renal pole that is malformed. Ectopic ureter and, to a lesser degree, ureterocoele, are the duplication anomalies that are relevant for this book.

The posterior urethral valve is a serious congenital malformation only affecting boys. As it may go undetected – in mild cases – until later childhood or adolescence, and poses difficult differential diagnostic problems, it will be dealt with in some detail below. Other anatomical causes of bladder outlet obstruction may also lead to incontinence and are therefore mentioned briefly.

UROGENITAL SINUS ANOMALIES

Failure of closure of the embryological urogenital sinus in girls may result in a urovaginal confluence. This means that the bladder drains into a common vaginal-urethral canal which is wide and lacks a functional sphincter. Incontinence is continuous and the appearance of the orifice is highly anomalous.

ECTOPIC URETER

In ureteric ectopy the ureteric orifice is congenitally displaced distally. If the ureter drains functional renal tissue and the orifice is located below the sphincter, a condition almost exclusively seen in girls, incontinence will ensue. As mentioned above, ureteric ectopy usually belongs to the spectrum of duplication anomalies, i.e. the malformed ureter is one of two draining the same kidney, but a minority of displaced ureters are single. In both cases the kidney or part of the kidney drained by the anomalous ureter is often dysplastic. The infrasphincteric ureteric orifice may be located in the vagina or the introitus.

Infrasphincteric ureteric ectopia typically presents with primary incontinence of a constant, dribbling type superimposed on a normal micturition pattern. The constant nature of the incontinence distinguishes it from, for instance, urge incontinence or voiding post-ponement, whereas the otherwise normal micturition habits serve to differentiate it from neurogenic bladder dysfunction. The picture may, however, be blurred by the following factors: (1) some girls with intravaginal ectopia may be able to remain dry for short periods of time, and some even manage to stay dry overnight; (2) the renal tissue drained by the ectopic ureter may be so dysplastic as not to produce more than minimal amounts of urine, in which case vaginal discharge may be the only symptom; and (3) excessive parental efforts in trying to make their child dry may provoke abnormal voiding patterns with urgency, frequency and so on. Needless to say, correct history taking is crucial here, if complications such as renal scarring are to be prevented.

Physical examination is often unremarkable, but in some cases the urinary leakage may actually be observed in the introitus.

All children with suspected ureteric ectopia should be examined with urography (one of the few remaining indications for this examination in children not suspected of having stones) and ultrasound. Further investigations include DMSA scintigraphy to assess differential renal function and MCU to detect VUR.

The *methylene blue test* is an ingenious investigation that may be undertaken in cases where ureteric ectopia is suspected but urography has turned out negative or inconclusive. A pad is placed upon the vulva after the intravesical instillation of methylene blue. If subsequent urine leakage makes the pad blue, then infrasphincteric ectopia is *not* the problem, and vice versa.

Incontinence due to ureteric ectopia is one of the few forms of incontinence that can be reliably eradicated by surgery. The ectopic ureter is ligated and reimplanted into the bladder if it drains enough functional renal tissue to be worth saving; otherwise heminephrectomy or nephrectomy is curative. The latter options are usually chosen.

URETEROCOELE

In ureteric duplication the ureter draining the upper kidney pole may be dilated and saccular upon entering the bladder. This condition affects approximately 0.02 per cent of the population, and 80 per cent of those affected are girls. The dilated portion of the anomalous ureter – the ureterocoele – may either lie entirely intravesically (orthotopic ureterocoele) or extend beyond the bladder neck (ectopic ureterocoele). VUR, obstruction of one or several ureters or disturbance of bladder function with the accumulation of residual urine may ensue

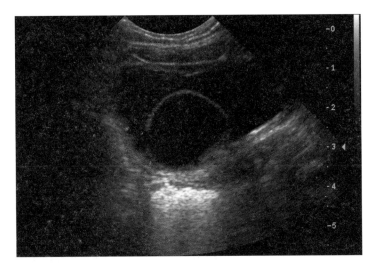

Fig. 8.1 Ureterocoele, as viewed by ultrasound.

(Abrahamsson et al 1998). Ureterocoeles are usually detected either by prenatal ultrasound or after UTI during infancy, but they may in rare cases present with UTI or chronic urinary retention in later childhood. Detection is by ultrasound and treatment is surgical.

Ureterocoeles that are *not* associated with ureteric duplication are more common in boys. In these cases the presenting symptom – if any – is usually UTI, and associated anomalies are rare. The condition may also be an incidental finding. Surgery is only indicated if the coele causes unequivocal UTIs, or in the rare cases where it leads to upper urinary tract obstruction.

Posterior Urethral Valves

The congenital posterior urethral valve (PUV) is the most common serious malformation of the urinary tract. It affects only boys, in whom the incidence is around 1 in 4000–8000. PUV is usually not associated with malformations of other organ systems, and the majority of cases are sporadic. The defect develops around the seventh week of gestation and will, if sufficiently severe, result in structural and functional changes in the bladder, the upper urinary tract and kidneys. These secondary changes include:

1 Increased bladder wall thickness and collagen component
2 Increased detrusor contractility (Holmdahl et al 1995)
3 Hydronephrosis
4 VUR (often grade V) (Holmdahl 1997)
5 Renal dysplasia with consequent polyuric kidney failure

Severity may vary between the extremes of neonatal death or early terminal uremia on the one hand, and UTIs or enuresis in the adolescent on the other. The relevance of PUV for

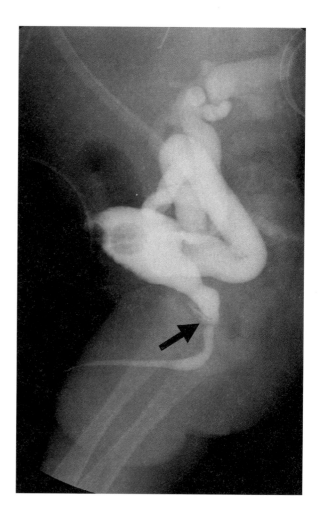

Fig. 8.2 Posterior urethral valve
(arrow), with dilatation of the
upper urinary tract.

this textbook is that it may in rare cases present with enuresis and/or daytime incontinence in childhood or adolescence.

It is important to remember that although the primary defect in PUV is the more or less complete membrane in the proximal urethra, much of the morbidity is due to the bladder disturbance and the mainly tubular kidney damage caused by this malformation.

Although the bladder of the foetus with PUV may be large postnatally, it is usually small and overactive in early childhood (Holmdahl et al 1995). Detrusor overactivity is thus common in these boys, even after surgical correction of the valve. As the child grows, the bladder volume usually increases and contractility decreases, with the accumulation of residual urine and risk for UTI. Interestingly, it has been shown that the bladder in children with urethral valves is usually only overactive during the daytime (Holmdahl 1997).

Kidney damage is caused by high intravesical pressure which is transmitted to the kidneys via VUR or hydronephrosis. The damage is mainly tubular, which results in decreased renal concentration capacity and polyuria; it can correctly be described as partial nephrogenic diabetes insipidus with concomitant reduction of filtration. Thus, a vicious circle is likely to develop: increased urine flow leads to high intravesical pressure, which in turn leads to tubular kidney damage, which leads to increased urine flow, and so on. This situation may worsen as the child gains nocturnal continence and has to accommodate ever larger amounts of urine in the bladder.

In the older child with previously undetected PUV, presenting symptoms may be related to either the bladder or the kidneys. Bladder-related symptoms are UTIs (cystitis or pyelonephritis) or incontinence, whereas kidney-related symptoms are enuresis, polyuria/ polydipsia or growth failure, nausea and other symptoms related to renal failure.

UTIs in boys with urethral valves, after infancy, present as other UTIs and are usually accompanied by residual urine. This is the reason why uroflowmetry with residual urine measurement should be performed during the follow-up of the first UTI in all boys after the first few years of life. Daytime incontinence may be due to detrusor overactivity, or it may be of the overflow type. It can be either primary or secondary. Enuresis in boys with PUV is usually of the polyuric type, but responds poorly to desmopressin treatment.

The case history may reveal that the boy is thirsty and needs to drink at night, that the urine stream is weak and/or that growth has been poor. It may also reveal that desmopressin treatment of enuresis has not been of any help. Physical examination is usually unremarkable.

When there is the slightest suspicion of PUV, two examinations should be performed without undue delay: uroflowmetry (with residual urine measurement) and ultrasound. The typical uroflow pattern in these patients is the plateau-shaped curve (see Fig. 8.3) or, in cases of long-standing polyuria and bladder enlargement, the interrupted curve. Residual urine is almost invariably present. The ability to void with a normal maximum flow speaks strongly against PUV. Ultrasound typically reveals an enlarged upper urinary tract and a thick bladder wall, but may in some cases appear normal. If, after these investigations, PUV has not been ruled out, an MCU with lateral views is mandatory.

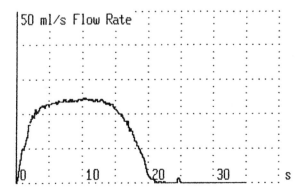

Fig. 8.3 Plateau uroflow curve due to outlet obstruction (residual urine 50 ml, voided volume 389 ml).

189

Urethral valves are ablated surgically, usually via the endoscopic route, but it should be remembered that this procedure only removes the valve and does little to improve the function of the bladder, ureter and kidney.

The incontinence in boys with urethral valves often responds favourably to anti-cholinergic medications such as oxybutynin. This may often not be a feasible strategy, however – at least not as monotherapy – since it entails a high risk of increasing residual urine. Urotherapy is therefore the first-line treatment. In many cases, however, residual urine cannot be eliminated, which means that drainage must be provided either by CIC – which is often difficult to perform in these children with intact urethral sensibility – or by the creation of a continent catheterizable channel such as a Mitrofanoff conduit. Long-term antibiotic prophylaxis may be needed to protect the kidneys from pyelonephritic damage while the residual urine is dealt with.

Hydronephrosis and/or VUR in PUV will often have to be corrected surgically in cases where pyelonephritic episodes occur or there is a suspicion of upper tract obstruction due to increased bladder wall thickness.

Treatment of renal failure due to urethral valves does not differ much from that due to other causes. It is of paramount importance for the preservation of kidney function that the bladder is properly drained so that it cannot generate high intravesical pressures or permit the occurrence of febrile UTIs.

Even though PUV is no longer a disorder with a significant mortality, long-term prognosis cannot be regarded as favourable (Lal et al 1999). The bladder disturbance tends, if anything, to worsen as the child grows, and the vicious circle of polyuria and high intravesical pressure mentioned above often leads to successively diminished kidney function.

STRUCTURAL BLADDER OUTLET OBSTRUCTION FOR OTHER CAUSES

In boys, strictures after hypospadias surgery, meatal stenosis and – in very rare cases – pathological phimosis, may cause bladder outlet obstruction which may lead to overflow incontinence. Girls are much less commonly affected: the usual cause here is haemato- or hydrocolpos due to imperforate hymen.

The incontinence of these children is usually due to obstructive detrusor overactivity. This means that incontinent episodes are usually associated with the sensation of urgency. If imperforate hymen is the underlying cause, then the incontinence starts at puberty and is accompanied by primary amenorrhoea.

Uroflowmetry, with measurement of residual urine, is the investigation of choice in these cases. Many patients do not describe their urinary stream as weak (they have nothing to compare it with), but this will be revealed by uroflowmetry, and residual urine is almost uniformly present. Ultrasound will often disclose a thick bladder wall, but the upper urinary tract is usually not dilated. Haemato- or hydrocolpos is always visible by ultrasound (if one knows what to look for). Cystoscopy is usually the next step, and treatment is surgical. As with PUV there is unfortunately a tendency for the bladder disturbance to persist, occasionally for an extended period of time (several years) after correction of the underlying cause. Treatment with anticholinergics and/or urotherapy is often helpful, however, and the overall long-term outcome is usually favourable.

EPISPADIAS

In children with epispadias the urethra is displaced anteriorly. In males this defect can be of variable extent, with the urethral orifice placed anywhere between the glans and the proximal penile shaft. Girls with epispadias always have a complete defect, which means that the orifice is located anterior to a bifid clitoris. In both sexes the defect is associated with a deficient urethral sphincter, and the consequent presentation is primary incontinence of the dribbling type. For obvious reasons, diagnostic problems only arise in girls, whose parents may not notice that the genitalia of their daughter look strange. But the defect should be clear to the doctor.

Neurogenic urinary incontinence

Urinary incontinence may be the presenting or predominant symptom of neuropathic bladder, i.e. bladder disturbance due to damage to the CNS or the innervation of the lower urinary tract. This poses no differential diagnostic problem in the case of myelomeningocele (MMC), the most common cause of neurogenic urinary incontinence in childhood, but there are other kinds of spinal dysraphism or damage to the lower spinal medulla that are not as obvious from the outside. Disease processes of supraspinal parts of the central nervous system may also cause neurogenic bladder disturbances. A list of causes of neuropathic bladder in childhood is provided in Table 8.1.

CONGENITAL CAUSES

Spinal dysraphism is a collective term denoting the partial failure of closure of the neural crest during early foetal life. In MMC this failure has resulted in neural tissue lying more or less exposed on the outside of the developing foetus. When this is not the case we talk about *spina bifida occulta*, a term that encompasses everything from the absence of a few vertebral arches in the lumbosacral area – a probably harmless abnormality, found incidentally on X-ray (Alhano et al 1996, Silveri et al 1997, Samuel and Boddy 2004) – to intraspinal cysts and lipomas that may cause bladder disturbances of a severity sometimes equalling that of overt MMC.

TABLE 8.1
Underlying causes of neuropathic bladder in children

Congenital	Acquired
Spinal dysraphism	Traumatic spinal injury
Myelomeningocele (MMC)	Spinal artery thrombosis
Spina bifida occulta	Prematurity/umbilical catheters
Diastematomyelia	Tumours
Lumbosacral lipoma	Neuroblastoma
Intraspinal cysts	Others
Tethered cord	Inflammatory
Sacral agenesis	Transverse myelitis
	Vertebral osteomyelitis
	Spinal abscess
	Multiple sclerosis
	Cerebrovascular insults

The tethered cord syndrome is a somewhat special case: the distal part of the spinal medulla is tethered to the inside of the spinal canal and gradually stretched as the child grows. This is a very common complication after lower spinal neurosurgery (such as the closure of the neural defect in MMC), but can also be a mainly congenital abnormality in itself, due to a thickened filum terminale.

Sacral agenesis, the congenital absence of the lowermost sacral segments, can either be part of complex anorectal malformations or occur in isolation; in the latter case it is often associated with maternal diabetes mellitus. The spinal malformation in sacral agenesis is incomplete, and peripheral neurological deficits are not proportional to the degree of bladder disturbance.

Neurogenic bladder dysfunction is also common in children with congenital anorectal malformations (Kakizaki et al 1994, Taskinen et al 2002), and may not become evident until after surgical correction of these. This association has often been overlooked, even though up to 20 per cent of these patients may suffer from urinary incontinence.

ACQUIRED CAUSES

The acquired causes of neurogenic bladder in childhood are much less common than the congenital causes. Spinal tumours may cause damage to the sacral medulla, as may localized infectious or inflammatory processes. In transverse myelitis, neurogenic bladder disturbance may be the one remaining sequela after other neurological deficits have abated. The rare cases of spinal artery thrombosis usually occur in very ill neonates or in association with advanced surgery.

As in adults, traumatic spinal injury in children predictably leads to disturbances of bladder function. The usual development in these cases is bladder areflexia, requiring drainage, during the initial phase of spinal shock, followed after six to eight weeks by detrusor hyperreflexia with or without detrusor sphincter dyssynergia.

URODYNAMIC FEATURES

The disturbance of the bladder-sphincter function in the neuropathic bladder is dependent on the level and the degree of damage to the spinal cord. Most of our knowledge and our classification of these bladder disturbances derives from studies on children with MMC, but it is applicable to children with spina bifida occulta as well. It has proven useful to differentiate between the contractile bladder, the acontractile bladder and intermediate bladder dysfunction (see Table 8.2).

The *contractile bladder* is seen when the motor neurons of the conus medullaris and the pathways between them and the bladder/sphincter are intact, but their proximal connections are severed. The spinal micturition reflex arch is therefore still functional but it is no longer subject to the tonically inhibiting influence from the pontine micturition centre, and marked detrusor overactivity is the consequence. The coordination between detrusor and sphincter contraction is also lost, so voidings – which only occur via involuntary, uninhibited detrusor contractions – are accompanied by detrusor–sphincter dyssynergia. We talk about dynamic sphincter obstruction when describing the outflow obstruction caused by sphincteric contractions that is present in these children. The voiding

192

TABLE 8.2
Characteristics of different types of neuropathic bladder

Type	Injury distribution	Detrusor function	Sphincter function	Voiding	Clinical characteristics
Contractile bladder	Suprasacral damage, conus medullaris intact	Overactivity Compliant	Detrusor–sphincter dyssynergia Dynamic sphincter obstruction	Only via detrusor hyperreflexia	Bladder volume small or normal Incontinence in discrete amounts Residual urine and UTI common
Acontractile bladder	Sacral damage, conus medullaris destroyed	Acontractile Non-compliance common	Varying degrees of sphincteric incompetence and/or static sphincteric obstruction	Either overflow or via increased abdominal pressure	Bladder and residual volumes determined by the degree of sphincteric obstruction Overflow incontinence common
Intermediate bladder dysfunction	Intermediate	Overactivity, but often low pressure Non-compliance common	Varying degrees of sphincteric incompetence Possible static sphincteric obstruction	Intermediate	Intermediate

is urodynamically similar to that seen in children with non-neurogenic voiding dysfunction. The bulbocavernous reflex is positive in these children and the radiographic appearance of the bladder may be normal. Approximately 25 per cent of children with MMC have this type of bladder disturbance.

The *acontractile bladder* is seen in the child whose conus medullaris is destroyed. This means that the innervation of the detrusor and the external sphincter – but not the sympathetically supplied internal sphincter – is lost. The result is that the detrusor cannot contract and the spincter shows varying degrees of incompetence. Voiding is accomplished either by simple overflow incontinence, when the often non-compliant bladder is stretched to its limits, or by increased abdominal pressure. Outflow obstruction, if present, is static (in contrast to the dynamic sphincter obstruction of the contractile bladder described above), and the degree of obstruction will determine bladder and residual volume. We can discern two extremes between which these two types of bladder fall:

1 Bladder volume is small and residual urine absent. Urine is more or less constantly leaking.
2 Bladder volume is large, with large amounts of residual urine. Incontinence is associated predominantly with straining or coughing or the child may even be continent.

These children have an absent bulbocavernous reflex, and the bladder often has a sacculated appearance on X-ray. The acontractile bladder afflicts about 15 per cent of children with MMC.

As in any classification of nature, there is always an intermediate and more vaguely defined category between the clear-cut cases. This is classified as *intermediate bladder dysfunction*. In this disturbance there is a combination of overactivity of the detrusor – usually not generating very high intravesical pressures – and varying degrees of sphincteric incompetence. Non-compliance of the detrusor is common, and obstruction, when present, tends to be more static than dynamic. This is the most common type of neurogenic bladder disturbance seen in children with MMC.

PRESENTATION, PRIMARY EVALUATION

As should be clear from the explanation above, neuropathic bladder leads to varying degrees of urinary incontinence. The following signs should raise suspicion of neurogenic bladder disturbance in an incontinent child:

1   Clues from history and voiding chart data: continuously dribbling incontinence made worse by straining or coughing. The need to strain in order to urinate. Interrupted or weak urinary stream. Slow motor development, especially as regards walking. Habitual toe-walking.
2   Physical signs: dimples or hairy area on the lower back, scoliosis, gluteal assymetry, flattening of the upper buttocks, leg length differences, reflex assymetria in the lower limbs, foot malformations, positive Babinski's sign, decreased leg muscle strength, decreased perineal sensibility. Observable incontinence elicited by bladder compression (almost pathognomonic).
3   Flowmetry data: any pathological flow curve that is consistently present on repeated examinations (with the possible exception of the tower-shaped curve without residual urine) and does not disappear with basic urotherapy. The most pathological in this respect is the interrupted curve with large residual urine volume.

Note that incontinence *per se*, unaccompanied by the signs listed above, is not an indication for cystometric evaluation, even if it proves to be resistant to standard therapy.

If there are grounds for suspecting neurogenic bladder disturbance, two examinations are unavoidable: ultrasound and cystometry.

Ultrasound is performed first in order to exclude upper tract dilatation or gross kidney damage. It also gives information regarding bladder wall thickness, residual urine and the presence of bladder diverticula.

Cystometry is the mainstay of diagnosis and classification of neurogenic bladder disturbance. Video-cystometry – if available – is superior to conventional cystometry, since the bladder can be visualized and VUR confirmed or excluded. If ordinary cystometry is used, an MCU is also required to obtain this information.

In any child with cystometrically confirmed neuropathic bladder MRI of the spine is mandatory. Plain X-ray is of little use here, since the anatomy of the soft intraspinal tissues needs to be assessed in detail. An MCU also needs to be performed (unless video-cystometry is available – see above), since children with neurogenic bladder disturbance often have VUR.

Both the type and severity of bladder disturbance in spinal dysraphism change, usually for the worse, during growth, and the condition therefore needs to be monitored by repeated ultrasound and cystometry. Extra care needs to be taken when following these children through puberty, since this is a time when the neuropathic bladder often deteriorates. Boys fare slightly worse than girls in this respect, possibly because of prostate growth.

The main goal of treatment is to preserve kidney function; achievement of continence is a secondary goal. It should always be remembered that the kidneys are the first priority. Increased urethral resistance may result in continence at the same time as it destroys the kidneys via raised intravesical pressure.

Clean intermittent catheterization (CIC: see Chapter 5) is the mainstay of treatment. Through regular emptying of the bladder, residual urine is abolished, and at the same time the risk for bladder overfilling (with concomitant high intravesical pressure) is reduced. Through CIC most children with neuropathic bladder can preserve good renal function, but only 10 to 20 per cent achieve continence by this measure alone. Further treatment depends on the type of urodynamic disturbance.

Neurogenic detrusor overactivity can usually, but not always, be brought under control with anticholinergic medication. Oxybutynin is most commonly used here, in dosages usually between 2.5 and 5.0 mg orally tid. The same dose can conveniently be instilled intravesically during CIC, which reduces the risk of side effects (Holland et al 1997). Side effects (constipation, dry mouth, vertigo, psychic alterations) do occur, but there is some hope that this problem may diminish if the newer drug tolterodine proves to be effective in this patient category. If detrusor overactivity is not brought under control by anticholinergics, or if medication brings unacceptable side effects, then the bladder may have to be surgically enlarged, using various kinds of augmentation cystoplasty.

Detrusor non-compliance cannot be corrected with drugs. So if the child has a small, non-compliant bladder which causes pressure that endangers the kidneys or makes continence unachievable with CIC, then we have to resort to surgery. Again, augmentation cystoplasty of one type or another will be needed.

For the treatment of *sphincter incompetence* the situation is less than satisfactory. Although the less severe cases can sometimes be handled medically, using α-adrenergic agonists such as ephedrine, the moderate to severe cases present a dilemma to the urologist. The unresolved dilemma is reflected in the large number of surgical procedures that have been tried: periurethral collagen or silicone injections, bladder neck suspension or muscular sling techniques, bladder neck obliteration or the implantation of an artificial sphincter. We will not delve further into the subject here.

Although many children with neurogenic bladder disturbance have bacteriuria, this does not in itself – in the absence of VUR – entail an increased risk for kidney scarring, and should *not* routinely be treated with antibiotics (Ottolini et al 1995).

Urinary tract infection

The presence of virulent bacteria in the bladder irritates the urothelium via unmyelinated C-fibre afferents, which may lead to uninhibited detrusor contractions and consequent

195

incontinence and/or enuresis as well as dysuria, which is a more specific symptom of UTI.

The causes behind UTIs in childhood are usually *not*, as commonly believed, hygienic shortcomings (Mazzola et al 2003), but rather anatomical factors such as VUR (in small children) or bladder/bowel disturbances (in later childhood and adolescence) (Moore et al 2000).

DIFFERENTIAL DIAGNOSIS

It is clear that incontinence can be a symptom of lower urinary tract infection/cystitis. The fact that an underlying bladder disturbance such as overactive bladder or voiding postponement may lead to both incontinence and UTIs is also well established. What is also true, although less well known, is that so-called asymptomatic bacteriuria (ABU) – that is, urinary colonization with apatogenic bacteria – is common in all ages (Kunin 1970, Wettergren et al 1985), and that such colonization may be even more common in children with bladder disturbances such as overactive bladder (Hansson et al 1990). The prevalence of ABU in school children is around 0.5–2.0 per cent (Kunin 1970, Yayli et al 2003). These circumstances make differential diagnosis quite difficult. Furthermore, it is not easy to take good urine cultures in children, and therefore a positive urine culture may just be caused by contamination of the sample.

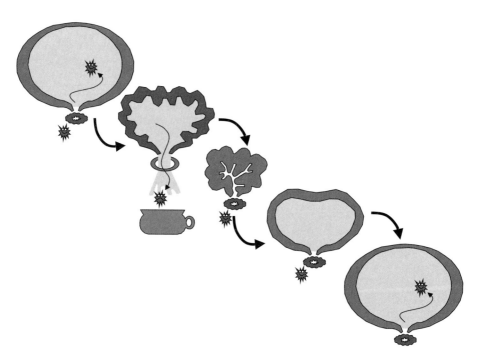

Fig. 8.4 The role of normal bladder function in UTI protection. Virulent bacteria are expelled before they have time to proliferate.

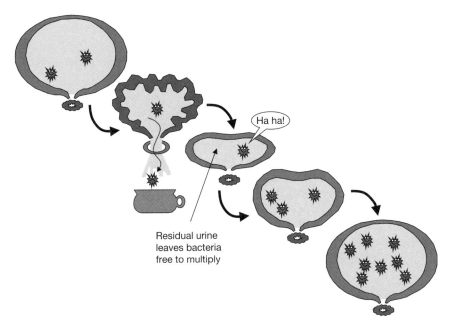

Fig. 8.5 The role of residual urine in the pathogenesis of UTI.

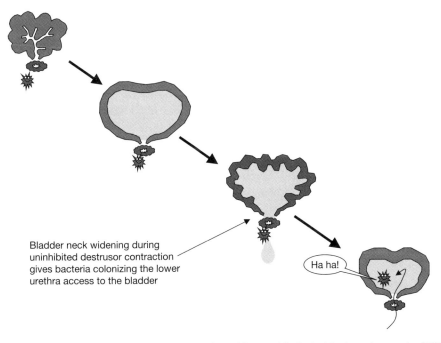

Fig. 8.6 The proposed role of detrusor overactivity (without residual urine) in the pathogenesis of UTI.

A.A., 8-year-old girl
Diagnoses: Urinary incontinence; bacteriuria

A. had had a febrile UTI at the age of 6 months. Ultrasound had been normal but a voiding cystourethrogram two months afterwards had revealed a vesico-uretheral reflux grade II on the right side. Antibiotic prophylaxis had been discontinued and a follow-up renal scintigram had detected no scarring. There had been no more febrile UTIs, general health and growth had been good, and A. was almost never ill.

A. had become reasonably daytime continent at age 3 and stopped using diapers at night one year later, but she had always had a 'troublesome bladder', with occasional urgency or episodes of slight incontinence when a toilet was not readily at hand. A.'s mother remembers that she herself also had some bladder problems during childhood. Since A. started school two years ago, the problems had accelerated, with periodic incontinence occurring approximately two to three times per week. She had been given at least eight antibiotic treatments because of bacteriuria without fever, which had only helped a little. When new urine cultures had been taken after treatment for suspected UTI there had often still been bacteria present and new antibiotics had been given. The parents were becoming increasingly frustrated and wondered if A. was becoming 'immune' to antibiotics. There were no bowel complaints.

Physical examination was normal except for slight perigenital eczema. Uroflow showed a normal curve without residual urine. The urine dipstick test was positive for bacteria and white blood cells even though she had had a 'good week' with no incontinence. The culture showed >100,000 E. coli per ml. The frequency-volume chart showed very irregular voidings with volumes between 50 and 400 ml and a low fluid intake. Bowel movements occurred most days.

The tentative conclusion was drawn that A. was suffering from a primary disturbance of bladder function combined with asymptomatic bacteriuria. The absence of prompt antibiotic effect, the abnormal voiding pattern and even the previous slight vesico-ureteric reflux and the positive heredity all supported this conclusion. Consequently, she was given proper bladder training by a urotherapist. The family physician was instructed not to take urine cultures or consider antibiotic treatment unless the girl had unexplained fever or bothersome dysuria. A weak cortisone ointment was given for the eczema. After a few weeks A. was reliably dry and after two years there has still been no need for antibiotics.

So, in the case of an incontinent child with a positive urine culture there are five possibilities:

1 *UTI with no underlying bladder disturbance*. The incontinence is caused by the bacteria alone and will quickly – within a maximum of two to three days – disappear with

antibiotic treatment, provided that the bacteria are not resistant to the drug used. The risk of recurrence is low.

2 *UTI because of an underlying bladder disturbance.* The incontinence is caused by the bacteria, but disturbed bladder function made the bacterial attack possible. The incontinence will disappear with proper antibiotic treatment, but there is a high risk of recurrence as long as the underlying bladder dysfunction is not treated.

3 *UTI and concomitant bladder disturbance.* The incontinence is caused by both the bacteria and the bladder. Antibiotic treatment may be needed, and may partially ameliorate the continence situation, but as long as the bladder dysfunction is not treated full continence will not be achieved and the bacteria will keep coming back.

4 *ABU in a child with disturbed bladder function.* The incontinence is caused by the bladder disturbance alone, and the bacteria are just innocent bystanders. The child needs treatment of his/her bladder. Antibiotics will not help at all and may even worsen the situation, since eradication of the harmless bacteria leaves the field free for virulent strains.

5 *Contaminated urine sample in a child with disturbed bladder function.* The incontinence is caused by the bladder disturbance alone. The bacteria in the urine culture have come from the prepuce, vulva or perineum. Obviously, antibiotics will not help.

Differentiating between these situations is not easy. Unnecessary antibiotic prescription is harmful *both* for the patient – because of side effects and the risk of actually causing UTIs via the removal of protective bacterial strains (Kunin 1970, Hansson et al 1989) – *and* for society at large – because of increasing bacterial antibiotic resistance. So, how do do we differentiate? The case history provides some clues.

Dysuria that is not caused by local irritation such as vulvitis or balanitis (remember to look at the genitalia) makes a diagnosis of cystitis likely (case 1, 2 or 3 above). The *absence of previous micturition symptoms* (urgency, incontinence, holding manoeuvres) or *previous UTIs* suggests a simple UTI without significant bladder disturbance (case 1 above). Conversely, incontinence that has persisted for months or years is not usually a symptom of an uncomplicated UTI. This is even more true for enuresis – monosymptomatic enuresis is only rarely caused by UTI. Furthermore, the results of previous antibiotic treatment for suspected UTIs are very interesting. If the treatment did not result in quick amelioration or disappearance of the incontinence, then the bacteria were not the main culprits and we should focus on the bladder.

Laboratory tests do not help here – apart from the simple direct urine test or urine sediment. If there are no white or red blood cells in the urine then UTI is very unlikely, and culture is not necessary, since bacterial growth would just mean that the test was contaminated (Hoberman et al 1994). On the other hand, if there are white or red cells in the urine, there may or may not be UTI, so a culture should then be taken. Since cystitis does not entail any risk for kidney damage, it is safe, and indeed often advisable, to wait for the culture results before considering antibiotic therapy, at least in unclear cases.

Finally, if the child has unexplained fever concomitant with incontinence of recent onset, *pyelonephritis* must be ruled out or confirmed without delay. Blood samples for

C-reactive protein (CRP), creatinine and electrolytes should be obtained. Cystatin C is an alternative to creatinine. The decision whether to regard the child's condition as pyelonephritis or not is based on the clinical picture, the urine quick-test (or sediment) and the CRP value. In these cases there is no time to wait for culture results, since even a few days' treatment delay may result in kidney damage.

TREATMENT

Urinary tract infections are, of course, treated with antibiotics (Keren and Chan 2002). From the discussion above it should be clear that far too much antibiotics are given today to incontinent children. Except for cases in which there are grounds for suspicion of pyelonephritis, it is advisable to be circumspect about prescribing these drugs.

That said, a short antibiotic treatment – say, five days – is of course warranted straight away in a clear-cut case of cystitis (Abrahamsson et al 2002) (case 1 above). Furthermore, children with symptomatic UTI secondary to, or concomitant with, an underlying bladder disturbance (cases 2 and 3 above), should also be prescribed antibiotics. However, one should not fool oneself into thinking that everything is solved by this; the bladder will also need to be treated (see below). If it is not treated, there will be recurrent UTIs, or the child will have bladder or bowel problems regardless of bacterial infection.

Finally, if the child belongs to the not insignificant group of individuals with ABU (case 4 above), antibiotics will not help at all and may – as mentioned above – even be slightly harmful (Hansson et al 1989). However, it is often difficult or impossible to know beforehand if the individual incontinent child with bacteriuria belongs to the ABU group or not. Therefore, a short *diagnostic* treatment course can be defended in uncertain cases. If this results in clear amelioration of the symptoms within a maximum of two to three days, it can be concluded that the child had cystitis (case 2 or 3 above); if it does not, the child has ABU.

A.E., 9-year-old girl
Diagnoses: Urinary incontinence due to recurrent cystitis;
voiding postponement; chronic constipation

A. had become daytime continent at the age of 4, and had stopped wetting her bed with the help of an enuresis alarm at the age of 7. Her father had been a bedwetter until early school age. During the last six months before admission A. had had six culture-proven UTIs, with incontinence, dysuria and enuresis – but no fever. She had received antibiotics every time, with prompt disappearance of symptoms. Ultrasound of the kidneys and urinary tract had been normal. Her family physician had then started treatment with daily low-dose antibiotic prophylaxis and had referred her to the paediatric clinic. Between the cystitis episodes A. was reliably dry, but the parents noted that from time to time she had to rush to the toilet and that sometimes, especially after meals, she complained of stomach pains. She admitted that she didn't use the toilets at school because they were dirty. Bowel movements were reported to occur most days and there was no encopresis.

General physical examination, including genital inspection, was normal, but rectal palpation revealed formed faeces in the ampulla. The urine dipstick test was negative. Uroflow showed a short, tower-shaped curve, and she was found to have 56 ml of residual urine. A frequency-volume chart revealed that she voided seldom and irregularly with large volumes (between 200 and 400 ml) and that she had bowel movements three times a week. The 'corn test' gave a suggested gastrointestinal passage time of 50 hours.

A. was suspected of having combined bladder and bowel dysfunction with voiding postponement and constipation. She was given basic urotherapeutic advice, bulk laxatives, and advice about bowel habits, and antibiotic treatment was discontinued. The urotherapist saw her after two months and she reported that there had been no more UTIs and that the stomach pains had disappeared. A. still had some residual urine but this was not treated in the absence of subjective complaints or UTIs.

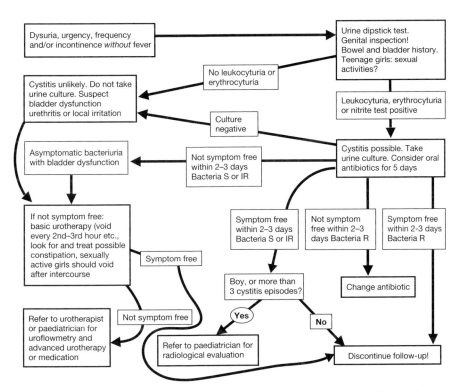

Fig. 8.7 Suggested flow-chart for the evaluation of cystitis in children after 2 years of age. S = sensitive, R = resistant, IR = intermediately resistant

The individual antibiotic drugs are described in some detail in Chapter 5 and listed in Table 5.3. The choice of which drug to use should be based on the resistance profile of the bacteria, if known. If the antibacterial spectrum is not known (because no culture was taken, or for one reason or another one wants to start treatment before obtaining the result), then one has to use clinical judgement. This requires knowledge of the antibiotic susceptibility of the strains that are common in the local community.

Intermediate bacterial sensitivity is quite sufficient in the treatment of cystitis, and bacteriostatic drugs are just as good as bacteriocidic ones. For ecological reasons, one should keep in mind that (1) broad-spectrum antibiotics should not be the first-line choice, and (2) one should not always use the same drug.

This leaves at least the following drugs as reasonable first-line alternatives in the treatment of cystitis in children after the first years of life: trimethoprim, nitrofurantoin, mecillinam and cefadroxil. The length of treatment should be short; five days is sufficient (Abrahamsson et al 2002).

In pyelonephritis the situation is different. Antibiotics need to be bacteriocidal, and broad-spectrum preparations are often needed, since there is no time to wait for culture results. The length of treatment should be expanded to ten days (Keren and Chan 2002).

PROPHYLAXIS, PREVENTION OF RELAPSE
Prevention of relapse is just as important as treatment of the initial UTI, otherwise the child might have to undergo numerous courses of antibiotic treatment, with all the associated side effects and ecological risks. For the same reasons, the use of antibiotic prophylaxis as a means of preventing relapse should only be considered either when everything else has failed or as a temporary measure while an underlying bladder disturbance is treated (Williams et al 2001). The focus should be on the bladder rather than on the bacteria.

The child with UTIs often suffers from an overt voiding disorder, such as urge incontinence, voiding postponement or constipation. These should be treated in accordance with the suggestions outlined in the relevant chapters. If treatment is successful, the risk of relapsing UTI is low.

But even children without bladder or bowel complaints before and after their UTIs often have a subclinically disturbed bladder function with, for instance, intermittent residual urine or uninhibited detrusor contractions. This holds true especially for children who have several UTI episodes. Thus, we suggest that all children above the age of 3 to 4 with UTIs be given basic bladder and bowel advice, and that this is intensified if UTIs recur. The advice that should be given is simple and straightforward:

1   Go to the toilet regularly, approximately six times per day, or every other hour.
2   Sit on the toilet and don't urinate in a hurry.
3   Drink extra water in the mornings and at lunch.
4   If a child has fewer than five bowel movements per week, he or she should be treated for constipation.

Sexually active teenage girls should also be advised to void after intercourse.

In the majority of cases, these measures are sufficient to prevent further infections, *if the advice is followed.* Compliance, however, is an issue here, since not all parents – not to mention teachers and preschool carers – have the time to help their children follow the doctor's advice properly. The help of a dedicated nurse is of immense value here.

Antibiotic prophylaxis is warranted in those children who still have UTIs, despite these interventions, but it should be regarded as a temporary measure. The idea is to keep the bacteria away while the child and family work with the main issue of bladder and bowel control. Consequently, the need for continued antibiotic prophylaxis should be reevaluated regularly, and it should in no way be seen as the definitive solution.

Antibiotics, when used prophylactically, can and should be given in lower than therapeutic dosage. Bacteriostatic preparations are suitable, but broad-spectrum antibiotics should emphatically *not* be used. This means that nitrofurantoin, trimethoprim and cefadroxil can be regarded as first-line choices.

The use of probiotics, and urinary antiseptics such as cranberry juice or methenamine hippurate, has been advocated as a way of reducing the need for antibiotics. These approaches have a clear logical appeal but evidence is so far lacking for their efficacy in children, with the possible exception of methenamine hippurate, which may perhaps be recommended in children who are difficult to wean off antibiotics.

The follow-up of children with UTI differs according to the underlying cause, and falls largely outside the scope of this book. Suffice it here to remind the reader that:

1   Boys with proven UTI may have urethral valve deformity and should be evaluated with ultrasound, uroflowmetry and residual urine measurement after the first UTI.
2   Kidney damage should be excluded (preferably with DMSA scintigraphy) after pyelonephritis, at least if the infection was severe (high CRP) or treatment effect was delayed.
3   Follow-up urine cultures are of limited value in the absence of new symptoms.

Vulvovaginitis

Vulvovaginitis in girls of preschool and early school age is one of the most common conditions mistakenly diagnosed as cystitis. The principal symptom is vulval soreness, which usually precedes the other symptoms, which often include vaginal discharge and dysuria. Frequency, urgency or secondary incontinence may also be present but are not typical. This diagnosis is one of the reasons why genital inspection should be part of the examination of every child with urinary symptoms. In girls with vulvovaginitis the vulva and perineum may be red and oedematous, in which case the diagnosis is clear. Urine analysis may show sterile pyuria or growth of non-typical bacteria such as *staphylococcus albus*.

Treatment is mainly supportive; the girl should avoid tight underwear or over-zealous washing (which may make the skin dry and sore). If the symptoms are severe, short-term antibiotic treatment may be useful and justified. In some cases streptococci are the offenders, and a perineal direct strepto-test, such as is commonly used in the throat in the diagnosis of tonsillitis, may turn out positive; penicillin may then be indicated. Long-term antibiotic prophylaxis should be avoided, even in the minority of girls who, for unknown reasons, tend to have many recurrences. The patient and parents should be reassured that the condition is self-limiting in the long run.

It is a common misconception that girls with a vulval and perineal rash suffer from an infection with *candida albicans* and need antifungal treatment. The fact is that candida needs either oestrogen or sugar to thrive. There are three situations in which such infection may occur: (1) infants, who still retain some oestrogen from the mother, (2) girls with glucosuria due to diabetes mellitus, and (3) pubertal girls who have oestrogen of their own. In the remainder of children, fungal genital infection is exceedingly rare. The reason why the commonly prescribed combined antifungal/steroid topical preparations often help is because either the condition would have receded spontaneously, or the girl suffered from eczema and was helped by the steroids.

Balanitis

Inflammation of the foreskin in prepubertal boys may cause dysuria and, rarely, incontinence. Urethral discharge and irritation are the central symptoms. This diagnosis will not be missed if a more than rudimentary history is taken and – again – if the genitalia are inspected.

Diabetes mellitus

To miss a diagnosis of diabetes mellitus in a child who presents with enuresis is every doctor's nightmare. The risk of it happening, however, is very small. Although it is true that nocturnal enuresis may be a presenting symptom of this disease (Alon et al 1992), most diabetic children have other symptoms as well. Thus, children with diabetes mellitus are usually tired, have lost weight, suffer from excessive thirst and have stomach pains. In a child who seeks medical help just for primary monosymptomatic enuresis, diabetes mellitus is a very unlikely cause.

The reason that enuresis may be a presenting symptom of this disease is of course the osmotic polyuria, which in turn is caused by heavy glucosuria. Thus, no blood glucose measurements are needed to screen for diabetes mellitus in the enuretic child – a urine sample is enough. If there is no heavy glucosuria, diabetes mellitus is not the cause of the child's wetting. Because this is such an easy and cheap test to perform, and it would be so potentially damaging to miss the diagnosis, we suggest that it be performed in every child who presents for the first time with nocturnal enuresis, even though the risk that a child who presents with *just* enuresis will turn out to have diabetes mellitus is slight.

On the other hand, in the child who has secondary enuresis of recent onset, who is thirsty and tired and who has lost weight, it is imperative to check for blood and urine glucose immediately, since in this case diabetes mellitus is very likely. Needless to say, enuresis that is caused by diabetes mellitus will cease as soon as the disease is brought under control (Alon et al 1992).

Since enuresis or incontinence – not caused by diabetes – is such a common disorder, it will certainly sometimes, by mere coincidence, occur in children with diabetes as well.

These children should basically be treated in the same way as other enuretic or incontinent children. No standard treatment of these disorders is contraindicated because of diabetes mellitus.

Central diabetes insipidus

Central, or hypophyseal, diabetes insipidus means polyuria and polydipsia due to lack of vasopressin secretion. For guidelines regarding this condition the reader is advised to consult other publications (Robertson 1995). Here we are concerned mainly with when to suspect or not suspect diabetes insipidus in an enuretic child.

PRESENTATION

Children with central diabetes insipidus suffer from polyuria and polydipsia and sometimes, but not uniformly (Feldman 1983), enuresis secondary to the polyuria. The patients often drink and void colossal amounts of fluid (amounts above 10–15 litres per day are not unheard of), and they need to drink regularly during the night as well. If the child is unconscious or denied free access to water, potentially life-threatening dehydration will ensue.

PATHOGENESIS AND AETIOLOGY

The neurohypophyseal hormone vasopressin is pivotal in the reuptake of water from the primary urine in the collecting duct. Its absence will consequently result in loss of large amounts of dilute urine and a corresponding thirst due to plasma hyperosmolality.

About 50 per cent of cases are idiopathic, whereas the rest are caused by various congenital, space-occupying or invasive lesions – including tumours or Langerhans cell histiocytosis – in the region of the hypothalamus or hypophyseal stalk (Maghnie et al 2000). Hereditary or autoimmune causes may be presumed in some of the idiopathic cases (Scherbaum et al 1985, Repaske et al 1990).

INITIAL DIAGNOSTIC INVESTIGATION

First, it is worth pointing out that the majority of enuretic children who are regarded as 'thirsty' by their parents do *not* have diabetes of any kind; they have just fallen into the habit of drinking a lot. As everybody knows, we drink not only because we are thirsty, but also because it gives comfort, because it tastes good or because we do not want to become thirsty.

Thus, a child who is regarded as thirsty and who drinks a lot during the daytime *but does not need extra fluids at night* is very unlikely to suffer from diabetes insipidus. The parents should also be asked about what happens if the child is not given a drink when he or she asks for it. If the child can be distracted for an hour or two without complaining of severe thirst, then the polydipsia is very probably habitual and not organically caused.

So-called 'psychogenic polydipsia' is a special disturbance which is not likely to cause differential diagnostic confusion in the paediatric age group. Those who suffer from this condition are psychiatrically disturbed patients who for unclear reasons compulsively drink huge amounts of water, sometimes enough to cause hyponatremia with convulsions (Illowsky and Kirch 1988, Ellinas et al 1993).

The first diagnostic step to take when the history makes one suspect diabetes insipidus is to record the child's fluid intake and urine production over a few days and nights at home (the weight of nappies or bedclothes can be measured to record enuresis urine volumes, but if fluid intake and daytime urine production are strictly noted this extra procedure may be omitted). Osmolality measurement in a morning urine sample is also advised, since a high value (say, above 600–700 units mOsm/kg) excludes the disease, although a low value in no way makes the diagnosis certain.

FURTHER DIAGNOSTIC PROCEDURES: THIRST PROVOCATION
If the measurements above strengthen the suspicion of diabetes insipidus, then blood tests for electrolytes and renal function (sodium, chloride, potassium and creatinine) need to be taken, in order to exclude kidney disease, and the patient should be submitted to an inpatient thirst provocation. For a description of this test see Chapter 4.

If these examinations reveal that an enuretic child (or any child) has central diabetes insipidus, more investigations are evidently needed. Several other hormones need to be screened and MRI of the area around the hypothalamus and hypophysis needs to be performed. But this falls outside the field of this book.

TREATMENT
Desmopressin, being an analogue of vasopressin, is the logical treatment for central diabetes insipidus (Aronson et al 1973, Robinson and Verbalis 1985). The usual doses are lower (5–10μg per day) than those required in nocturnal enuresis (20–40μg per day). The treatment is safe (Fjellestad-Paulsen et al 1993b), effective and can be given intravenously, intranasally or orally (Fjellestad and Czernichow 1986).

Nephrogenic diabetes insipidus
Nephrogenic diabetes insipidus means polyuria and polydipsia due to lack of renal tubular response to vasopressin secretion.

PRESENTATION
In the case of isolated nephrogenic diabetes insipidus without kidney failure or compound tubular defects, the symptoms are only related to polyuria and indistinguishable from isolated central diabetes insipidus (see above). Thus, these children have polyuria, polydipsia and enuresis or nocturia. If the diabetes insipidus is part of a more generalized tubular disorder or polyuric kidney failure then the polyuria and polydipsia are usually accompanied by other signs and symptoms, such as growth failure, nausea, malaise, rickets or hypertension.

AETIOLOGY AND PATHOGENESIS
Inability of the renal collecting duct to respond to vasopressin may be due to several causes. The primary defect may be in the renal vasopressin receptors, as in familial, X-linked nephrogenic diabetes insipidus, or it may reside in the aquaporins – i.e. the water-channel-forming proteins that aggregate on the luminal side of the tubular cells in response to vasopressin receptor activation – as in other hereditary forms of the disease (Deen and

Knoers 1998). Apart from these genetic variants, nephrogenic diabetes insipidus may result from other inborn tubular disorders or from structural or toxic tubular damage.

Among the latter kinds of renal polyuria, it is especially important to mention obstructive uropathy. Polyuric renal failure is common in urinary tract malformations causing obstructed urine flow, such as posterior urethral valves. The reason for this is that a disproportionate part of the kidney damage in these conditions is located in the tubules and medullary interstitium. Other disorders that can have a similar presentation are cystic kidney diseases such as nephronophthisis.

DIAGNOSTIC INVESTIGATION

If the child shows signs and symptoms of kidney failure or other renal disease, such as anorexia, nausea, dehydration, hypertension or growth failure, blood samples (creatinine, electrolytes, calcium, phosphate, blood gases), urine evaluation and renal ultrasound are needed without delay. These initial findings will dictate further investigations.

On the other hand, if the symptoms are just related to the polyuria, then the diagnostic investigation will be identical to that described for central diabetes insipidus above, until and including the thirst provocation test and the urinary concentration test with desmopressin (see Chapter 4). Polyuria with increased plasma osmolality and inability to concentrate the urine during thirst provocation indicates a diagnosis of diabetes insipidus; absence of amelioration on desmopressin medication specifies the diagnosis as nephrogenic.

Every child with nephrogenic diabetes insipidus needs a full evaluation of renal function and morphology, to exclude kidney damage or metabolic disease.

TREATMENT OF THE POLYURIA

Obviously, since the kidneys do not respond to vasopressin, there is no use treating these children with desmopressin. If the polyuria is caused by structural damage such as obstructive kidney failure, then there is no effective treatment for the polyuria *per se*. As renal failure progresses and glomerular damage becomes more prominent, polyuria will decrease, but this is no great comfort.

If the child suffers from hereditary nephrogenic diabetes insipidus, then at least partial reduction of polyuria can, paradoxically, be achieved with thiazide diuretic treatment. The treatment is complicated, however, and requires frequent follow-up. Usually potassium supplementation or combination therapy with amiloride is needed as well, and fully normal urine volumes should not be expected. Furthermore, all these children need to undergo regular kidney function evaluation and renal ultrasound, since the increased urine flow may cause upper urinary tract dilatation with consequent kidney damage.

TREATMENT OF THE ENURESIS

In the enuretic child with nephrogenic diabetes insipidus, bedwetting is caused by the combination of polyuria and the inability to wake up when the bladder is full. Since the polyuria cannot be more than partially treated, the arousal defect is the obvious factor to address when trying to help the child become dry. Thus, the enuresis alarm may be worth trying.

The problem is that some children produce such huge amounts of urine that they would need to wake up several times every night in order to stay dry. In these cases sleep would be so much disrupted that daytime alertness would be diminished. The only way to make these children dry would be either if they wore a transurethral urinary catheter every night or if they were surgically provided with a continent urinary diversion such as a Mitrofanoff stoma.

The intriguing possibility that desmopressin may still help, even though the patient has no renal response to the drug, has recently been illustrated by case reports of two children with no functioning vasopressin receptors due to hereditary nephrogenic diabetes insipidus who became dry on desmopressin treatment even though urine production was not affected (Jonat et al 1999, Muller et al 2002). These are exceptional cases that are very difficult to explain (see the discussion on possible CNS effects of desmopressin in Chapter 5), but it may be worth testing the drug for a week or two to see if the experience can be repeated.

K.R., 7-year-old boy
Diagnoses: Monosymptomatic nocturnal enuresis;
nephronophthisis (kidney disease)

K. was admitted because of nocturnal enuresis which was resistant to desmopressin treatment. He was the first child of two of non-consanguineous parents and had no family history of enuresis or incontinence. His cognitive and neurological development had been normal but his weight and height gain had slowed down over the previous year in spite of eating with a good appetite. He had also been slightly more tired than expected and needed to drink approximately two litres of fluid each day. He had hardly ever had a dry night. He had no daytime bladder complaints and no symptoms suggesting constipation.

Physical examination, including blood pressure, was unremarkable except that his height and weight were –2.5 SD for his age (parental measures were –1.0 and –0.5 SD). The urine dipstick test revealed traces of protein but nothing else. A voiding chart revealed normal voided volumes but high fluid intake and high urine production. The investigation was widened due to suspicion of kidney disease. Plasma creatinine and cystatin C were elevated and a Chr-EDTA clearance confirmed that K. had a glomerular filtration rate of 50 ml/min, corrected for body surface. Urine analysis showed tubular proteinuria; and renal ultrasound, performed by a skilled radiologist, revealed abnormal echogenicity of the renal medulla and a slightly dilated renal pelvis on the right side. An inpatient thirst provocation test revealed an inability to concentrate the urine to more than 450 mOsm/kg, despite borderline hypernatremia.

Given these data, a kidney biopsy was performed, yielding tissue that was consistent with, although not diagnostic for, nephronophthisis, a hereditary kidney disease characterized by tubular fibrosis, micro-cysts and progressive renal failure. K. was followed up by the paediatric nephrology team and was put on the waiting list for an enuresis alarm.

Epilepsy

It is well known that epileptic seizures may lead to involuntary loss of urine. Incontinence may also less frequently occur during syncope (Hoefnagels et al 1991) or pseudo-seizures (Meierkord et al 1991). This does not usually pose any problems of differential diagnosis.

In fact, bedwetting in children with known epilepsy usually occurs not during seizures but between them (St Laurent et al 1963, Gastaut et al 1964) – a fact that may reflect either coincidental coexistence of enuresis and epilepsy in the same child, or decreased CNS bladder control during the postictal phase. The general clinical impression (which has not to our knowledge been tested scientifically), that enuresis is not more prevalent among children with epilepsy than among the normal population, favours the former explanation. *Frontal lobe epilepsy* is an exceptional case, since seizures in this disorder are usually confined to the night and are frequently misdiagnosed as all kinds of parasomnias, including nocturnal enuresis (Oldani et al 1998). Age of onset is any time during childhood, seizures are brief (30 seconds to 2 minutes), stereotypic, and frequent (3–22/night). Clinical features include explosive onset, screaming, agitation, stiffening, kicking or bicycling of the legs, and incontinence. Daytime EEG is usually normal (Sinclair et al 2004). So, in a child with secondary enuresis and frequent attacks of strange pavor nocturnus-like behaviour, video-EEG examination may be indicated.

Upper airway obstruction

There is a definite association of enuresis with obstructed upper airways during sleep, but how many enuretic children have upper airway obstruction, and how many otherwise therapy-resistant children would be helped by airway treatment, is unknown. The problem here is that the detection of upper airway obstruction during sleep requires costly inpatient sleep monitoring; and the available treatments, whether surgical or orthodontic, are significant and definitive interventions which one would not want to undertake without being certain they were needed.

Ordinary, everyday snoring is not more common among enuretic children than among dry children (Nevéus et al 1999a). In carefully performed evaluations of children with polysomnographically documented upper airway resistance, enuresis prevalence has ranged between 5 per cent (Guilleminault et al 1996), which is no more than in the general population, and 40 per cent (Brooks and Topol 2003), which clearly is. It is clear that there are children and adults who become enuretic as they develop sleep apnoeas, and who become dry when these are alleviated (Everaert et al 1995, Kramer et al 1998).

PATHOGENESIS

The probable mechanism behind the association between enuresis and sleep apnoeas is polyuria secondary to increased secretion of atrial natriuretic peptide, which in turn is secondary to the negative intrathoracic pressure that is the consequence of respiratory effort against closed upper airways (Krieger et al 1991, Ichioka et al 1992, Umlauf and Chasens 2003). An alternative or contributing explanation may be that the repetitive arousal stimuli that the apnoeas constitute may cause a paradoxical low arousability – in other words, the organism tries to protect the integrity of sleep in the face of frequent interruptions (Chugh et al 1996).

PRESENTATION, ASSESSMENT

Snoring or disordered breathing at night is common among normal children; rates between 5 and 25 per cent are reported (Owen et al 1996, Nevéus et al 2001a). There is currently no way of knowing which subgroup of bedwetting snorers deserves further evaluation for sleep apnoeas and upper airway obstruction.

Although future research may change the picture, we suggest that a child should be referred only if the following criteria are fulfilled: habitual heavy snoring (not just during upper respiratory tract infections) with audible sleep apnoeas, mouth breathing or daytime sleepiness, together with enuresis resistant to standard therapy.

Sleep monitoring for the evaluation of upper airway obstruction usually takes place at an otorhinolaryngological clinic and involves the measurement of chest movements, nasal/oral airflow and percutaneous oxygen saturation. If upper airway obstruction is confirmed, it may or may not be causing the enuresis. The only way to find out is to remove the obstruction and see if the enuresis disappears as well.

TREATMENT

Tonsillectomy or adenoidectomy are the treatments of choice for obstructed upper airways due to enlarged tonsils or adenoids.

In one study by Weider et al it was found that 76 per cent of 115 severely enuretic children with upper airway obstruction were cured of their enuresis when the obstruction was removed (Weider et al 1991). All these children were nocturnal mouth-breathers, and the prognosis was best for those with secondary enuresis. Similar results were found by Cinar et al (2001), but in a smaller study (Elsherif and Kareemullah 1999) it was found that 76 children operated on for obstructed breathing showed improvement for all symptoms *except* the enuresis.

The use of nasally applied continuous positive airway pressure (CPAP) is a common treatment for sleep apnoeas not attributable to tonsillar or adenoidal hypertrophy, predominantly among obese adults. Concomitant enuresis or nocturia is common in this population as well, and it has been clearly shown that CPAP treatment solves these problems as well as the apnoeas (Everaert et al 1995, Kramer et al 1998). The curious orthodontic procedure known as *rapid maxillary expansion*, which was mentioned in Chapter 6 (see page 125), may have its possible antienuretic effects via correction of sleep-disordered breathing as well.

Allergies

The evidence for a causal relationship between enuresis or incontinence and food is mostly anecdotal. There are reports of children who become dry when treated for food allergy (Jakobsson 1985, Oei et al 1989), but comparisons between bedwetters and dry children have failed to show any increased prevalence of allergies in the former (Siegel et al 1976, Kaplan et al 1977).

As for the mechanism behind this proposed association, we can only guess; it may act via constipation or sleep-disordered breathing (i.e. subclinical asthma).

Cow's milk intolerance is a special case, since it is a clear risk factor for constipation and encopresis (see Chapter 10). It is conceivable that it may also cause incontinence or enuresis via constipation.

There is probably a group of enuretic and allergic children who need anti-allergenic treatment to become dry, but this group is very small, so we suggest that elimination diets or anti-allergenic treatment should not be instituted if enuresis is the only symptom. Cow's milk intolerance is the possible exception here; a one-week elimination followed by provocation may be tested in therapy-resistant enuretic children with concomitant gastrointestinal symptoms or an atopic disposition.

Other causes of organic urinary incontinence

URINARY INCONTINENCE IN CHRONIC PAEDIATRIC ILLNESS

Any disease that is severe enough to make the child incapable of getting out of bed or using the toilet will cause enuresis or incontinence; this goes without saying. It is also probable that there are disorders that lead to an increasing risk of wetting regardless of the level of physical incapacitation incurred, but very little research has been done in this field.

Cystic fibrosis may be such a disease. It has been shown that adolescent girls suffering from this disease have a high risk of daytime incontinence, which in many cases is severe enough to affect their quality of life negatively (Nixon et al 2002). The cause of this association is obscure.

URINARY INCONTINENCE IN PHYSICAL DISABILITY

In other incapacitating chronic conditions, such as *spinal muscular atrophy* (SMA), the rate of associated incontinence is high. In one study, 29 per cent of patients wetted at night and/or during the day, mostly younger children with SMA types I and II. The types of incontinence varied, including nocturnal enuresis, voiding postponement, dysfunctional voiding, stress, and neurogenic incontinence. Many patients were also constipated, soiled or had UTIs (von Gontard et al 2001b).

As in the case of chronic illness, physical disability may make it impossible for children to use the toilet or get out of bed without help. Despite this, at the age of 6, the prevalence of incontinence among children with tetraplegia was just 46 per cent, and those with di- or hemiplegia 20 per cent (Roijen et al 2001).

Children with *cerebral palsy* often suffer from disturbances of bladder function. It is unclear whether this should be regarded as neurogenic bladder disturbance or not, and the distinction is perhaps not important. The aetiology is central nervous damage, resulting in sphincter and/or detrusor malfunction. Detrusor overactivity is the most common urodynamic finding (Mayo 1992). Most children can achieve dryness with urotherapy and/or anticholinergic treatment (Decter et al 1987, Reid and Borzyskowski 1993). Low IQ is a prognostically unfavourable factor in children with cerebral palsy (Roijen et al 2001), whereas in larger, unselected groups of children with learning and/or motor disability, mobility was found to be more important than intelligence for the achievement of continence (Van Laecke et al 2001).

Boys with *Duchenne's muscular dystrophy* probably have enuresis and daytime incontinence in excess of what can be explained by their physical disability alone (Caress et al 1996). Detrusor overactivity is the probable pathogenic mechanism (MacLeod et al 2003), and it may be caused either by abnormalities of smooth muscle or by abnormalities of the CNS.

Parkinson's disease and multiple sclerosis – both of which are exceedingly rare among children – are characterized by an increased risk for detrusor overactivity and/or polyuria with consequent incontinence or enuresis (Rabey et al 1979, Suchoversky et al 1995). Desmopressin has been shown to be beneficial in treating the polyuria of these patients (Suchoversky et al 1995, Valiquette et al 1996).

URINARY INCONTINENCE IN SYNDROMES OF MENTAL RETARDATION
The rate of urinary incontinence is increased in patients with mental retardation. Thus, in a population-based study, 38.1 per cent of 7-year-olds wet at night and 39.0 per cent during the day (von Wendt et al 1990). The rates remain high even at the age of 20 years, with 20 per cent wetting at night and during the daytime. The risk for incontinence increases with the severity of mental retardation and is lowest in mild mental retardation (IQ 50–70).

In recent years, specific behavioural profiles have been identified for different genetic syndromes of mental retardation. Although voiding problems constitute a major burden in everyday life, they have been neglected in most research on 'behavioural phenotypes' – with only a few exceptions. Children with fragile-X syndrome, for example, have a high rate of urinary incontinence (27 per cent) (Backes et al 2000).

Treatment strategies have to be adapted according to the cognitive abilities of the child and any associated behavioural problems. One behavioural treatment is 'response restriction': children are allowed to approach the toilet, lower their pants, sit on the toilet and void – all other behaviours such as stereotypic, repetitive acts, walking about and putting hands on the toilet are interrupted or prevented (Duker et al 2001). In addition, diapers are withdrawn and children are prompted at regular intervals. Continence is reinforced by praise and other rewards. Accidents are followed by so-called 'positive practice' procedures (sitting on the toilet repeatedly). Follow-up measures aim to maintain the results achieved.

Another procedure described by Smith et al (2000), aimed at treatment-resistant children with combined encopresis and urinary incontinence, uses the technique of 'transfer of stimulus control' – i.e. the substitution of an inappropriate stimulus (nappy) with an appropriate one (toilet) for voiding. Shaping and fading are mainly employed in this programme and all aversive techniques avoided.

In conclusion, children with all degrees of mental retardation can be trained successfully to achieve continence by adapting standard behavioural techniques. Some, however, do require long-term training – lasting up to two years (Smith et al 2000). Also, some children will not achieve self-initiated continence but will continue to require prompting (Duker et al 2001). Individual treatment seems to have better long-term effects than group approaches (Hyams et al 1992).

9
FUNCTIONAL FAECAL INCONTINENCE (ENCOPRESIS)

Classification and definitions

According to the standard classification schemes – the ICD-10 of the World Health Organization (WHO 1993) and the DSM-IV of the American Psychiatric Association (APA 1994) – functional faecal incontinence (encopresis) is generally defined as both voluntary and involuntary passage of faeces in inappropriate places in a child aged 4 years or older after organic causes have been ruled out. Despite major similarities between the two classification systems, they differ regarding essential points, especially the definition of subtypes. The diagnostic criteria of ICD-10 and DSM-IV will therefore be discussed separately; the major differences are shown in Tables 9.1 and 9.2.

DEFINITIONS ACCORDING TO ICD-10

Further specifications can be found in the clinical criteria according to ICD-10, which, unfortunately, are both imprecise and confusing (Remschmidt et al 2001). Thus, ICD-10 does not differentiate exactly between primary and secondary forms of encopresis. In most, but not all, studies, the definition using an interval without encopresis of six months or longer is used. In addition, ICD-10 does not differentiate clearly between encopresis with constipation (retentive encopresis) and encopresis without constipation (solitary encopresis).

Also, the restrictions regarding the comorbidity of enuresis and urinary incontinence are not very useful for clinical practice. Thus, only encopresis should be diagnosed if several forms of incontinence coexist. If one were to follow the specifications exactly, the full

TABLE 9.1
Definition of non-organic encopresis according to ICD-10 (WHO 1993)

A. The child repeatedly passes faeces in places that are inappropriate for the purpose (e.g. clothing, floor) either involuntarily or intentionally (the disorder may involve overflow incontinence secondary to functional faecal retention).
B. The child's chronological and mental age is at least 4 years.
C. There is at least one encopretic event per month.
D. Duration of the disorder is at least six months.
E. There is no organic condition that constitutes a cause for the encopretic events.

A fifth character may be used, if desired, for further specification:

F98.10 Failure to acquire physiological bowel control
F98.11 Adequate bowel control with normal faeces deposited in inappropriate places
F98.12 Soiling that is associated with excessively fluid faeces, such as with retention with overflow

TABLE 9.2
Diagnostic criteria according to DSM-IV (APA 1994)

A. Repeated passage of faeces in inappropriate places (e.g. clothing or floor) whether involuntary or intentional.
B. At least one such event a month for at least three months.
C. Chronological age is at least 4 years (or equivalent developmental level).
D. The behaviour is not due exclusively to the direct physiological effects of a substance (e.g. laxatives) or general medical condition except through a mechanism involving constipation.

Code as follows:

787.6 With constipation and overflow incontinence
307.7 Without constipation and overflow incontinence

---

spectrum of comorbidity could not be assessed. Therefore, it is much more useful to diagnose the type of encopresis, and, if present, any comorbid type of wetting disorder.

In contrast, the DSM-IV criteria are more precise in specifying the subtypes and are therefore more applicable for both clinical and research purposes.

DEFINITIONS ACCORDING TO DSM-IV

The specific differentiation into these two subtypes (with and without constipation) is of utmost importance as they differ decisively according to pathophysiology, clinical features and especially treatment (the first type does not respond to laxatives, while in the second type laxatives are essential in treatment). The diagnostic criteria (according to DSM-IV) for these two subtypes are specified in more detail in Table 9.3.

These two subtypes will be dealt with in detail in later sections. But other definitions and subtypes have to be considered.

ICCS TERMINOLOGY

The International Children's Continence Society (ICCS), an international, multi-professional organization dealing with children with enuresis and urinary incontinence, has recently compiled a new standardization of terminology (Nevéus et al 2006). This has included definitions for encopresis, as wetting and soiling problems often coexist and have to be diagnosed and dealt with.

TABLE 9.3
Specific diagnostic criteria for encopresis with and
without constipation according to DSM-IV (APA 1994)

Encopresis with constipation and overflow incontinence (787.6): there is evidence of constipation on physical examination or by history. Faeces are characteristically (but not invariably) poorly formed and leakage is continuous, occurring both during the day and during sleep. Only small amounts of faeces are passed during toileting, and incontinence resolves after treatment of the constipation.

Encopresis without constipation and overflow incontinence (307.7): there is no evidence of constipation on physical examination or by history. Faeces are likely to be of normal form and consistency, and soiling is intermittent. Faeces may be deposited in a prominent location. This is usually associated with the presence of oppositional defiant disorder or conduct disorder, or may be the consequence of anal masturbation.

Encopresis: The ICCS recommends adhering to the internationally established usage of the term encopresis, as it has been defined by the ICD-10 and the DSM-IV. There is basically no reason to change this term. Encopresis therefore means any type of functional passage of faeces in inappropriate places, of any size and consistency.

Soiling: In contrast, soiling is a confusing and ill-defined term that should not be used, in view of established international definitions of encopresis (ICD-10, DSM-IV). Soiling is generally defined as 'making dirty by defecating in or on' (*New Oxford English Dictionary*). Some authors in the UK and Australia define soiling as an 'involuntary' passage of faeces (in contrast to a 'voluntary' passage in encopresis). Others define soiling by stool consistency as 'the involuntary seepage of faeces which is often associated with faecal impaction, and reflects staining of underwear' (Benninga et al 1994: 187). Still others define soiling by the volume of stool as 'the leakage of small amounts of stool' – in contrast to the 'expulsion of normal bowel movement' in encopresis (Di Lorenzo and Benninga 2004). To avoid this confusion, the term soiling should be avoided as a definition of any specific condition, and should only be used in a general way.

Faecal incontinence: Faecal incontinence is an umbrella term encompassing any sort of inappropriate deposition of faeces – both functional and organic. The terms functional faecal incontinence and encopresis can be used interchangeably.

Anal incontinence: Anal incontinence is a general term encompassing both inappropriate passage of faeces and flatulence – both functional and organic. The use of this term is not recommended.

ROME-II CRITERIA

A set of definitions regarding functional gastrointestinal disorders in children was compiled by paediatric gastroenterologists in 1997 (Rasquin-Weber et al 1999). The three most important conditions in this context are listed in Table 9.4.

The Rome-II criteria are considered too restrictive and do not identify many children who would be diagnosed by clinicians (Loening-Baucke 2004). On the other hand, some children fulfil the Rome-II criteria who would not be diagnosed by traditional clinical criteria. The overlap is greatest for functional non-retentive faecal soiling. As the Rome-II criteria are difficult to use in clinical practice, a revision is recommended (Voskuijl et al 2004a).

PACCT GROUP CRITERIA

Recently, revised suggestions were published by a group of paediatric gastroenterologists meeting in Paris – hence the name 'Paris consensus on childhood constipation terminology' (PACCT 2005). The main recommendations are summarized in Table 9.5.

The PACCT Group also advises dropping the terms functional faecal retention, soiling and encopresis. As these recommendations reflect the view of only one paediatric sub-specialty, and as other disciplines and specialties (such as child psychiatry) are happy with the ICD-10 and DSM-IV terminology and would be reluctant to discard these terms altogether, we have chosen to use the terms encopresis and functional faecal incontinence interchangeably.

216

TABLE 9.4
Rome-II criteria (Rasquin-Weber et al 1999)

G4b. Functional constipation

In infants and preschool children, at least two weeks of:

1   scybalous, pebble-like, hard stools for a majority of stools; or
2   firm stools two or less times/week; and
3   there is no evidence of structural, endocrine, or metabolic disease.

G4c. Functional faecal retention

From infancy to 16 years old, a history of at least 12 weeks of:

1   passage of large-diameter stools at intervals <2 times per week; and
2   retentive posturing, avoiding defecation by purposefully contracting the pelvic floor. As pelvic floor muscles fatigue, the child uses the gluteal muscles, squeezing the buttocks together.

G4d. Functional non-retentive faecal soiling

Once a week or more for the preceding 12 weeks, in a child older than 4 years, a history of:

1   defecation in places and at times inappropriate to the social context;
2   in the absence of structural or inflammatory disease; and
3   in the absence of signs of faecal retention (listed in G4c).

TABLE 9.5
PACCT Group criteria

Chronic constipation

The occurrence of two or more of the following symptoms, during the last eight weeks:

• frequency of bowel movements less than three per week
• more than one episode of faecal incontinence per week
• large stools in the rectum or palpable on abdominal examination
• passing of stools so large that they may obstruct the toilet
• display of retentive posturing with holding behaviours
• painful defecation

Faecal incontinence

• passage of stools in an inappropriate place

Organic faecal incontinence

• faecal incontinence resulting from organic disease (e.g. neurological damage or sphincter abnormalities)

Functional faecal incontinence

• non-organic disease which can be subdivided into:
  constipation-associated faecal incontinence
  non-retentive (non-constipation-associated) faecal incontinence

PRIMARY AND SECONDARY ENCOPRESIS

Primary and secondary encopresis are defined according to the longest continuous interval without soiling. Most clinicians and researchers endorse the use of an interval of six months: i.e. if a child has been free of soiling for less than six months, this would be considered a primary form of encopresis; if a relapse occurs after six months or more, a secondary type of encopresis would be diagnosed. Whether or not this symptom-free interval is achieved by treatment is of no relevance, nor is the age at which it occurs.

Other definitions of primary and secondary encopresis have been used. Thus Bellman (1966) as well as the former DSM-III-R (1987) classification scheme employed a long period of twelve months in their definition. Unfortunately both DSM-IV and ICD-10 no longer specify an exact period of time. Thus, primary encopresis is described as a type 'in which the individual has never established faecal continence', and secondary encopresis as a type 'in which disturbance develops after a period of established faecal continence' (APA 1994). This imprecise definition makes comparisons between studies more difficult.

Despite these difficulties, most studies have shown that the prevalence of primary and secondary encopresis is almost the same. In the only population-based study, over half (57 per cent) of the boys studied were affected by primary encopresis (Bellman 1966). In clinical studies the rates have ranged from 51 per cent (Mehler-Wex et al 2005), to 54 per cent (Foreman and Thambirajah 1996) and 59 per cent (Bellman 1966, pilot study). For encopresis with constipation, 25 per cent of children had a primary type; for encopresis without constipation the rate was higher at 47 per cent (Benninga et al 1994). The peak for a relapse (secondary encopresis) is between the ages of 6 years (Benninga et al 1994) and 10 years (Largo et al 1978).

In nocturnal enuresis, subtyping into primary and secondary forms is of great clinical relevance. While the two forms do not differ regarding genetic and somatic factors, the rate of concomitant psychological symptoms and disorders differs greatly. Thus, in population-based studies, primary nocturnal enuresis was not associated with psychosocial factors or with higher rates of behavioural disorders (McGee et al 1984, Fergusson et al 1986). In contrast, a relapse was often precipitated by stressful life events such as separation and divorce of parents (Järvelin et al 1990a). Also, children with secondary nocturnal enuresis had a higher risk for emotional and behavioural disorders – both in population-based (Feehan et al 1990) and in clinical studies (von Gontard et al 1999a).

In contrast, children with primary and secondary encopresis do not differ regarding behavioural symptoms (Bellman 1966). Only in a highly selected group of 66 children in a child psychiatric setting, primary encopresis had higher rates of developmental disorders (68 per cent), while secondary encopresis had higher rates of psychosocial risks (69 per cent) and conduct disorders (54 per cent) (Foreman and Tharambirajah 1996).

In summary, there are no clear-cut differences between primary and secondary encopresis that could be of clinical relevance. Therefore, this subtyping is not useful in clinical practice.

ENCOPRESIS WITH AND WITHOUT COMORBID PSYCHIATRIC DISORDERS
In contrast, the assessment of comorbid behavioural and emotional disorders is of great relevance. If a child has encopresis only, symptom-oriented treatment will suffice and compliance with treatment will, in general, be much better. If behavioural or emotional disorders coexist, these often require additional treatment and children will often be less

compliant in adhering to symptom-oriented treatment schedules. It is therefore very important to assess both subclinical symptoms and manifest psychological disorders. In essence, the subtyping into two forms, with and without constipation and with and without mental disorders, is of great practical consequence (Table 9.6).

OTHER SUBTYPES

The comorbidity of *encopresis and wetting* is of great importance and will be dealt with later in this chapter (see pages 262–266).

The *toilet refusal syndrome* describes the behaviour of children who use the toilet for micturition but not for defecation. They insist adamantly on being given a diaper when wanting to pass faeces. This common syndrome in infancy has been shown to be a major risk factor for later encopresis.

Toilet phobia is basically an isolated phobic disorder. Children develop a generalized anxiety towards the toilet and refuse both micturition and defecation. Again, such avoidant and retentive behaviour can predispose towards encopresis.

Epidemiology

Only a very few population-based studies have addressed the general prevalence of encopresis. The most important studies are the study by Bellman (1966) and the two longitudinal Swiss studies (Largo and Stützle 1977, Largo et al 1978, 1996). Bellman conducted a cross-sectional epidemiological study of 8683 7-year-olds, of whom 132 soiled at least once a month. Retrospectively, prevalence rates for ages 2 to 6 years were compiled (see Table 9.7).

The two longitudinal Swiss studies reported on 413 representative newborns born in 1954 to 1956 (Largo and Stützle 1977, Largo et al 1978), and 320 infants born in 1974 to 1984 (Largo et al 1996). As both studies adhered to an identical design, the effects of different toilet-training practices on the prevalence of encopresis can be analysed. The prevalence rates are shown in Table 9.7.

As shown in Table 9.7, continence was achieved at a much earlier age in the 1950s, with a major decline in soiling from the age of 2 to 3. In the 1970s, nearly all children were

TABLE 9.6
**Classification of encopresis according to presence of constipation
and comorbid emotional/behavioural disorders**

	Constipation	No constipation
With emotional/behavioural disorder	Encopresis with constipation and emotional/behavioural disorder	Encopresis without constipation but with emotional/behavioural disorder
Without emotional/ behavioural disorder	Encopresis with constipation but without emotional/behavioural disorder	Encopresis without constipation and without emotional/behavioural disorder

TABLE 9.7
Prevalence of encopresis in Swiss longitudinal studies and Swedish cross-sectional study

Age (years)	1 **Zurich longitudinal study** (Largo and Stützle 1977, Largo et al 1978)	2 **Zurich longitudinal study** (Largo et al 1996)	**Swedish cross-sectional study** (Bellman 1966)
	Percentage in year of life: male, female (both)	Percentage in year of life: male, female	Percentage at birthday: male, female (both)
Infancy			
1	68%, 61%	99%, 99%	
1½	43%, 35%	99%, 99%	
2	27%, 17%	97%, 90%	56.9%, 43.2% (50.2%)
3	4%, 2%	46%, 18%	11.0%, 5.2% (8.1%)
Definitional age of encopresis			
4	2%, 3%	8%, 1%	4.3%, 1.4% (2.8%)
5	2%, 1%	7%, 1%	3.5%, 1.0% (2.2%)
School age			
6	1%, 1%	4%, 3%	2.9%, 0.8% (1.9%)
7	1.9%, 0.6% (1.3%)		2.4%, 0.7% (1.5%)
8	3.9%, 0.7% (2.3%)		
9	1.9%, 0.6% (1.3%)		
10	1.9%, 1.4% (1.7%)		
11	3.9%, 2.1% (3.1%)		
12	4.2%, 1.4% (2.8%)		
13	2.8%, 0.0% (1.4%)		
Adolescence (>14 years)	0%		

soiling up to the age of 4, with a gradual decline afterwards. At the definitional age of encopresis (4 years), 2 to 8 per cent of all boys and 1 to 3 per cent of all girls were still soiling. The sex difference remains constant over all age groups, with three to four times more boys being affected than girls.

Throughout the preschool years, school age and early adolescence, the rate of encopresis remains relatively stable, affecting 2 to 4 per cent of all boys and 1 to 2 per cent of all girls. In contrast to nocturnal enuresis, which shows a spontaneous remission rate of 13 to 15 per cent per year, no gradual decline occurs; the rate of children becoming continent is more than compensated for by those children experiencing a relapse, so that the general prevalence remains the same. After the age of 14, there were no adolescents affected by encopresis in the first Swiss study (Largo et al 1978). Clinical reports show that encopresis can occur in adolescents, often with a complicated, protracted course (Rex et al 1992, Fennig and Fennig 1999).

In adulthood, encopresis is described in patients with learning disability (Smith 1996) or co-occurring with psychiatric disorders (Bellman 1966, Fraser and Taylor 1986).

The underreporting of encopresis in adolescence and adulthood is partly due to the fact that the term encopresis is not used in adult medicine or adult psychiatry. Instead, the term faecal or stool incontinence is used as an umbrella term that includes not only functional but also medical forms of incontinence (Jameson and Scott 1997). Generally, the prevalence of faecal incontinence is high among adults (aged 18 or older); 2.7 per cent of all adults soil on a daily, 4.5 per cent on a weekly and 7.4 per cent on a monthly basis (Johanson and Lafferty 1996). Women soil more often than men and the prevalence increases drastically in older age (Roberts et al 1999). Due to the terminological differences in childhood (i.e. encopresis) and adulthood (i.e. faecal incontinence) the exact course of childhood encopresis in older age is not known. In long-term follow-up studies, 30 per cent of adolescents were still constipated (Van Ginkel et al 2003).

Nearly all children with encopresis soil during the day. Only 2.7 per cent soiled at night in the Swedish epidemiological study (Bellman 1966). In clinical studies, 30 per cent of children with constipation and only 12 per cent of children without constipation soiled at night (Benninga et al 1994).

Comorbid behavioural disorders

Children with encopresis have an extremely high rate of additional, co-occurring behavioural and emotional disorders. The rate is much higher than among children with nocturnal enuresis or even daytime wetting. This has been shown consistently in epidemiological as well as clinical studies in both paediatric and child psychiatric settings. Despite this high rate of comorbidity there is no evidence of any encopresis-specific psychopathology; in fact, a wide variety of behavioural and emotional disorders can co-exist. Also, no clear causal relationship can be identified. Thus, behavioural disorders can be a consequence of encopresis; they can precede and precipitate a relapse in secondary encopresis; the comorbidity can be due to common neurobiological factors; and in individual cases mental health disorders and encopresis can co-occur by chance without a causal association. As in previous chapters, clinically relevant disorders will be discussed first, followed by descriptive subclinical signs and symptoms.

CLINICALLY RELEVANT BEHAVIOURAL AND EMOTIONAL DISORDERS

As many studies have used the Child Behavior Checklist (CBCL; Achenbach 1991), the results can be compared easily. As shown in Table 9.8, 35 to 50 per cent of all children with encopresis had a total behavioural score in the clinical range on this parental questionnaire. Compared to the rate in the normative population (10 per cent), 3.5 to 5 times more children with encopresis have total behavioural scores in the clinical range. As all studies were conducted in a paediatric setting, this rate cannot be due to selection effects of mental health clinics. Children with behavioural maladjustment are less compliant than children without psychological disorders (71 per cent vs. 38 per cent non-compliant) – so, if these problems are not addressed, treatment will be less successful (Nolan et al 1991).

Encopretic children with constipation have the same rate of behavioural scores in the clinical range as children without constipation: 39 per cent vs. 44 per cent (Benninga et al 1994); and 37 per cent vs. 39 per cent (Benninga et al 2004). There was also no correlation between behavioural scores (CBCL) and colon transit time or defecation dynamics (Benninga et al 2004).

TABLE 9.8
Comorbidity of clinically relevant behavioural scores
(percentage of children with CBCL total score >90th percentile)

Study	Total N	Percentage in the clinical range (CBCL total score >90th percentile (norm: 10%))
Gabel et al 1986	55	49%
Young et al 1995	76	51%
Nolan et al 1991	169	43%
With constipation		
Loening-Baucke et al 1987	38	42%
Benninga et al 1994	111	39%
Benninga et al 2004	135	37%
Without constipation		
Benninga et al 1994	50	44%
Van der Plas et al 1997	71	35%
Benninga et al 2004	56	39%

Internalizing clinical behavioural scores (32 per cent) were twice as common as externalizing ones (17 per cent) in one study (Van der Plas et al 1997). In other studies, single behavioural items, denoting oppositional behaviour and attentional problems, predominated (Gabel et al 1986, Johnston and Wright 1993). Compared to controls, children with encopresis scored significantly higher regarding anxious/depressed behaviour, attentional difficulties and disruptive behaviour on the CBCL subscales. For example, the rate of attentional problems in the clinical and borderline range was six to seven times higher than in controls (20 per cent vs. 3 per cent; norm 5 per cent; Cox et al 2002). Again, the heterogeneity of behavioural symptoms is apparent.

Only a few studies have assessed behavioural and emotional disorders according to standardized child psychiatric criteria. These too show a high general rate and heterogeneity of comorbid disorders. Thus, 34 per cent of 41 children with encopresis had an emotional disorder, 12 per cent a conduct disorder and 10 per cent a hyperkinetic syndrome according to ICD-10 criteria (Steinmüller and Steinhausen 1990). In another study of 85 highly selected child psychiatric inpatients with encopresis, 83 per cent fulfilled the criteria for at least one ICD-10 diagnosis; 32 per cent had a hyperkinetic syndrome; and 21 per cent an emotional disorder (Mehler-Wex et al 2005).

SUBCLINICAL SYMPTOMS
In addition to clinical disorders or behavioural scores, subclinical symptoms are prevalent among children with encopresis. The only population-based study addressing this question was conducted in the 1960s long before the advent of ICD-10 and DSM-IV. In the study, 75 boys with encopresis were compared with 73 matched controls, as shown in Table 9.9 (Bellman 1966).

A high rate of heterogeneous behavioural symptoms was evident among boys with encopresis compared to controls. Specifically, encopretic boys showed higher rates of food refusal, general negativism, strong anxiety reactions, lack of self-assurance, poor tolerance of stress, both inhibited and aggressive behaviour, a strong fixation to their mother and difficulties in relationships.

Four different subclinical symptom constellations can be identified (Krisch 1985): increased aggressivity; inhibited compulsive behaviour; social withdrawal, introversion and depressive symptoms; and increased anxiety.

Unfortunately, these behavioural problems have not been investigated systematically in newer studies. For example, only two studies have addressed the construct of self-esteem in encopretic children, which has proven to be an important area of concern – and with contradicting results (Moffat et al 1987, Longstaffe et al 2000). Children with encopresis tended to feel less in control of positive life events and had a lower sense of self-esteem than children with other chronic conditions (Landman et al 1986). In the other, more recent study, self-esteem did not differ between children with encopresis and controls on the Piers–Harris questionnaire (Cox et al 2002). Although some of these subclinical symptoms will diminish under successful treatment (Van der Plas et al 1997, Benninga et al 2004), it is not known which ones will persist and become chronic.

Specific psychological disorders in children with encopresis

INTELLIGENCE

In general, children with encopresis do not have reduced intelligence. In one study the mean IQ was 105 for children with encopresis and 106 for controls (Bellman 1966). In another study, children with encopresis showed poorer school performance (TRF questionnaire), especially regarding reading and spelling (WRAT-R test), compared to controls (Cox et al 2002).

TABLE 9.9
Behavioural symptoms in 75 representative boys with
encopresis and 73 controls (Bellman 1966)

Symptoms	Children with encopresis n=75	Controls n=73
Food refusal	21%	7%
General negativism	12%	3%
Pilfering	43%	26%
Strong anxiety reactions	44%	18%
Lack of self-assurance	43%	11%
Poor tolerance of stress	31%	15%
Inhibited aggression	33%	12%
Aggressive behaviour	11%	1.4%
Fixation to mother	46%	18%
Difficulties in peer relationships	20%	1.4%

On the other hand, there is no doubt that children with learning disability are more likely to have problems with soiling. In a population-based Finnish study, 35.5 per cent of 7-year-olds and 19.0 per cent of 20-year-olds with learning disability soiled. This rate is much higher than the general prevalence of encopresis. The rate of encopresis correlates directly with the degree of learning disability; thus only 2.8 per cent of those with mild, 32.4 per cent of those with moderate, 38.1 per cent of those with severe, and 85.7 per cent of those with the most severe learning disability had encopresis (von Wendt et al 1990). Regarding specific syndromes of learning disability, 20 per cent of children and adolescents with fragile-X syndrome and 6 per cent of those with tuberous sclerosis soiled (Backes et al 2000).

OTHER DISORDERS

A whole variety of both internalizing and externalizing disorders can be present in children with encopresis. Irrespective of whether these occur before or after the onset of encopresis, they often require additional treatment. Also, treatment of encopresis can be difficult due to refusal and lack of compliance on the part of the child (Buttross 1999).

OPPOSITIONAL DEFIANT DISORDER

One typical disorder in encopretic children is oppositional defiant disorder, according to DSM-IV (313.81) (APA 1994). The typical sign of oppositional defiant disorder (ODD) is a pattern of negativistic, hostile and defiant behaviour. The child often loses his or her temper, argues with adults, actively defies or refuses to comply with adults' requests or rules, annoys people deliberately, blames others for his or her mistakes or misbehaviour, is often touchy or easily annoyed by others, is angry and resentful, spiteful or vindictive.

ODD usually begins before the age of 8 years and affects approximately 3 per cent of all children. It is seen as a milder form or developmental precursor of conduct disorder, which is defined as a 'repetitive and persistent pattern of behaviour in which basic rights of others or major age-appropriate societal norms and rules are violated'. The main aetiological factors are parental psychopathology, family dysfunction and problematic temperament (high reactivity, difficulty being soothed), combined with a genetic disposition. The main lines of treatment are parental guidance and cognitive-behavioural treatment. It clearly follows that if a child does not comply with rules in general, he or she will also refuse to comply with toilet programmes and laxatives.

ATTENTION DEFICIT HYPERACTIVITY DISORDER (ADHD)

Another externalizing disorder in encopretic children is ADHD (attention deficit hyper-activity disorder). This is characterized by symptoms of inattention; thus a child often has difficulty sustaining attention at school or in play, is easily distracted by external stimuli, does not seem to listen, does not follow through on instructions, and has difficulty organizing tasks and activities. In addition, symptoms of hyperactivity-impulsivity can be present, such as fidgeting with hands or feet, leaving their seat in the classroom, interrupting others, and having difficulty awaiting their turn. ADHD affects 5 to 10 per cent of all children, often from infancy onwards, and has a high tendency to persist into adolescence and even adulthood. The main lines of treatment are parental guidance, cognitive-behavioural therapy and stimulant medication. Again, a child with ADHD might not react adequately to, or might ignore, the need for defecation and might have difficulty in adhering to treatment regimes for encopresis.

INTERNALIZING DISORDERS

Of the internalizing disorders, both anxiety and depressive disorders are typical for children with encopresis.

Separation anxiety disorder, as well as *generalized anxiety*, is often associated with embarrassment and avoidance of going to the toilet when necessary. This can enhance retentive behaviour, increasing the risk for constipation. Toilet phobia – a specific phobia directed towards the toilet – will be discussed later in this chapter (see page 267) as a separate entity, again associated with avoidant and retentive behaviour.

Depressive disorders are common and affect up to 6 per cent of all children and adolescents. They are characterized by a depressed or irritable mood, diminished interest and pleasure, loss of activity, feelings of worthlessness, problems in concentrating, and a variety of physical symptoms such as loss of appetite, tiredness and insomnia. The main lines of treatment comprise cognitive-behavioural, psychodynamic and family therapies, often combined with antidepressant medication. It is easy to see that a depressed child may be too preoccupied with other thoughts and emotions to show sufficient motivation in the treatment of encopresis. On the other hand, encopresis may quite possibly be the cause or aggravating factor behind depressive symptoms, and a depressed child may be excessively preoccupied with feelings of guilt or low self-esteem associated with the soiling.

SEXUAL ABUSE

One specific often overlooked and underreported association with encopresis is sexual abuse, especially if associated with anal penetration. The physical trauma can lead to painful defecation and this, in turn, induces stool retention. In some cases, posttraumatic stress disorder can follow the immediate emotional trauma and complicate the course of encopresis.

The co-occurrence of encopresis and sexual abuse has been described by several authors (Dawson et al 1990, Boon 1991, Feehan 1995). In one study, 36 per cent of abused boys had encopresis (Morrow et al 1997). Other symptoms can also be present: thus, among males with repeated abuse, 24 to 90 per cent had signs and symptoms of encopresis, enuresis, dysuria, rectal impaction, anal erythema, fissures, tears and hyperpigmentation (Holmes and Slap 1998). In girls, vaginal pain, dysuria and frequency were common (Kleran and De Jong 1990). It is very important for the clinician to identify these children, protect them from possible ongoing abuse and provide professional child psychiatric care.

M.T., 10-year-old boy
Diagnoses: Secondary encopresis with constipation;
atypical eating disorder (F 50.8); moderate depressive
episode (F 32.1); recurrent sexual abuse

M. had started to soil again at the age of 8 years. He was constipated and the stool was of hard consistency. He refused to eat and lost weight. He withdrew socially, daydreamed and was very depressed affectively. His father was in prison after having sexually abused M. and his sister over several years.

On physical examination, abdominal masses were palpable, the anus was abnormally relaxed, and the rectum was filled with stool masses, which could be seen on ultrasound as well. His mental state examination showed overt signs of depression. Intelligence was in the normal range (IQ 93).

Because of the eating problems, as well as the depressive disorder, inpatient child psychiatric treatment became necessary. Disimpaction was initiated with three enemas. M. was sent to the toilet regularly and was given one tablespoon of lactulose three times a day. Intensive play therapy was conducted, with a marked reduction of emotional symptoms. After his father was convicted, M. was able to relax further. Due to neglect and inconsistent child rearing practices, M. could not return to his mother after leaving hospital. He was therefore placed in a children's home.

In this case, the psychiatric disorder, as well as the constipation and encopresis, was a consequence of the sexual abuse – a connection which is often overlooked.

Other psychological interpretations and models

Without any doubt, mental health disorders and psychological factors play an important role in the development and course of encopresis – much more so than in nocturnal enuresis and daytime urinary incontinence. The comorbid disorders are heterogeneous, i.e. there is no disorder that is specific for encopresis, nor is there any personality type typical for this disorder. Due to this heterogeneity, different models are needed to understand the association of encopresis and psychological factors.

LEARNING THEORY

The most common model is that of learning theory. Put simply, encopresis is seen as acquired, learned behaviour in disposed individuals. Once a certain behaviour is elicited, this is reinforced by positive effects (such as not having to go to the toilet during play), as well as by evading negative consequences (such as avoiding pain by postponing defecation). Encopresis can also elicit negative parental reactions, which means the child gets more attention. This 'vicious cycle' of interaction can be perpetuated by increasing intrafamilial conflicts.

Most treatment approaches for encopresis are based on learning theory. Cognitive-behavioural treatments have been shown to be the most effective for the symptoms of encopresis.

PSYCHODYNAMIC THEORIES

Psychodynamic theories interpret encopresis as an expression of unconscious conflicts. Psychoanalysts have seen encopresis as a manifestation of unconscious aggression or anxiety, as a sign of regression (returning to an earlier stage of cognitive development), as separation anxiety and as a drive for autonomy (Krisch 1985). In an interesting series of cases, it was shown that encopresis can be a conscious act in some children, who use the faecal masses for self-stimulation or 'anal masturbation' (Aruffo et al 2000).

These hypotheses are no longer tenable as general explanations for all cases of encopresis. They can, in individual cases, be helpful in understanding possible intrapsychic and intrafamilial dynamics. But even if the original conflict can be understood in these terms, once the symptom is present it often becomes an acquired, learned habit that persists even after the original conflict has been resolved (Krisch 1985, Cox et al 1998). Psychodynamic treatment approaches are indicated when comorbid emotional (internalizing) disorders coexist. An understanding of psychodynamics can also be very useful therapeutically in comprehending the subjective experience of the child – even if cognitive-behavioural approaches are being used as the mainline treatment.

FAMILY DYNAMICS

Family dynamics theories try to understand and interpret encopresis in terms of family interaction. Parents of children with encopresis are usually stressed and worried about the problem (Bernard-Bonnin et al 1993). But are families with encopretic children more disturbed? In one study, children with encopresis had family environments with less expressiveness and poorer organization than the family environments of controls (Cox et al 2002).

In another study of 104 families, nearly half (51) had no unusual family problems; 23 families had severe and widespread difficulties, including sexual abuse; 11 families described moderate difficulties and 18 a single traumatic event (Silver 1996). In other words, the atmosphere was warm and supportive without major difficulties in at least half of the families.

Without a doubt, families need to be included in treatment. In a retrospective study, the inclusion of family therapy techniques led to a better outcome in treating encopresis than treatment without these techniques in controls (Silver et al 1998).

Aetiology

Encopresis is clearly a heterogeneous disorder with a multifactorial aetiology. This involves psychological, genetic and somatic factors. In this section, the basic aetiological and pathophysiological mechanisms for encopresis in general will be reviewed. Specific aspects of the subtypes of encopresis will be discussed in later sections.

GENETICS

So far, no molecular genetic studies have been conducted for encopresis. Formal genetic approaches have included several empirical family studies and only one twin study (Bakwin and Davidson 1971). Formal genetics have shown four definite tendencies:

1   Encopresis has a clear genetic basis and is not a purely acquired disorder.
2   The penetrance (i.e. the proportion of those with a genetic predisposition actually expressing the phenotype of encopresis) shows a clear sex difference: not only are more boys affected by encopresis, but male relatives more often have a history of soiling than females.
3   Encopresis with constipation seems to have a higher genetic basis – the genetically determined phenotype is most likely to be constipation and not the encopresis itself. Recently, genetically determined subtypes such as 'slow transit constipation' have been identified (Hutson et al 2004).
4   Finally, although no systematic segregation analyses have been performed, a polygenic-multifactorial mode of transmission is most likely (i.e. there is no evidence for a clear monogenic mode of inheritance). In other words, several genes act in interaction with environmental factors. If a sufficient number of genes are involved and the threshold for a disease is transgressed, the phenotype becomes apparent. If the additive genetic effect is below the threshold, the disorder is not manifested (Harper 1982). As the threshold can vary between the sexes, this could explain why boys have a higher rate of encopresis.

EMPIRICAL FAMILY STUDIES

In a pilot study of 186 children, 6.9 per cent of fathers, 1.1 per cent of mothers and 1.6 per cent of brothers also soiled (Bellman 1966). In a population-based 'clientele study' of 75 boys, encopresis was reported among 15 per cent of fathers, 1.3 per cent of mothers and 8.7 per cent of brothers, while none of the relatives of the 73 controls were affected (Bellman 1966). In a study of 50 children with encopresis without constipation, 15 per cent of all relatives were constipated (Benninga et al 1994). In another study of 71 children, 23 per cent of all relatives showed a 'positive family history' (Van der Plas et al 1997).

The rates of affected relatives for children with encopresis with constipation were higher. In a study of 111 children, 42 per cent of relatives were constipated (Benninga et al 1994). And finally, in a study of 234 children, there was a 'family history' of nocturnal enuresis in 14 per cent, of encopresis in 15 per cent, and of constipation in 26 per cent (Loening-Baucke 1997).

TWIN STUDY

The genetic predisposition towards constipation was addressed in the only twin study to date (Bakwin and Davidson 1971). The study found that 59 (8.7 per cent) of 676 twins were constipated. The concordance rate for monozygotic twins was 70 per cent, and for dizygotic twins 18 per cent – a highly significant difference (p <0.005). The recurrence risk for a child to be affected was high, if the parents had constipation. The recurrence risk was 26 per cent if one parent was affected, 46 per cent if both parents were affected, 40 per cent if the father, and 19 per cent if the mother was affected – compared to 3.2 per cent if neither of the parents had been constipated. These formal genetic results show clearly that the primary phenotype is most likely to be constipation – with the soiling representing a secondary effect of stool retention.

METABOLIC AND ENDOCRINOLOGICAL FINDINGS

To discover if gastrointestinal motility was influenced by gastrointestinal hormones, 10 encopretic patients were compared to controls (Stern et al 1995). There were two significant differences: in encopretic children, postprandial levels of pancreatic polypeptide remained consistently higher and peaked earlier, while the motilin response was significantly lower. It is not known if these differences are a cause of encopresis by lowering gastrointestinal motility, or if they are a secondary result of the condition.

Encopresis also seems to affect breath methane production. Methane is an odourless gas, which is produced solely by colonic anaerobic bacteria. Most children do not excrete methane until their teenage years. In one study, 65 per cent of children with encopresis, but only 15 per cent of controls, excreted methane (Fiedorek et al 1990). After successful treatment, this was reversible, with many children no longer excreting methane. In contrast, the prevalence of methane production among constipated children (11 per cent) was not very different from that of healthy subjects (7 per cent). In this case the phenotype of encopresis (but not of constipation) is associated with methane production, possibly due to differences in colonic flora.

MANOMETRY

Ever since the 1980s, manometric studies have been conducted, especially among children with encopresis and constipation (Loening-Baucke and Cruikshank 1986). The main, consistent parameter that could be shown repeatedly in studies was a paradoxical contraction of the external anal sphincter during defecation. This sphincter spasm correlates highly with the frequency of faecal soiling, age at onset and duration of symptoms (Borowitz et al 1996). In addition to this main finding, other parameters were affected in children with encopresis and constipation: the gradient between rectal and sphincter pressure during attempted defecation, the critical distending volume for faecal urgency, and the ability to defecate a water-filled balloon (Sutphen et al 1997).

Again, it is not clear if these differences are a cause or a secondary effect of encopresis and constipation. Following these promising diagnostic results, manometric biofeedback programmes were instituted for children with encopresis. Unfortunately, the outcome results were far less positive than anticipated, and biofeedback is no longer recommended as a first-line treatment for children with encopresis.

In fact, not even the presence of a paradoxical constriction of the external anal sphincter has an influence on treatment outcome (Brooks et al 2000). The results and recommendations will be discussed later in this chapter, under the specific syndromes.

PERIPHERAL AND CENTRAL NERVOUS SYSTEM FACTORS

In addition to local gastrointestinal factors, the central nervous system (CNS) plays a decisive role in functional disorders of the gastrointestinal tract. In contrast to other organ systems, the gastrointestinal system has a separate local 'enteric nervous system' (ENS) (Wood 1994). This is an independent integrative system with structural and functional properties similar to those of the central nervous system – a 'mini-brain' placed in close proximity to the effector system it controls (Wood 1994).

Only 10 per cent of the interaction between the CNS and ENS is efferent; 90 per cent represents sensory pathways activated by the mechano-, chemo- and thermo-receptors, projecting to the dorsal root ganglion of the vagus nerve, the nucleus tractus solitarius (NTS) and the dorsal motor vagus nucleus (DMVN). From the brainstem, information is led to higher centres of the CNS (hypothalamus and limbic system) and finally to the cortex (Frieling 1993). This extensive interaction between the ENS and CNS is responsible for the bidirectional influences of emotions and gut: emotions can have a direct influence on the gastrointestinal tract; conversely, even primary organic diseases can affect psychological well-being (Frieling 1993).

The neurophysiological methods employed so far have been relatively unspecific but have nonetheless provided interesting insights. Thus, the rate of pathological electroencephalograms (EEGs) among encopretic children ranged from 21 per cent (Bellman 1966) to 37 per cent (von Gontard and Hollmann 2004), 40 per cent (Mehler-Wex et al 2005) and 78 per cent (Fehlow 1991). The EEG abnormalities consisted mainly of general anomalies of background frequency, abnormal beta or theta activity, and focal changes, and only rarely of spikes and sharp waves (von Gontard et al 1999e). The differences between the studies are due to selection effects, and technical and evaluation differences. They indicate an involvement of the CNS in a very unspecific way.

Regarding afferences, the function of peripheral somatic nerves is not affected. The pudendal nerve latency did not differ in encopretic children compared to controls (Sentovich et al 1998). In contrast, afferences measured with somato-sensory evoked potentials are affected. Thus, evoked potentials (measured over the centrally placed electrode Cz) did not differ in encopretic children compared to controls if the posterior tibial nerve was stimulated, but did differ with electrical stimulation of the anal canal, suggesting that rectal mucosal perception might be disturbed in children with chronic constipation (Kubota et al 1997). Cerebral evoked potentials (measured from Cz to Fz) were also evoked by rapid balloon distension in the rectum (Loening-Baucke and Yamada 1995). Children with encopresis and chronic constipation had significantly prolonged latencies of both the early-onset evoked potentials (N1 and P2) and the late-onset evoked potentials (NI, PI, NII). The results suggest a defect in the afferent pathway from the rectum in children with chronic constipation and encopresis (Loening-Baucke and Yamada 1995).

In addition, the processing of afferent stimuli in the brainstem has been investigated in animal studies. Thus, the distension of bladder, colon, rectum and even stomach can elicit electrophysiological activity of the noradrenergic neurons of the locus coeruleus (Elam et al 1986). This finding was replicated by Lechner et al (1997), showing that mechanical stimulation of the colon leads to specific activation of the locus coeruleus. The locus coeruleus contains 70 per cent of all noradrenergic neurons of the CNS and is involved in the activation of arousal and also attentional processes. It plays a decisive role in the pathophysiology of nocturnal enuresis, which is characterized by a deficit of arousal during sleep. In addition, children with nocturnal enuresis show a failure to inhibit micturition during sleep, which is transmitted by the pontine micturition centre (PMC). Another interesting animal study showed that the PMC is activated by distension of the colon as well (Pavcovich et al 1998). According to these findings, there is not only an extensive interaction between the brain and gut, but also between the brain, gut and bladder, which might explain the high comorbidity of enuresis, urinary incontinence and encopresis.

General approaches in assessment
The assessment of children with encopresis should be as short and as non-invasive as possible, and as thorough as necessary. Parents or other caregivers should always be included. For most children, a basic approach is sufficient. In complicated cases, further diagnostic procedures may be necessary. If indicated, these should be performed promptly and should not be postponed.

In the assessment of encopresis with constipation, one should bear in mind that an organic cause is responsible for a maximum of 5 per cent of all cases of faecal incontinence. The rate is even lower in children with encopresis without constipation, possibly as low as 1 per cent. In other words, in more than 95 per cent of children their encopresis will not have an organic cause, and the figure is 99 per cent in the case of encopresis without constipation. On the other hand, 40 per cent of children show clinically relevant comorbid emotional and behavioural symptoms and disorders. The assessment should focus on both somatic and psychological aspects, with the following goals:

1   Identification of the subtype of encopresis
2   Exclusion of organic faecal incontinence
3   Diagnosis of comorbid urinary incontinence or enuresis
4   Diagnosis of comorbid psychological symptoms or disorders
5   Formulation of a treatment plan
6   Motivation of child and family to comply with treatment

Standard assessment
The standard assessment steps, which should be included in every case, and the extended assessment, if there are special indications, are shown in Table 9.10.

HISTORY OF ENCOPRESIS
The history is the most important aspect of assessment. If conducted correctly and empathically, the most relevant information will be gathered through the history. Therefore history taking will be discussed in greater detail.

Both parents and child are usually present during history taking. This not only saves time, but gives the opportunity to hear both the child's and the parents' point of view, which

TABLE 9.10
Standard and extended assessment of encopresis

Standard assessment (sufficient for most cases of encopresis)
History
Physical examination
Sonography (not available in all centres)
Questionnaires and charts
Screening for behavioural disorders

Extended assessment (only if indicated)
Stool bacteriology
Radiology:
    Plain abdominal X-ray
    Colon contrast X-ray
    MRI of colon
Manometry
Endoscopy and biopsy
Full child psychiatric assessment

---

can differ greatly. Also, the parent–child interaction can be observed. The history follows the same sequence as the encopresis questionnaire (see Appendix 4) so that the two can be compared.

- *Reason for presentation*: Does the child knows why he is here? Is it because he soils his pants? Does he want to talk about it?
- *Frequency of encopresis*: Does the child soil during the day? How often does he soil during the day (i.e. how many days per week; days per month)? How many times does he soil per day? At what time of day does the child usually soil (during the morning, around noon, in the afternoon, evening)? Does the child soil during the night? How often does he soil during the night?
- *Encopresis symptoms*: If the child soils, how large are the stool masses (only smearing; smearing and stool masses; only stool masses)? What is the consistency of the child's stool (hard, soft, watery – or seven different consistencies according to the Bristol Stool Form Scale – see Fig. 9.1)? In which situations does the child soil? Does he soil in stressful situations? Can he postpone defecating if no toilet is available, e.g. while travelling in the car? If yes, how long?
- *Relapses*: Has the child ever had a period without soiling? If yes, what was the longest period? At what age did it occur? Was there a reason for the relapse (e.g. constipation, diarrhoea, pain while defecating, going to kindergarten, going to school, birth of a sibling, separation of parents, other life events)?
- *Toileting behaviour*: Does the child wear a diaper? If yes, when (during the daytime, night-time, both day- and night-time)? On how many days per week does the child pass stools into the toilet? How many times a day does the child defecate? How large are the stool masses in the toilet? Does the child have to be sent to the toilet? If yes, how does he react? Does the child take enough time going to the toilet? If yes, how long? Does the child play or read while sitting on the toilet?

- *Associated symptoms*: Does the child go to the toilet regularly at certain times of the day? If yes, when? Does the child have difficulty passing stools? Does he have to strain? Is it possible that the child is actively resisting the urge to defecate? Is defecation painful for the child? What is the consistency of the stools in the toilet (hard, soft, watery, with different consistencies, with blood – see Bristol Stool Form Scale)? Does the child have stomach or abdominal pains? How often does he have abdominal pains? How strong are the abdominal pains? When does he experience stomach pains? Before or after meals? Are they relieved after going to the toilet? Does the child pass wind?
- *Perceptions and reactions after soiling*: Does the child notice when he has soiled? Do the parents notice when the child has soiled? How do they notice it? Does the child tell his parents when he has soiled? If no, does the child try to conceal it? Does the child hide his underpants? How does the child react when he has soiled (indifferent, no reaction, sad, anxious, disappointed, ashamed, desperate, angry, other reactions)? Who removes the stools from the clothing (or the bed)? Does the child suffer emotionally due to the soiling? If yes, how intensely? How does this distress show? Is the child motivated for treatment?
- *Reaction of parents and others in the child's environment*: How do the parents react when the child has soiled? Are they distressed by their child's soiling? If yes, how intensely? Have they punished the child because of his soiling? Do they think that the child soils on purpose? Who else knows that the child soils? Has the child been rejected because of his soiling? If yes, how? How often does this occur? Has the child not been able to take part in activities because of his soiling? If yes, which activities (school outings, swimming, others)? Does the child engage in sports? If yes, what types of sports?
- *Eating and drinking habits*: How much fluid does the child drink per day? Does the child prefer to eat low-fibre foods? If yes, which? Does the child prefer to eat other specific types of foods? If yes, which?
- *Previous forms of treatment*: Does the child take laxatives? If yes, which? How long has he been taking them? Has the child been examined because of his soiling? If yes, where and when? Has the child been operated on because of his soiling? If yes, where and when? What have the parents done personally to treat the soiling?
- *Family history*: Has anyone else in the family soiled? Has any member of the family been affected by constipation? Night-time or daytime wetting? Has anyone had illnesses of the kidneys, stomach or gut?

The history should then follow the format outlined for enuresis and functional incontinence regarding comorbid wetting, as well as behavioural and emotional symptoms and disorders.

ENCOPRESIS QUESTIONNAIRES

The information gathered in the history taking can be complemented by questionnaires specifically designed to assess encopresis. In the Appendices, there are examples of two different questionnaires: a longer questionnaire that contains all relevant questions (Appendix 4), and a screening questionnaire that contains the most important questions (Appendix 5; von Gontard 2004).

Recently, the Virginia Encopresis Constipation Apperception Test (VECAT), a validated, picture-based questionnaire for children and parents, was shown to differentiate well regarding bowel-specific problems (Cox et al 2003). A health-related quality of life questionnaire with good psychometric properties has also been described. The Defecation Disorder List (DDL) consists of 37 items and can be used in children with all types of encopresis and/or constipation (Voskuijl et al 2004b).

The Bristol Stool Form Scale has been very useful in clinical practice (Fig. 9.1). Seven types of stool forms are described, ranging from 'separate hard lumps, like nuts (hard to pass)' (type 1) to 'watery, no solid pieces, entirely liquid' (type 7). The scale enables parents and children to identify the predominant type of stools very easily, without lengthy descriptions. The course of treatment can also be monitored using this scale.

CHARTS

If a child has both encopresis and enuresis/urinary incontinence, a toilet protocol can be very useful. Parents are asked to measure the volume of fluids drunk, as well as the volume of urine passed. The volumes are documented on a chart (see Appendix 2). Also, any episodes of wetting, defecation on the toilet, and soiling, as well as other symptoms, are documented.

BEHAVIOURAL QUESTIONNAIRES

Because of the high comorbidity, we recommend that psychological symptoms be screened in all children with encopresis. The most widely used questionnaire is the Child Behavioral Checklist (CBCL/4–18) by Achenbach (1991). This questionnaire comes in different versions for preschool children (CBCL/1½; C-TRF), for adolescents (YSR), for teachers (TRF) and even for young adults (YABCL and YASR).

MENTAL STATE EXAMINATION

Again, because of the high comorbidity, the child's behaviour, parent–child interaction and any other psychopathological signs should be observed and documented by trained professionals. One widely used instrument is the CASCAP (Döpfner et al 1999).

PAEDIATRIC EXAMINATION

Every child should undergo a complete paediatric and neurological examination. Abdominally, spleen and liver should be palpated; distension of the abdomen, abdominal sounds and palpable stool masses should be noted. The perianal and perigenital region should be examined in detail. A rectal examination may be indicated in order to differentiate between encopresis with and without constipation. The child should be informed and prepared before rectal examination. In some situations it may be appropriate to postpone the rectal and perianal examination to a later time. Neurologically, the spinal cord, reflex differences and asymmetries of the buttocks should be looked for. If indicated, the anal and cremaster reflex can be elicited, but this is not necessary routinely.

THE BRISTOL STOOL FORM SCALE

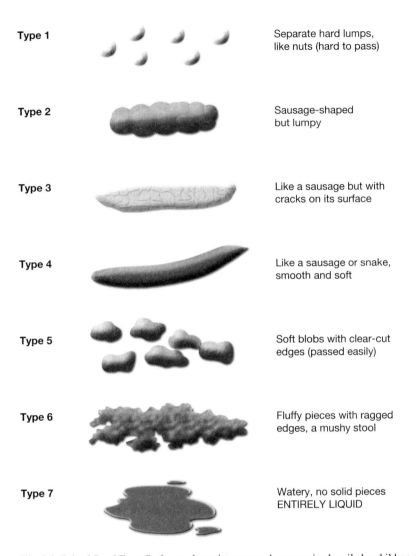

Type 1		Separate hard lumps, like nuts (hard to pass)
Type 2		Sausage-shaped but lumpy
Type 3		Like a sausage but with cracks on its surface
Type 4		Like a sausage or snake, smooth and soft
Type 5		Soft blobs with clear-cut edges (passed easily)
Type 6		Fluffy pieces with ragged edges, a mushy stool
Type 7		Watery, no solid pieces ENTIRELY LIQUID

Fig. 9.1 Bristol Stool Form Scale: stool consistency can be recognized easily by children and parents.

Ultrasound

As in the case of urinary incontinence/enuresis, traditions and strategies differ between countries and centres regarding the question of whether or not to use abdominal ultrasound routinely in the evaluation of encopresis or constipation. Not all experts consider ultrasound indispensable, but useful information can certainly be obtained. The liver, spleen, kidneys, urinary tract and bladder are all visualized by abdominal ultrasound, but the retrovesical area is of special interest. If a child is constipated and has retained stools, retrovesical impressions can often be seen. Also, the diameters of the rectum and sigmoid are often enlarged and can be measured. If urinary incontinence coexists, the bladder wall may be thickened and the child may show signs of residual urine.

Sonography can also be used therapeutically as a form of biofeedback training. Children can be shown how distended their rectum is. After treatment with laxatives and stool regulation, the reduction of the rectal diameter can be seen.

Extended assessment

Usually, these basic steps are sufficient in the assessment of children with encopresis. If there is any sign of a possible organic cause of faecal incontinence, further diagnostic steps may be necessary. Children with encopresis and constipation may require a more detailed and invasive type of diagnostics than encopretic children without constipation, as organic causes are more common in the former.

Possible signs that may be indicative of organic disease have been listed by Baker et al (1999): failure to thrive, abdominal distension, lack of lumbosacral curve, pilonidal dimple covered by a tuft of hair, midline pigmentary abnormalities of the lower spine, sacral agenesis, flat buttocks, anteriorly displaced anus, tight empty rectum in the presence of palpable abdominal faecal mass, gush of liquid stool and air from rectum on withdrawal of finger, occult blood in stool, absent cremaster reflex, decreased lower extremity tone and/or strength, absence or delay in relaxation phase of lower extremity deep tendon reflexes. In these cases a detailed assessment is necessary.

LABORATORY EXAMINATIONS

Depending on history and other physical signs, laboratory tests, including electrolytes, thyroid parameters and gliadin or transglutaminase antibodies (if celiac disease is suspected), as well as sweat tests or the measurement of elastase in faeces (cystic fibrosis), can be indicated (Buderus 2002). Stool bacteriology is recommended if a gastrointestinal infection is suspected. If a child has additional wetting problems, urine screening, as well as urine microscopy and bacteriology, may be necessary.

RADIOLOGICAL EXAMINATIONS

To measure transit time, radio-opaque markers can be given and an abdominal X-ray is performed on the first and fourth day (Benninga et al 2004). The transit time is calculated from the distribution of the markers (Buderus 2002). Only a few authors recommend plain abdominal X-rays to detect coprostasis (Youssef and Di Lorenzo 2001). Generally, plain abdominal X-rays should not be performed routinely, as the information from transit-time examinations is more relevant, and coprostasis alone can usually be detected by a good clinical examination.

Finally, radiological examination of the lower gastrointestinal tract with contrast media can be indicated in the assessment of Hirschsprung disease and in other malformations. It is no longer performed routinely in encopresis with constipation but only if organic causes of faecal incontinence or constipation are suspected (Buderus 2002).

236

MRI

If tethered-cord syndrome, spinal dysraphism or other malformations of the spinal cord are suspected or need to be excluded, MRI of the spinal canal is indicated. Routine MRI examinations in children with encopresis are not indicated or useful, as rectal dilatation and stool impaction can be detected by other means.

BIOPSY AND ENDOSCOPY

To exclude Hirschsprung disease and other intestinal diseases, a biopsy can be indicated. Also, endoscopy is indicated if other diseases of the lower gastrointestinal tract need to be excluded.

MANOMETRY

Anorectal manometry is performed by inserting balloon-catheters. Pressure curves and elicited rectoanal reflexes are documented. The most important and consistent manometric finding in children with constipation is a paradoxical contraction of the external anal sphincter during defecation. Manometry is not routinely indicated in encopretic or constipated children, but is needed when Hirschsprung disease is suspected.

OTHER FORMS OF ASSESSMENT

In certain cases, specific investigations such as 8-canal manometry, electromyography and endorectal sonography can be indicated (Schuster and Kellnar 1997). In comorbid, complicated forms of urinary incontinence, a detailed urodynamic investigation may be necessary.

ADDITIONAL PSYCHIATRIC ASSESSMENT

If a manifest emotional or behavioural disorder is present, a more detailed assessment should be performed by a child psychiatrist. In addition to a detailed history regarding behavioural symptoms and a mental state examination, general and specific questionnaires regarding behaviour can be useful. Specific instruments include questionnaires regarding depression, tics, obsessions and compulsions, as well as general domains such as self-esteem.

Formal psychological testing is necessary to assess general cognitive level, as well as specific developmental aspects. This may be indicated in case of school failure or if specific developmental disorders such as dyslexia or dyscalculia are suspected. In addition, projective tests, family assessment and other tests may provide important information.

All of these diagnostic steps should be performed in an outpatient setting, if possible. Day-clinic or inpatient care may become necessary in severe cases with comorbid emotional or behavioural disorders, or in certain situations such as suspected sexual abuse.

General approaches to treatment

Treatment should be symptom-oriented and tailored specifically to the type of encopresis, which means that a detailed diagnostic assessment is mandatory. The specific therapeutic steps will be presented in each section separately. However, certain general principles should be followed in all forms of encopresis. The basic approach in treatment has been outlined in several sets of guidelines (Baker et al 1999, Felt et al 1999, von Gontard et al 2006b). The essential points are psychoeducation, demystification and stool regulation.

The provision of information regarding the type of encopresis is of great importance. Many children and parents are not aware that constipation and retention of stool can be the main cause of encopresis – rather than an insufficiency of the anal sphincter, as they presume. The fact that genetic factors can play a role in constipation is a source of great relief to parents. Many parents are also unaware of the possible association with behavioural and emotional disorders in many, but not all, children. In addition to the provision of information, feelings of guilt, parental attributions ('my child is doing this on purpose') and parental frustration or anger can be verbalized. Ineffective parental interventions such as punishment or non-indicated medication can be discussed with parents. Feelings of shame and low self-esteem in children are often relieved when they talk about them. Real information can be provided during this process and erroneous ideas corrected. Levine (1991) described this approach as a process of demystification.

The main treatment approach is that of stool regulation. Children are asked to go to the toilet three times a day after mealtimes. This period of time is especially useful as the postprandial defecation reflexes are then most active. Children are asked to sit on the toilet in a relaxed manner for five to ten minutes. To be relaxed, it is important that their feet touch the floor when they sit on the toilet. A foot-stool should be provided if needed. These toilet sessions should be a positive experience: children should be allowed to read comics and books, play with game-boys, sing songs, etc. They do not need to pass urine or stools every time. The toilet sessions are documented on a chart (see Appendix 14). If necessary, the child's cooperation can be enhanced by a simple token system with small rewards. All negative criticism or punishment should be avoided.

If the child's food intake is restricted to low-fibre foods, or he or she drinks an excessive amount of cow's milk, a change in diet can be useful. Also, the amount of fluids may need to be increased, as many children do not drink enough during the day.

These simple measures are highly effective and should be started directly after the diagnostic steps have been completed. A simple 'baseline' with observation but without intervention, which is very useful in nocturnal enuresis, is not recommended in encopresis. In a study of 54 children aged 5–14 years with encopresis with and without constipation, these measures were recommended: eight (15 per cent) of the children became completely free of soiling within six weeks – after a single contact with the doctor. Six of these eight children remained free of soiling even after one year (Van der Plas et al 1997).

Additional treatment components

If encopresis with constipation is present, laxative treatment is indicated and useful in most children. If, however, no constipation or retention is present, laxatives are contraindicated as they can worsen the soiling (Benninga et al 1994). Biofeedback treatment is not effective in encopresis, with or without constipation (Brazelli and Griffiths 2002).

If a manifest behavioural or emotional disorder is present, child psychiatric assessment and specific treatment are indicated. In all cases, even with behavioural comorbidity, encopresis should be treated in a symptom-oriented way. However, in the case of the behavioural disturbances, compliance with treatment may be lower (Nolan et al 1991). The behavioural or emotional disorder will therefore require separate treatment.

In contrast, routine general psychotherapy is not effective in the treatment of encopresis, according to a systematic review (Brooks et al 2000). All symptom-oriented approaches basically represent cognitive-behavioural types of treatment. The addition of other, even short-term, focal forms of psychotherapy does not yield better results than the basic treatment approaches alone (Brooks et al 2000).

Most studies on the treatment of encopresis are non-randomized, non-controlled studies with positive effects between 43 and 100 per cent. Nine randomized, controlled studies (RCT) have been conducted in school-age children, but none so far in preschool children. In general, medical-behavioural or behavioural approaches alone are similarly effective in RCTs, according to the meta-analysis of Brooks et al (2000). The paradoxical contraction of the external anal sphincter had no predictive value for treatment outcome. In another meta-analysis of 42 randomized, controlled studies, four types of treatment were categorized as 'probably efficacious', and three were identified as 'promising' methods of treatment (McGrath et al 2000). No specific type of therapy fulfilled the criteria for the highest category of 'empirically supported therapies' according to Chambless and Hollon (1998).

In summary, only a few treatment recommendations are based on the highest level of evidence (i.e. at least one good randomized, controlled study); many recommendations are still based on the lowest grade of evidence, such as clinical experience, descriptive studies and recommendation of experts (Baker et al 1999). Specific treatment recommendations will be presented in the following sections.

Functional faecal incontinence (encopresis) with constipation

DEFINITION
(Other terms used to describe this condition are: encopresis with constipation and overflow incontinence; constipation-associated faecal incontinence; and retentive encopresis.)

One of the two most important forms of soiling is encopresis with constipation or stool retention. Encopresis with constipation is defined as voluntary or involuntary passage of faeces in non-appropriate places after the age of 4 years with clear evidence of comorbid constipation. Specifically, chronic (and not acute) constipation is associated with soiling.

Acute constipation is quite common in infancy and affects up to 16 per cent of all 22-month-old children (Loening-Baucke 1994). This type of constipation is transitory and resolves spontaneously in most children. A few, however, develop a chronic course. Thus, 3 per cent of all preschool children and 1–2 per cent of all school children are affected by chronic constipation. In younger children there is no major sex difference, while more boys are affected from school age onwards. In many cases, this development is overlooked and constipation is not diagnosed until one to five years later on average (Felt et al 1999). Fortunately, children are now being referred at an earlier age. Thus, the average age for referral has fallen from 9.7 years to 6.5 years in the past 20 years (Fishman et al 2003). As will be outlined in this section, the diagnosis of constipation is very important since specific treatment is required.

DEFINITION OF CHRONIC CONSTIPATION

As has been shown in epidemiological studies, most children from the age of 4 onwards pass stools once a day on average – with great interindividual variability (Weaver 1988). Therefore, constipation was originally defined as passing stools three times or less per week. This purely frequency-based definition is not sufficient, as some children are heavily constipated, but still go to the toilet regularly every day. Therefore, other clinical signs are needed as additional criteria, such as painful defecation, palpable abdominal masses, hard stool masses during rectal examination, abdominal pain, and typical ultrasound findings such as enlarged rectal diameter and retrovesical impressions.

In summary, constipation is a clinical diagnosis, based on multiple symptoms, as reflected by the definition of the American Association of Pediatric Gastroenterology: constipation is defined as 'a delay or difficulty in defecation, present for two or more weeks and sufficient to cause significant distress' (Baker et al 1999). The most practical definition was proposed by the PACCT Group, as summarized in Table 9.5 (PACCT 2005).

Constipation in different age groups

Differences between constipation in children and adults have to be considered before arriving at a diagnosis. As shown in Table 9.11, there are major differences regarding various aspects of symptoms (Youssef and Di Lorenzo 2001).

In children, more boys are affected; constipation typically starts during toilet training or when starting school. During defecation, children retain stools and soiling is common; constipation is only rarely due to medical diseases or pharmacological side effects. Hirschsprung disease has to be excluded. Dietary changes are often not sufficient as the only mode of treatment; biofeedback is seldom effective; and surgery is usually not indicated. But even in childhood there are major changes in the developmental course from infancy to adolescence. The official classification of defecation syndromes (Rome-II criteria) is set out in Table 9.12. This represents preliminary attempts at classification by paediatric gastroenterologists.

Infant dyschezia begins in infants aged 6 months or younger (Rasquin-Weber et al 1999). Despite soft or fluid stools, they cry and scream for at least 10 minutes a day – probably due to a dyscoordination of increased intra-abdominal pressure and relaxation of the pelvic floor. As this disorder usually resolves without further treatment, parental counselling and advice is sufficient treatment.

Functional constipation starts in children under 5 years of age with a stool frequency of two times, or less, per week. Quite often, symptoms begin at the end of breast feeding when cow's milk products are introduced. Functional constipation is treated by stool softeners such as lactulose or fruit juices, thus avoiding painful defecation.

TABLE 9.11
Comparison of children and adults with constipation (Youssef and Di Lorenzo 2001)

	Children	Adults
More common in	Males	Females
Initial presentation	Toilet training, starting school	Adolescence, young adulthood
Defecation behaviour	Withholding	Straining
Encopresis	Common	Rare
Secondary to systemic disease or use of medications	Rare	Common
Indication for barium enema	To rule out Hirschsprung disease	To rule out intraluminal lesion
Effect of high-fibre diet	Rarely helpful	Helpful
Role of biofeedback	Controversial	Benefit in pelvic floor dyssynergia
Role of surgery	Not indicated in functional defecation disorders	May help in slow transit constipation (selected patients)

TABLE 9.12
Childhood functional defecation disorders: Rome-II diagnostic criteria
(according to Youssef and Di Lorenzo 2001 and Rasquin-Weber et al 1999)

Infant dyschezia	Functional constipation	Functional faecal retention
Age less than 6 months	Infants and preschool children	Infants to 16 years of age
At least 10 minutes of straining and crying	For at least 2 weeks, majority of stools hard, rock-like; stools are	For at least 12 weeks, passage of large-diameter stools at intervals of
Successful passage of soft stools in an otherwise healthy infant	passed <=2/wk; no evidence of structural, endocrine, or metabolic disease	<= 2/wk; retentive posturing, avoiding defecation using both pelvic floor and gluteal msucles

Finally, *functional stool retention*, i.e. chronic constipation, is typical for the whole of childhood and adolescence. It quite often develops as a result of acute constipation, especially if associated with painful defecation. Children avoid passing stools and enter into a vicious cycle of retention and accumulation of stool masses. The soiling is a consequence of the retention.

Differential diagnosis of constipation
Constipation in children is due to organic causes in only 5 per cent of cases. In other words, in the overwhelming majority (95 per cent) it is a purely functional disorder with no underlying medical disease. The diseases that need to be excluded in these 5 per cent of children are summarized in Table 9.13. The broad categories to be considered are anatomical, metabolic, endocrine, neurogenic, neuropathic and pharmacological causes.

The most common medical cause is anal fissures associated with painful defecation. In one retrospective study of children with chronic constipation, 63 per cent had a history of painful defecation (Partin et al 1992). Anorectal malformations need to be excluded, but are much less common, with a prevalence of 1 in 8000. Rarely, idiopathic congenital megacolon

241

TABLE 9.13
Differential diagnosis of organic causes of chronic constipation
(according to Youssef and Di Lorenzo 2001, Felt et al 1999, Hatch 1988)

Anatomic
Anal fissures, abscess, skin tags, dermatitis, anal stenosis, other anorectal malformations (e.g. anterior displaced anus), acquired strictures from inflammatory bowel disease or necrotizing enterocolitis, idiopathic megacolon

Metabolic
Hypokalemia, hypomagnesemia, hypophosphatemia, hypercalcaemia, cystic fibrosis, celiac disease, cow's milk intolerance/allergy

Endocrine
Diabetes mellitus, multiple endocrine neoplasia IIb, hypothyroidism, hyperparathyroidism, diabetes insipidus

Neuropathic
Cerebral palsy, spina bifida

Colonic neuropathies
Hirschsprung disease, intestinal neuronal dysplasia, pseudo-obstruction, others

Drugs
Anticholinergics, antidepressants, antihypertensives, opiates, iron, chemotherapeutic agents (vincristine), anticonvulsants, lead intoxication

---

can affect children with constipation from infancy onwards (Gattuso and Kamm 1997, Gattuso et al 1997). In addition, constipation can be caused by a variety of metabolic and endocrine diseases, such as diabetes mellitus and hypothyroidism. Neurogenic diseases such as spina bifida and tethered-cord syndrome need to be excluded. Intestinal disorders of motility (Koletzko 2002), as well as secondary pharmacological effects, should also be considered.

The most important differential diagnosis, however, is Hirschsprung disease. This congenital aganglionosis is the most common neuromuscular disease of the gastrointestinal tract. It affects 1 in 5000 of all newborns, four to five times more boys are affected, and in 95 per cent of cases the disease is limited to the rectosigmoid. While 80 per cent are sporadic cases, the remaining 20 per cent follow autosomal dominant, recessive and polygenic modes of inheritance. Without doubt, the importance of Hirschsprung disease has been over-emphasized in the differential diagnosis of encopresis, for several reasons:

1   Encopresis is defined as a disorder from the age of 4 years onwards. By this age, most cases of Hirschsprung disease have already been diagnosed: 61 per cent of cases are diagnosed at the age of 12 months and 82 per cent by the age of 4 years (Felt et al 1999). In other words, in only 18 per cent of cases of Hirschsprung disease (or 1 in 25,000 children in total) has the diagnosis not been made by this time.

2   Children 4 years and older are likely to have milder variants of Hirschsprung disease – and not the severe forms that are typical for the neonatal age, with abdominal distension, vomiting, obstruction and failure to grow.

242

TABLE 9.14
Differential diagnosis of encopresis/chronic constipation and Hirschsprung's disease
(according to Hatch 1988, Levine 1991, Youssef and Di Lorenzo 2001)

	Encopresis/constipation	Hirschsprung disease
Soiling	Always	Rare
Constipation	Common, may be intermittent	Always present
Symptoms as newborn	Rare	Almost always
Infant constipation	Sometimes	Rare
Late onset (after age 3 years)	Common	Rare
Problem in bowel training	Common	Rare
Avoidance of toilet	Common	Rare
Failure to thrive	Rare	Common
Anaemia	None	Common
Obstructive symptoms	Rare	Common
Stool in ampulla	Common	Rare
Rectal ampulla	Dilated	Narrow
Loose or tight sphincter tone	Rare	Common
Palpable abdominal stool masses (scybala)	Common	Rare
Distended abdomen	Common	Occasional
Large calibre stools	Common	Never
Preponderance of males	86%	90%
Prevalence	1.5% at age 8 years	1 in 5000 live births
Anal manometry	Paradoxical contraction of sphincter during defecation, otherwise variable	Always abnormal

3　Finally, as shown in Table 9.14, encopresis is not a typical symptom of Hirschsprung disease. In fact, encopresis and Hirschsprung disease differ regarding most clinical signs (see Table 9.14) and can easily be differentiated.

If, however, Hirschsprung disease is suspected, further gastroenterological and surgical assessment and treatment should not be postponed.

In summary, considering the wide variety of possible medical causes, it is evident that every child with encopresis should be examined in detail with special attention paid to the examination of the abdomen, rectum, perianal and perigenital region, as well as the spinal cord. A complete neurological examination should always be part of the diagnostic process. Laboratory tests should be performed only if indicated.

EPIDEMIOLOGY
Chronic constipation affects 1 to 2 per cent of all school-aged and adolescent children. Some authors, such as Levine (1991), believe that all children with encopresis are automatically also constipated, and they have even coined the term 'occult constipation'. This term implies that even if there are no overt signs of constipation present, it is just a matter of not having looked closely enough. This extreme view is no longer tenable in view of newer studies.

In the meantime it has become evident that not all children with constipation soil – and conversely, not all children with encopresis have constipation. Of those children with constipation, 68 to 90 per cent (Arhan et al 1983, Partin et al 1992, Van der Plas et al 1997) also soil during the day, and 27 per cent at night (Van Ginkel et al 2003). Regarding the group of children with encopresis, an even greater variability has been documented in different studies. This is probably due to selection effects, differences in definitions, and differences in the clinical procedures in diagnosing constipation. In 15 early studies of 890 encopretic children in total, 44 per cent were also constipated – with a great variability, from 5 per cent to 94 per cent, in different studies (Krisch 1985). In the only population-based study, 24 per cent of children with encopresis, and 16 per cent of the controls, had constipation (Bellman 1966). In paediatric settings, the rate of constipation among encopretic children was 63 per cent (Van der Plas et al 1997) and 69 per cent (Benninga et al 1994), respectively. In a child psychiatric inpatient setting, the rate of constipation was even higher at 78 per cent (Mehler-Wex et al 2005).

In summary, the terms encopresis and constipation should not be used synony-mously. They can, but do not need to, coexist. Thus, 70 to 90 per cent of all constipated children will have soiling problems. In turn, 40 to 80 per cent of children with encopresis are also constipated. In the only population-based study, the rate was much lower at 24 per cent.

AETIOLOGY

As was outlined above (see pages 228-229), genetic factors play a major role in encopresis with constipation. Thus, the concordance rate was significantly higher for monozygotic (70 per cent) compared to dizygotic twins (18 per cent) (Bakwin and Davidson 1971). In family studies, a high proportion of relatives, especially male relatives, were affected by constipation. Molecular genetic studies have not been conducted yet, so possible candidate genes are not known.

It is most likely that these genetic factors have an effect on function of the colon, as has been shown in various transit studies. While the orocaecal transit time (OCTT) did not differ between children with encopresis with constipation and controls, the colon transit time (CTT) was significantly prolonged (Benninga et al 1994). Again, children with a prolonged colon transit time are likely to represent different heterogeneous groups; thus, 13 per cent had a prolonged transit time of the entire colon, 20 per cent only of the rectal sigmoid, while 56 per cent had a completely normal transit time (Benninga et al 1994). Prolonged CTT is associated with low defecation frequency and high frequency of encopresis (de Lorijn et al 2004). As there is a significant association between abnormal colon transit time (CTT) and prolonged rectosigmoid transit time (RSTT), it was hypothesized that in some children withholding behaviour induces a delay in RSTT, which, in turn, leads to a secondary prolongation of CTT (de Lorijn et al 2004).

Slow transit constipation

Efforts have been undertaken to identify specific subtypes. Using radio-opaque markers, Cook et al (2002) identified three subgroups:

1   Children with a prolonged transit time, in 51 per cent of cases (slow transit constipation)
2   Children with retention, but a quick passage of 30 hours or less, in 37 per cent of cases (functional faecal retention due to psychological factors)
3   Children with increased radioactivity exclusively in the rectum, in 13 per cent of cases (stool retention due to physiological factors not yet specified)

Of these three, slow transit constipation has been identified as a specific disease entity. Typical features are: delayed passage of the first meconium stool beyond 24 hours of age; symptoms of severe constipation within a year, or treatment-resistent encopresis at 2–3 years; soft stools despite infrequent bowel actions and delayed colonic transit. Genetic factors play a major role and some children have signs compatible with intestinal neuronal dysplasia (IND) (Hutson et al 2001). In contrast to functional faecal retention, large, soft stools, abdominal distension and bloating and a lower stool frequency are typical (Hutson et al 2004, Shin et al 2002). Psychological symptoms do not seem to play a major role in the aetiology in childhood, but adults with slow transit constipation had significantly lower behavioural scores on a questionnaire (Hopkins Symptom Checklist) than patients with normal transit constipation (Wald et al 1989).

If these findings are replicated by other studies, these subtypes may be of great importance, as they might imply specific treatment approaches in the future. At the present time, transit-time examinations are not performed as part of routine practice.

Toilet training and encopresis
The effect of parental toilet training practices on the development of encopresis has been a matter of great debate. This question was addressed by two Swiss longitudinal studies, which followed a similar design (Largo and Stützle 1977, Largo et al 1978, 1996). In the first Swiss study (1954–1956), 96 per cent of all parents started toilet training their children before the age of 12 months; 3 per cent of parents began training even at the age of 1 month – long before voluntary sphincter control is possible. These early and rigid child-rearing practices have to be understood in the historical context of the 1950s: other ideals regarding cleanliness and continence were prevalent, cloth diapers were used and many households did not have washing machines. In the second Swiss study (1974–1984), parents started toilet training at the age of 19 to 21 months on average. This was probably due to the availability of disposable diapers and a more relaxed and liberal attitude towards children.

While these different toilet training practices had no effect on the attainment of dryness during the night and only temporary effects on dryness during the day, they did have an impact on achieving stool continence. As can be seen in Table 9.7, more children achieved stool continence at an earlier age with a stricter toilet training regime. In fact, more children raised in the 1970s and 1980s continued soiling up to the age of 6 years. In other words, of the three types of continence, the control of defecation is the area that is most likely to be influenced by environmental factors.

However, this process seems to be influenced by the congruence in the interaction between parents and children. In the 1950s, parents started prompting children long before they showed active signals of wanting to be put on the potty. In the 1970s, however, there was a congruence between the active signalling by the children and parental prompting. In other words, most parents are able to react intuitively and reinforce their children positively when they want to become dry and clean.

The Swiss studies did not address the question of what effect toilet training would have on the later development of encopresis in children. The Swedish study by Bellman (1966) showed that it was not the time of toilet training *per se*, but the quality of the interaction that was decisive. Thus, 31 per cent of children with encopresis had undergone forceful toilet training with high parental pressure, but only 5 per cent of controls. On the other hand, toilet training which is too unstructured, too late or too passive also seems to have a negative effect. Eight per cent of parents of encopretic children had never trained actively, compared to none of the control parents (Bellman 1966). In another study, early toilet training was not associated with constipation, stool withholding or stool toileting refusal. Early training takes longer to complete, so there is 'little benefit in beginning intensive training before 27 months of age in most children' (Blum et al 2003: 810).

In summary, stool continence can be influenced by environmental factors. Ideally, parents should react to their children's signals and reinforce their wish to achieve continence, which is a major developmental step in infancy. Forceful toilet training too early, and a *laissez-faire* attitude without training, are both equally problematic for the child's development. In other words, the quality of the interaction has the greatest effect on later encopresis.

Development of encopresis with constipation

Encopresis with constipation often develops in infancy and preschool years as a result of acute constipation. It can be triggered by a wide variety of psychological as well as somatic factors (Hatch 1988, Levine 1991, Loening-Baucke 1994). The most important trigger is painful defecation, e.g. following anal fissures in up to 63 per cent of cases (Partin et al 1992). In some patients, constipation starts at a very early age, probably due to congenital or genetic factors. Thus, 40 per cent of patients had their first signs of constipation under the age of 1 month (Arhan et al 1983). Most had a prolonged colon transit time. Another risk group is preterm infants. At the age of 6 years, 60 per cent of former preterm infants (birthweight 750 g) had signs of stool retention, and there were signs of encopresis in 53 per cent, painful defecation in 60 per cent, ritualized toilet behaviour in 27 per cent and wetting in 53 per cent of cases (Cunningham et al 2001). In another study, 8 per cent of preterm boys and 7 per cent of preterm girls soiled at the age of 4 years (Largo et al 1999).

At a later age, constipation can be elicited by psychological factors, such as specific toilet phobias (see page 267). Dietary changes, irregular daily routines, and behavioural disorders such as hyperactivity, as well as a variety of precipitating life events, can also trigger encopresis. Typical difficult life events for children are parental separation and divorce, birth of a sibling, and starting kindergarten and school (Levine 1991, Cox et al 1998). Whatever the trigger may be, a similar vicious circle develops: stool is retained, faecal masses begin to accumulate in the colon, peristaltic activity and sensibility are reduced, and this in turn leads to further accumulation of faecal masses, which become hardened in the process. Fresh stool passes around and in between the old faecal masses and leads to soiling.

The most differentiated model of the development of constipation was outlined by Cox et al (1998) – see Table 9.15. Basically, 10 steps in the development of encopresis with constipation can be differentiated. An episode of acute constipation due to various triggers leads to painful defecation; this in turn elicits a paradoxical contraction of the external anal sphincter with further avoidance of defecation. Stool retention increases, leading to chronic constipation and loss of rectal sensitivity. These processes lead to soiling, and this in turn leads to interaction problems and intrapsychic conflicts.

CLINICAL SIGNS AND SYMPTOMS

Many of the clinical signs and symptoms can be understood in the context of the patho-physiology of faecal retention. The specific clinical picture is best described in the study of Benninga et al (1994), who compared 111 children with encopresis and constipation with 50 children with encopresis without constipation (Table 9.16).

In the constipated group, there were more girls; only half of the children had had any sort of toilet training. They passed stools on the toilet less often than the group without constipation – twice a week on average. The stool masses were large, and the stool consistency was normal in only half of the children. They soiled nearly every day; 50 per cent experienced pain during defecation, 40 per cent complained about abdominal pain. Rectal sensibility and appetite were reduced. Colon transit time was prolonged in contrast to the transit time from the oral cavity to the colon. In 40 per cent of children abdominal masses could be palpated; the manometric results were abnormal in 60 per cent. Laxative treatment was effective.

In summary, children with encopresis and constipation have a profile of clinical symptoms which, if evaluated carefully, will point towards the diagnosis.

PSYCHOLOGICAL ASPECTS

Approximately 40 to 50 per cent of all children with encopresis and constipation have clinically relevant behavioural symptoms or disorders – the same rate as in children with encopresis without constipation (Benninga et al 1994). In other words, the two major types of encopresis cannot be differentiated according to behavioural comorbidity. More importantly, regarding the aetiology, there is no evidence that one type (i.e. with constipation) has a more somatic aetiology, while the other type (i.e. without constipation) has a more psychogenic aetiology. Again, there is no specific psychopathology typical for encopresis – all types of behavioural and emotional disorders can coexist.

Major findings from studies are summarized in Table 9.8. Looking at specific studies, 42 of 55 children had encopresis with constipation in the study by Gabel et al (1986). Overall, 49 per cent had behavioural problems in the clinical range, i.e. a rate five times higher than in the normative population. Twenty per cent of the children had a total score above the 98th percentile, a tenfold increase compared to the normal population rate of 2 per cent. The most common single items of the CBCL were signs of oppositional behaviour

TABLE 9.15
Steps in the development of encopresis with constipation (adapted from Cox et al 1998)

Steps	Mechanisms
1	Acute constipation
	Acute constipation is triggered by pain, transition from liquid to solid foods, intensive toilet training, medication, emotional trauma, and psychological conflicts such as birth of a sibling
	▼
2	Painful defecation
	The acute constipation causes painful defecation, muscular bracing, and avoidance of defecation, inducing a paradoxical contraction of the external anal sphincter
	▼
3	Paradoxical contraction of the external anal sphincter
	The paradoxical contraction is maintained to avoid pain and becomes a habitual behaviour
	▼
4	Avoidance of toilet and of defecation
	Defecation is avoided by not spontaneously seeking the toilet, by not straining sufficiently to expel the stool on the toilet, and by paradoxically contracting the external anal sphincter to prevent stool from passing
	▼
5	Faecal impaction
	Avoidance of bowel movement leads to accumulation of faecal material in the rectum, where fluid withdrawal culminates in large, hard faecal masses
	▼
6	Chronic constipation
	Defecation avoidance leads to chronic constipation
	▼
7	Rectal insensitivity
	Habitual retention of large stool masses stretches the rectal capacity, resulting in acquired megacolon. Through the enlargement of the rectum, larger stool masses are necessary to induce defecation and sensitivity diminishes
	▼
8	Encopresis
	Soiling develops either as overflow ('interflow') incontinence, or because the child waits too long before seeking out a toilet and the external anal sphincter is unable to retain the faecal matter
	▼
9	Interpersonal consequences
	Soiling can trigger interpersonal conflicts with peers and parents. Adults might attribute the child's behaviour to laziness or interpret it as a purposeful act. Struggles about when to use the toilet develop as a result of the child's avoidance. Public soiling can trigger peer rejection and teacher alienation
	▼
10	Intrapersonal conflicts
	These experiences can lead to feelings of humiliation, poor self-esteem, social withdrawal and other behavioural problems

TABLE 9.16

Differences between encopresis with and without constipation (Benninga et al 1994)

	Constipation/encopresis with constipation N=111	Encopresis without constipation N=50
Boys	68%	86%
Age (mean)	8.0	9.0
Toilet trained	56%	69%
Age at which toilet training started (years)	1.5	2.0
Bowel movements/week (mean)	Seldom (2x/week)	Often (7x/week)
Large amounts of stools	Yes (61%)	No (0%)
Normal stools (consistency)	54%	82%
Daytime soiling	77%	68%
Episodes/week	7x/week	3.5x/week
Night-time soiling	33%	6%
Episodes/week	Seldom	Seldom
Pain during defecation	50%	30%
Abdominal pain	41%	22%
No rectal sensation	18%	6%
Good appetite	58%	78%
Colon transit time	Long (62.4 h)	Normal (40.2 h)
Orocaecal transit time	No difference	No difference
Palpable abdominal mass	39%	0%
Palpable rectal mass	31%	0%
Normal defecation dynamics	41%**	54%**
Daytime urinary incontinence	12%	7%
Nocturnal enuresis	29%	10%
CBCL total score in the clinical range*	38.5%	44.2%
Laxative therapy	Helpful	Not helpful, even worsening

* 10% in normative population (cut-off: 90th percentile)
** controls: 93%

(3/4 children), followed by shyness and attention problems (2/3 children). Only 12 per cent had presented to mental health services.

In the study by Loening-Baucke et al (1987), most children had additional constipation. Fifty per cent of the girls and 38 per cent of the boys had a total behavioural score in the clinical range (norm: 10 per cent – so four to five times higher than would be expected). Twelve per cent of the boys and 17 per cent of the girls had clinical behavioural scores even above the 98th percentile (norm: 2 per cent – so six to eight times higher than would be expected).

Young et al (1995) found a CBCL total score above the 90th percentile in 51 per cent of all children (norm: 10 per cent). The rate of comorbid behavioural symptoms had a decisive influence on treatment success: 36 per cent of those treated successfully had an initial CBCL total score in the clinical range; whereas in the group with treatment failure, 75 per cent of the children had an initial CBCL total score in the clinical range.

In summary, a large proportion of children with encopresis and constipation are affected by behavioural symptoms and disorders – much more so than non-soiling children or even children with urinary incontinence and enuresis. The types of disorders are heterogeneous, with internalizing as well as externalizing problems prevailing. If these additional behavioural disorders are not addressed properly, there will be a higher likelihood of treatment failure. Therefore, it is essential to diagnose both the type of encopresis and the type of comorbid behavioural disorder. A symptom-oriented approach is needed for the soiling problem. Some of the behavioural symptoms will disappear if constipation and encopresis resolve. If the behavioural problems persist after the encopresis has remitted, or if they are clearly evident at the beginning, they will need additional professional treatment.

ASSESSMENT

The assessment should follow the guidelines outlined for encopresis in general. Special attention should be given to the perigenital and perianal region. A rectal examination is indicated. The abdomen should be palpated for abdominal masses. An ultrasound examination of the abdomen is very useful. Constipation shows itself in an enlarged diameter of the rectum and sigmoid, as well as retrovesical impressions. As these will remit during treatment, ultrasound can be used to document the progress of treatment. Also, it can be employed therapeutically as a variant of 'biofeedback' training. Children can be shown their ultrasound pictures and the changes in the rectal diameter can be demonstrated.

TREATMENT

The treatment recommendations here follow the American (Felt et al 1999) and German guidelines (von Gontard et al 2006b) and are similar to many other recommendations (Levine 1991, Loening-Baucke 2000). Primary physicians still tend to undertreat childhood constipation, however, so that many children remain symptomatic from the start (Borowitz et al 2005).

Basic therapy

The main line of treatment is the stool regulation regime as outlined previously. Provision of information and psychoeducation play an even greater role in encopresis with constipation than without. Levine (1991) called this process a form of 'demystification' and recommended the use of diagrams (see Fig. 9.2). One has to remember that many children and parents are not aware of the associations of retention and soiling. They often think that the soiling problem is due to leakage (insufficiency of the sphincter) and not a consequence of the retention. Therefore, simple information will enhance their understanding of the pathophysiology and increase their compliance regarding treatment.

In this process of counselling, parental attributions, worries and possible guilt feelings should be explored and addressed. Emotional distress and anxieties of the children should be discussed. As bullying by peers is not uncommon, this too should be addressed.

As outlined previously, children are asked to sit on the toilet three times a day in a relaxed manner for five to ten minutes. The situation should be approached in as positive a way as possible. Toilet sessions, as well as passed urine and stool, should be documented on a chart (see Appendix 14). If a child adheres to a low-fibre diet, a change in diet can be useful. Also, it is important to record fluid intake, as many children do not drink sufficient amounts of fluids. If this is the case, they should be encouraged to drink larger amounts. One

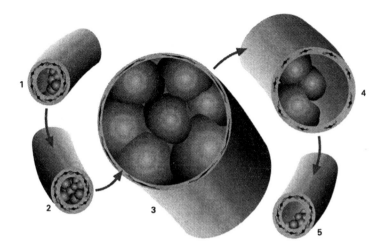

Fig. 9.2 Stool retention: from initial acute constipation, chronic stool retention, megacolon and chronic constipation develop (reprinted with permission from von Gontard 2004); treatment consists of evacuation of faeces (disimpaction) and prevention of relapse by toilet training programmes and oral laxatives.

way to encourage drinking is the 'empty bottle technique'. A bottle holding the designated amount is filled with water in the morning. The children are allowed to pour out the same amount of water every time they drink – until the bottle is empty by evening time. This basic approach has been shown to be effective and should be continued throughout the entire treatment, including the maintenance period of up to 24 months. To gain continuing compliance, positive reinforcement with simple behavioural token systems can be useful.

Laxatives: general aspects
Laxatives are an important treatment component if constipation is present. In a randomized, controlled study, children treated with additional laxatives achieved a significantly higher rate of complete remission than those treated with behavioural modification alone. The complete remission rate was 39 per cent vs. 12 per cent after three months, and 49 per cent vs. 30 per cent after six months (Nolan et al 1991). However, only 31 per cent of children were constipated on abdominal radiographs and, according to newer studies, only these should receive laxatives. Laxatives are not indicated in encopresis without constipation, as symptoms can even worsen (Benninga et al 2004).

Disimpaction
If large amounts of faecal masses have accumulated in the course of chronic constipation, toilet scheduling on its own will not be sufficient. The faecal masses need to be evacuated initially, in a process called disimpaction.

In most cases, disimpaction is possible only by rectal enemas. The most widely used and recommended form is enemas containing phosphates such as sodium hydrogen phosphate and sodium monohydrogen phosphate. Recommended doses are 30 ml per 10 kg bodyweight, or half an enema for preschool children, and between three-quarters and a whole enema in school children.

Before applying a rectal enema, it is important to explain the process to the child in detail. The enema should be shown to the child. One can remind them that they have tolerated stools with much wider diameters than the applicator of the enema. They should be informed that the first evacuation can be painful, but that the long-term relief will be of great benefit. Children are asked to lie on their side and pull up their knees, and the enema is applied. They are asked to hold the fluid for 15 to 20 minutes and then go to the toilet. One should make sure that younger children do not retain the enema fluid because phosphate intoxication has been detected (Harrington and Schuh 1997). In children under 2 years of age and in those with kidney problems, enemas containing sorbid can be used as an alternative (Keller 2002).

Clinical practice shows that often enemas are required repeatedly. In some children, the application of enemas has to be repeated during the first days of treatment, while in others regular enemas once or twice a week may be necessary to avoid new accumulation of masses.

If these simple enemas are not sufficient, children should be referred to a department of paediatric gastroenterology. In rare cases, higher and antegrade enemas and even surgical evacuation may be necessary.

Due to the advent of new oral laxatives, rectal disimpaction can be avoided in children in the early stages of chronic constipation. The laxative of choice is polyethylene glycol (PEG) or Movicol®. In less severe cases oral treatment can be tried first.

Maintenance
After the disimpaction, a sufficiently long maintenance period has to be adhered to to avoid reaccumulation of faecal masses. Felt et al (1999) recommend a maintenance period of at least six months and possibly up to 24 months. Laxatives should be discontinued slowly with a reduction of the dose every six months. During this time, the basic stool regulation regime should be continued. To enhance compliance and avoid drop-outs and complications, regular attendance at the clinic should be continued. Felt et al (1999) recommend attendance after two weeks, one, three and six months. Loening-Baucke (2000) recommends visits at monthly intervals. These appointments do not necessarily need to be with a doctor; a dedicated and trained nurse will suffice in many centres. During the maintenance period, regular, daily laxatives should be given. The two most widely used laxatives are lactulose and polyethylene glycol (Movicol®). These two laxatives will be discussed in detail.

Lactulose. Previously, lactulose was the first-line oral laxative. It is an osmotic laxative, a non-absorbable disaccharide that binds fluids in the colon. It can be given in powder or fluid formulation. The dose is 1–3 ml per kg bodyweight per day in one to three doses (Baker et al 1999), or globally 20–30 ml in preschool children, 30–90 ml in school children, one to three times a day (Keller 2002). The doses must be adjusted in light of clinical symptoms, i.e. if diarrhoea occurs, the dose must be reduced. Although lactulose is generally tolerated, some children complain about flatulence, abdominal pain and diarrhoea. Other children do not like the sweet taste. In that case the powder is usually better tolerated than the syrup.

Polyethylene glycol (Movicol®). The most important new laxative of recent years is polyethylene glycol (PEG or Movicol®), which is likely to become the standard form of therapy in the future (Bishop 2001). PEG is an osmotic laxative and consists of a long, linear polymer that binds water molecules through hydrogen bridges in the intestinal lumen. It is classified as a nutritional additive by the FDA in the United States. In the UK it is licensed as Movicol®. PEG is not yet licensed for children in Germany and other countries. Because of the very positive effects, however, off-label use is recommended even in young children.

PEG is not resorbed, and not metabolized, but has a purely physical action by increasing the osmotic pressure and hydration of stool. PEG contains no electrolytes or sugar and can be dissolved in water or other fluids.

The side effects consist of abdominal pains and flatulence, but are extremely rare. The contraindications are abdominal pain of unclear aetiology and severe gastrointestinal diseases such as gastrointestinal obstruction, danger of perforation, and chronic inflammatory diseases such as Crohn's disease or ulcerative colitis, as well as general medical diseases.

Several dose-finding studies have been conducted. In one study, the aim was to achieve more than three stools per week. The optimal dose was 11.7 g per day among 4 to 7-year-olds and 60 g per day among 8 to 15-year-olds (Dupont et al 2000). In another study, the aim was to achieve two soft stools per day (Pashankar and Bishop 2001). The optimal dose was 0.84 g per kg bodyweight a day in two doses, with a large therapeutical range from 0.27 to 1.24 g per kg per day. Marked changes could be documented during the first week in half of the children. Eight weeks later, the rate of painful defecation had diminished from 75 to 0 per cent, blood on stools from 40 to 0 per cent, anxieties regarding defecation and retention from 70 to 5 per cent, abdominal masses from 44 to 0 per cent, rectal masses from 83 to 22 per cent and rectal dilatation from 78 to 11 per cent.

In another study, PEG was compared to milk of magnesia (Loening-Baucke 2002). The dose was 0.5 g per kg per day without stool masses and 1 g per kg per day if stool masses were present. In this study, PEG was not more effective than milk of magnesia. The main difference was that PEG was tolerated by all children, while 30 per cent did not like the taste of the traditional laxative.

In the first long-term study, over eight months, with an average dose of 0.7 g/kg/day, symptoms improved significantly. In the children with encopresis, soiling ceased completely in half and was reduced in all others (Pashankar et al 2003a). PEG was well tolerated with no major clinical adverse effects (Pashankar et al 2003b).

In a double-blind, randomized, controlled trial, PEG was more effective and had fewer side effects (less abdominal pain, straining and pain on defecation) than lactulose in children with functional constipation. After eight weeks, the success rate was 56 per cent for PEG and 29 per cent for lactulose. The recommended dose was lower than in previous studies (0.26 g/kg/day) (Voskuijl et al 2004c).

In summary, PEG has become the first-choice oral laxative for chronic constipation in children. The recommended doses vary from 0.26 to 0.84 g/kg/day and are adjusted according to clinical signs. PEG is highly effective, shows few side effects and is well tolerated. It can be dissolved in various fluids and foods. Long-term compliance seems to be better than with other laxatives.

R.K., 7-year-old boy
Diagnosis: Encopresis with constipation

R. had secondary encopresis, having being continent from the age of 2½ to 4 years. He was currently soiling large amounts of faeces one to three times per day. This occurred during the day after school at home. He retained stool, complained of abdominal pains and was constipated for a maximum of two days. Defecation was not painful. Ultrasound showed a marked increase in rectum diameter (44 × 41 mm) and the bladder wall was thickened. There were no signs of behavioural problems.

R. was sent to the toilet three times a day. During the first three weeks, enemas were given twice a week, then once a week. The encopresis disappeared completely. He needed no further treatment.

This is a case of encopresis with constipation. Even though R. went to the toilet regularly, stool was retained with typical symptoms. The parents were *laissez-faire* in their child-rearing practices and profited positively from counselling. Except for toilet training and laxatives no further treatment was needed. Nowadays, one would choose PEG (Movicol®) for both disimpaction and maintenance therapy.

Other laxatives. For most clinical cases, these two basic laxatives are sufficient. Other laxatives are still in use, especially in the USA. As there are major differences in laxative treatment between Europe and the USA, other laxatives will be mentioned briefly. Details can be found in previews by Keller (2002), Baker et al (1999) and Price and Elliott (2002), who have compiled a Cochrane Review. The grade of evidence for laxatives is relatively low. Most recommendations rely on open, clinical studies, or even just clinical experience.

Other laxatives include suppositories in smaller doses for infants and young children, which are not useful in the treatment of chronic constipation in school-aged children and adolescents. These are mini-enemas containing citrate, glycerol, sodium hydrogen carbonate, or phosphate suppositories, leading to CO_2 production.

Another laxative is paraffin oil given in a dose of 30 ml per 10 kg bodyweight. This should not be used in children under 2 years of age, nor in children with learning disability, due to a higher risk of aspiration and pneumonia (Keller 2002). In the USA Senna laxatives are used. These should not be given to children under 12 years of age because of possible electrolyte imbalances and disorders of motility. Bisacodyl and magnesia-containing laxatives are not regularly used in Europe. Other laxatives, such as propulsive prokinetics (cisapride), have shown positive effects but are no longer available in many countries (Germany, UK, Canada) because of cardiac side effects (Keller 2002).

Changes in diet, such as increasing the fibre load, can be helpful, even though the empirical evidence for its effect is low (Keller 2002). In a recent RCT, fibre (glucomannan) was shown to be beneficial in the treatment of constipation with and without encopresis. It led to a marked reduction of symptoms compared to placebo (Loening-Baucke et al 2004). In addition, increasing fluid intake, especially in the form of fruit juices, can have a positive laxative effect. In general, laxatives do not affect the nutritional status of children (McClung et al 1993).

Biofeedback
Manometry has been shown to be an important diagnostic tool, with paradoxical contraction of the external anal sphincter being the most consistent finding in encopretic children. Other findings have included dyscoordinated defecation dynamics, reduced sensibility and changes in pressure gradients. The logical consequence of these manometric findings was to try to develop techniques to normalize these functional changes. One approach considered in many studies was that of biofeedback. Biofeedback is defined as a collection of therapeutical methods by which autonomic, physiological processes are registered and 'fed back' in real time visually or acoustically, so that they can be perceived and processed consciously. Biofeedback methods are usually combined with other types of treatment, such as psychoeducation, relaxation, physiotherapy or cognitive-behavioural therapy.

Different types of biofeedback have been employed in children with encopresis and constipation: using either intrarectal measurement of pressure, or EMG activity registered by surface electrodes. These measurements are presented acoustically or visually – for example by means of a coloured ellipse on a monitor (Iwata et al 1995). In one of the first studies, 86 per cent of children achieved normal defecation dynamics after only two to six sessions. Twelve months later, 50 per cent of the biofeedback group were free of symptoms, compared to 16 per cent of those who had been conventionally treated (Loening-Baucke 1990).

All other later studies, however, were unable to replicate these initial positive results. In a four-year follow-up, 86 per cent of children with conventional treatment and 87 per cent of children with biofeedback treatment had a reduction of their symptoms of constipation and encopresis; 62 per cent of the conventionally treated children were completely symptom-free – compared to 50 per cent of the successfully treated biofeedback group and 23 per cent of the non-successfully treated biofeedback group (Loening-Baucke 1995). These disappointing results could be due to the fact that the abnormal defecation dynamics might not be a primary pathophysiological cause of constipation but a consequence of stool retention. Also, positive effects could be due to unspecific treatment components such as increased attention to the children (Loening-Baucke 1996).

In a large randomized, controlled study, again, there were no differences between conventionally treated children and those who received biofeedback in addition to conventional treatment. After one year, 59 per cent of the conventionally treated and 50 per cent of the biofeedback group were classified as treated successfully. These results remained constant in the 18-month follow-up. In addition, there was no association between success and abnormality of defecation dynamics. The authors therefore concluded that additional biofeedback training does not lead to a higher success rate and that abnormal defecation dynamics are not decisive in the pathogenesis of childhood constipation. The traditional intensive treatment, including laxatives, should therefore remain the main line of treatment (Van der Plas et al 1996a). Similarly, Nolan et al (1998) found no evidence of a lasting benefit in clinical outcome for biofeedback training.

In another randomized study three groups were compared: the first group was treated by laxatives alone; the second by laxatives plus extended toilet training (ETT); and the third by laxatives, ETT and biofeedback. The ETT was conducted by a clinical psychologist and contained the following components: intensive psychoeducation, individual doses of laxatives, token plans, and detailed instruction in and demonstration of optimal defecation. Children were asked to sit on the toilet for at least 12 minutes twice a day, to adhere to standardized relaxation and contraction exercises during the first 4 minutes, to play for 4 minutes, and strain for 4 minutes. Biofeedback was conducted with a non-invasive surface EMG which was applied perianally. The biofeedback measurements were presented visually via a computer game. The results were astonishing: 19 per cent of the laxative group, 71 per cent of the laxative and ETT group, and 64 per cent of the combined group with biofeedback showed a significant reduction of soiling. 'Outcome was significantly predicted by improvement during the initial 14 days of treatment' (Cox et al 1996: 659). The authors concluded that behavioural ETT should remain the treatment of choice.

The same design was replicated in a second study (Cox et al 1998). Again, after three months, 44 per cent of the laxative, 85 per cent of the ETT and 61 per cent of the biofeedback group had a significant reduction of soiling episodes. In other words, again, behavioural treatment alone (ETT) was far more effective than with the additional component of biofeedback. Possibly, the application of electrodes and preoccupation with the biofeedback apparatus divert attention from the essential components of therapy, i.e. toilet training, direct instruction and personal relationship to the child.

In summary, biofeedback training cannot be recommended as a first-line treatment for children with encopresis and constipation. Cognitive-behavioural components, stool regulation and laxatives are far more effective and should be the mainstay of treatment. It is not clear if subgroups of children might profit from biofeedback training, such as children with highly abnormal defecation dynamics and treatment resistance.

COURSE AND PROGNOSIS

The course and prognosis of encopresis with constipation is not very promising, mainly due to the fact that many of these children are not followed up regularly, as recommended in the guidelines (Felt et al 1999). After one year, 50 per cent of girls and 70 per cent of boys were treated successfully for constipation (de Lorijn et al 2004). A good outcome was associated with a faecal mass on rectal examination; a poor outcome with a prolonged transit time (CTT) of over 100 hours.

In a 6 year 8 month follow-up of 43 children, 70 per cent had no encopresis, while 30 per cent continued soiling (Sutphen et al 1995). Of 418 patients with constipation, 40 per cent remained constipated after one year and 20 per cent after eight years. Treatment success was associated with onset of constipation after 4 years of age and low encopresis frequency. In other words, constipation plus encopresis is more difficult to treat than constipation alone (Van Ginkel et al 2003).

SUMMARY AND CLINICAL GUIDELINES

Chart 9.1 provides an overview of the diagnostic aspects of functional faecal incontinence (encopresis). The differential diagnosis, as well as the assessment of comorbid disorders, is shown in Chart 9.2. The treatment steps, if encopresis with constipation is diagnosed, are outlined in Chart 9.3.

Information, including guidelines on changes in diet and drinking habits, should be provided. Large amounts of faecal masses should be evacuated by enemas initially (disimpaction). In less severe cases, disimpaction by oral laxatives (PEG) can be tried. Maintenance therapy consists of regular toilet sessions three times a day after main meals. Children are asked to sit on the toilet in a relaxed manner for ten minutes. Charts are filled out. If required, this toilet training can be enhanced by a simple token system (rewards). In addition, oral laxatives (preferably PEG) are given and regular follow-up visits are arranged. Maintenance therapy should continue for at least six months (and up to 24 months) to avoid the reaccumulation of faecal masses. Due to the common and severe coexisting behavioural and emotional disorders, additional counselling, psychotherapy and other child psychiatric interventions are often required.

Functional faecal incontinence (encopresis) without constipation

(Other terms used to describe this condition are: solitary encopresis; functional non-retentive encopresis; and non-retentive (non-constipation-associated) faecal incontinence.)

This type of incontinence has been defined as 'encopresis or soiling without any sign of constipation' (Benninga et al 1994). It has also been called 'solitary encopresis' (Van Ginkel et al 2000) or 'functional non-retentive encopresis' according to the Rome-II criteria (Rasquin-Weber et al 1999). In contrast to the ICD-10 and DSM-IV criteria, a soiling frequency of at least once a week in the last 12 weeks is required under the Rome-II criteria. Interestingly, it is interpreted as an emotional disorder, as an 'impulsive act' or as 'a mani-festation of unconscious anger'. The goal of treatment according to the Rome-II document is to educate parents to accept that there is no underlying organic disease and to make sure that their child is seen by a mental health care professional (Rasquin-Weber et al 1999). This assumption certainly needs to be revised: children with this disorder do not have more psychiatric disorders than those with constipation and should be referred only if coexisting behavioural disturbances are present. With the exception of laxatives, assessment and treatment are the same as in children with encopresis with constipation.

257

As has been shown previously, 31 to 84 per cent of all encopretic children do not have constipation. Encopresis without constipation is therefore probably just as common as encopresis with constipation. The great variability in these prevalence figures is again due to selection effects and differences in diagnosing constipation. Possibly, paediatric centres are more likely to see children with constipation, while child psychiatrists or general practitioners might see more children without constipation.

CLINICAL SIGNS AND SYMPTOMS

The main clinical symptoms have been outlined in the classic paper by Benninga et al (1994), who compared children with encopresis with and without constipation (see Table 9.16).

There appear to be more boys among children with non-retentive encopresis. Children pass stools regularly every day, the stool masses are small, the consistency is more often normal, and they soil less often – only 3.5 times a week on average. They complain of painful defecation and abdominal pains less often; rectal sensation is normal, appetite unchanged, and colon transit time is not prolonged on average, although some patients show a prolonged transit time of over 62 hours. Stool masses cannot be palpated. In the 1994 study, only 54 per cent had normal defecation dynamics, compared to 93 per cent of controls. In a recent study, 91 per cent of children had a normal colon transit time, but only 48 per cent had normal defecation dynamics (Benninga et al 2004).

DIFFERENTIAL DIAGNOSIS

The differential diagnosis of non-retentive encopresis is not based on high-evidence studies. Diarrhoea and spina bifida occulta have to be ruled out as possible organic causes (Hyman and Fleisher 1994). Encopresis without constipation can also occur as a long-term effect of rectal pull-through operations (Hyman and Fleisher 1994). But non-retentive encopresis is mainly interpreted, even by paediatricians, as a psychogenic form of encopresis. From clinical impressions, inadequate or ambivalent toilet training as well as prolonged use of diapers are often involved. Intrafamilial conflicts and emotional disorders are also often present. These associations are not based on empirical research, but on clinical observations only.

AETIOLOGY

The hypothesis of some paediatric gastroenterologists that encopresis without constipation is a psychogenic condition (Hyman and Fleisher 1994, Rasquin-Weber et al 1999) cannot be substantiated by empirical research, as the rate of comorbid behavioural and emotional symptoms and disorders is no different in children with or without constipation. Thus, 44 per cent compared to 39 per cent had a CBCL total score in the clinical range (norm: 10 per cent) (Benninga et al 1994); and in a recent study the rates were 39 per cent and 37 per cent (Benninga et al 2004). In another study, 35 per cent had a CBCL total score in the clinical range (Van der Plas et al 1997). Regarding the type of behavioural problems, 32 per cent of the children had a clinical score regarding internalizing behaviour, and only 17 per cent regarding externalizing behaviour (norm: 10 per cent). In other words, internalizing problems seem to predominate.

Looking at specific syndrome scores, one has to bear in mind that a different cut-off – the 98th percentile – is used, i.e. only 2 per cent of children in the normative population would have a score on these scales in the clinical range. In those children with encopresis without constipation, the percentages with clinical scores were: 12 per cent for social withdrawal, 3 per cent for somatic complaints, 13 per cent for anxiety/depression, 10 per cent for social problems, 5 per cent for schizoid/compulsive behaviour, 7 per cent for attentional problems, 3 per cent for delinquent behaviour, and 8 per cent for aggressive behaviour. It can clearly be seen that the internalizing components of social withdrawal, anxiety and depression predominate.

In summary, 35 to 50 per cent of all children with non-retentive encopresis show clinically relevant behaviour and emotional problems or disorders. This means that not all children show behavioural problems and so a purely psychogenic aetiological model is no longer tenable. The psychiatric comorbidity is heterogeneous, with internalizing disorders predominating. In some cases non-retentive encopresis can be understood as a symptom of an externalizing oppositional defiant disorder; in many other cases as a symptom of an internalizing disorder with signs of anxiety and depression. The high, heterogeneous psychiatric comorbidity does not allow a general explanation of the aetiology of non-retentive encopresis, so one has to conclude that the cause is not known (Benninga et al 1994).

ASSESSMENT

The assessment does not differ from that used in other forms of encopresis. The rate of possible organic causes is bound to be lower than in encopresis with constipation.

TREATMENT

The treatment approach should focus on the symptom of soiling. The main approach is the standard toilet training programme, as outlined previously. Laxatives are contra-indicated, as symptoms can worsen (Benninga et al 1994). In a single case report of a 20-year-old patient with childhood-onset encopresis with retention, an opioid antagonist (loperamide) was successful at a dose of 5 mg one to two times a day (Voskuijl et al 2003). Loperamide inhibits peristaltic movement by reducing the release of acetylcholine and prostaglandin during distension. It also increases anal sphincter pressure. Although promising, this approach requires systematic studies before it can be generally recommended for children.

Otherwise, medication is not indicated. Screening for possible comorbid behavioural and emotional disorders should be undertaken in every case. If additional psychological disorders are present, these should be treated, in addition to the symptom-oriented therapy of the soiling. Some psychological symptoms can resolve under successful treatment (Van der Plas et al 1997). If, however, a manifest disorder is present, it will require professional diagnostic assessment and treatment. If the psychological problems and disorders are severe, these may need treatment first, so that children are motivated and open for treatment of their soiling problems. In these cases, an interdisciplinary approach, with child psychiatrists and psychologists, is needed.

S.E., 14-year-old girl
Diagnoses: Encopresis without constipation; dysfunctional voiding;
secondary nocturnal enuresis; recurrent urinary tract infections;
VUR grade I to II left; conduct disorder (F 91.2)

S. soiled on three days per week, hid her underwear and refused to deal with her problem. Her bowels were regular and there were no signs of constipation. She had become dry at the age of 1½ years and had relapsed at the age of 4 during the night. She postponed micturition, wet during the day, and urinary tract infections occurred repeatedly. As a child, she had undergone play therapy because of oppositional, defiant behaviour.

The paediatric examination was normal. The bladder wall was thickened to 4.1 mm, and residual urine was up to 370 ml. The uroflow showed an interrupted curve with EMG contractions. According to the frequency-volume chart, the first micturition occurred at 5 p.m. with large volumes, between 300 and 600 ml. In the mental state examination S. was dysphoric and oppositional towards her parents.

Therapeutically, the micturition frequency was increased, S. had regular toilet visits and antibiotic prophylaxis was continued. Daytime wetting and soiling ceased completely, and nocturnal enuresis was reduced. Psychotherapy was started again because of the behavioural problems. Two years later, conduct problems such as truancy, school refusal, stealing and lying re-occurred, and child psychiatric inpatient treatment became necessary. No further signs of encopresis re-occurred at this time.

Specific treatment
Other forms of treatment are not effective in children with non-retentive encopresis. Thus, children treated with biofeedback do not show better results on follow-up than conventionally treated children: 18 months after treatment, 47 per cent, compared to 48 per cent of controls, were free of soiling (Van der Plas et al 1996b).

In another prospective, randomized study, children with non-retentive encopresis were treated either with laxatives and biofeedback or with biofeedback alone (Van Ginkel et al 2000). The combined group with biofeedback and laxatives had less successful results after 12 months. In other words, laxatives are not indicated in the treatment of non-retentive encopresis. This study also showed that the main treatment effects emerged before the actual biofeedback training started, which means that psychoeducation and provision of information, as well as emotional support, are the decisive elements in treatment (Van Ginkel et al 2000).

In summary, neither biofeedback nor laxatives are indicated in children with non-retentive encopresis.

COURSE AND PROGNOSIS
The long-term prognosis of encopresis is not very positive, probably due to the fact that children are not followed up for long enough, and comorbid disorders are not given adequate attention. Table 9.17 lists several studies that have reported follow-up results. Unfortunately, most include mixed groups of encopretic children. The overall prognosis for children to continue having encopretic episodes lies between 24 and 64 per cent in follow-ups of one to seven years.

Van der Plas et al (1997) followed up children with encopresis without constipation: 20 months later more than 50 per cent were still soiling. After two years, 70 per cent, and after four years, 30 per cent of the children continued to soil. In 24 per cent of cases, the incontinence persisted into adulthood (Voskuijl et al 2002).

SUMMARY AND CLINICAL GUIDELINES
The treatment of encopresis (functional faecal incontinence) without constipation is purely non-pharmacological. Laxatives are contraindicated and can lead to a worsening of the condition.

Provision of information and regular toilet sessions for ten minutes after main meals three times a day are the main lines of treatment. Motivation sometimes needs to be enhanced by a simple token system (rewards). Because of the high rate of coexisting psychological problems and disorders, additional counselling, psychotherapy and other child psychiatric interventions are often required.

Combined functional faecal incontinence (encopresis) and wetting
Wetting, urinary tract infections, encopresis and constipation commonly coexist and children with this condition require especially careful assessment and treatment. This

TABLE 9.17
Prognosis of encopresis

Study	Total number	Duration of follow-up	Success: no encopresis
Bernard-Bonnin et al 1993	28	3 years 5 months	36%
Rockney et al 1996	45	4 years 5 months	58%
Sutphen et al 1995	43	6 years 8 months	70%
Steinmüller and Steinhausen 1990	41	3 years 6 months	76%
Van der Plas et al 1997 (encopresis without constipation)	67	1 year 6 months	47% biofeedback 48% laxatives
Mehler-Wex et al 2005	35	5 years 5 months	40%

association has been called 'complicated enuresis' by some authors (Issenman et al 1999) and even 'elimination syndrome' by others. For obvious reasons, both terms are not very well chosen, and it would be preferable to describe and diagnose each voiding disorder separately as common comorbidities. This is the basic approach that has been endorsed throughout this book.

Combined problems of wetting and encopresis have only recently gained the attention they deserve, although children with these problems have always existed. This could be due to the fact that paediatric urologists and nephrologists have tended to ignore bowel problems, whereas paediatric gastroenterologists have shown a tendency to ignore problems of bladder function. At last, the necessity of a multidisciplinary approach is being realized, and it is hoped that this will lead to an integrated approach to this problem in the future (Chase et al 2004).

PREVALENCE OF WETTING PROBLEMS IN CHILDREN WITH ENCOPRESIS
Quite a few children with encopresis also show wetting problems, as can be seen in Table 9.18. Approximately one-third of all encopretic children have additional wetting problems, with a range of 10 to 50 per cent across different clinical studies. Day and night wetting occur at similar rates – and, even more surprising, the rates do not really differ between encopresis with and without constipation (see Table 9.18).

TABLE 9.18
Rate of enuresis/urinary incontinence in children with encopresis

Study	Total number (N)	Percentage of children with wetting problems
Bellman 1966 (clientele study)	75	37% total; controls 5.3%
Foreman and Thambirajah 1996	63	36.5% total
Benninga et al 1994 (encopresis with constipation)	111	12% DW 29% NW
Benninga et al 1994 (encopresis without constipation)	50	7% DW 10% NW
Van Ginkel et al 2000 (encopresis without constipation)	48	46% DW 40% NW
Gabel et al 1986 (42 of 55 with constipation)	55	31% total
Freunek 1993	29	55% total 31% DW
Steinmüller and Steinhausen 1990	41	59% total
Mehler-Wex et al 2005	85	45% total
Loening-Baucke 1997 (encopresis with constipation)	234	34% NW 29% DW 46% total
Loening-Baucke 2002 (encopresis with constipation)	49	29% DW 41% NW

DW: daytime wetting
NW: night-time wetting

The only epidemiological study in the table is the clientele study of Bellman (1966): 37 per cent of encopretic children but only 5.3 per cent of controls showed wetting problems. In addition there is a high association between secondary encopresis and secondary enuresis, which means that if a relapse occurs, this can affect both types of voiding disorder. Of those children with secondary encopresis (n=37), 2.6 per cent had primary and 18.9 per cent secondary enuresis. In contrast, of those children with primary encopresis (n=38), 31.6 per cent had primary and 21.1 per cent secondary enuresis, i.e. no great difference (Bellman 1966). In a recent Swedish population-based study, there was a highly significant association of faecal incontinence with daytime wetting, but not with nocturnal enuresis (Söderström et al 2004).

All other studies are based in different clinical settings with possible confounding effects due to selection and referral biases. Interestingly, the comorbidity rate of encopresis and wetting problems does not really differ in clinical (compared to population-based) studies. In a highly selected group of child and adolescent psychiatric patients, 37 per cent with encopresis also wetted (Foreman and Thambirajah 1996). In the classic study of Benninga et al (1994), children with encopresis and constipation had higher rates of wetting (12 per cent daytime, 29 per cent night-time) than children without constipation (7 per cent daytime, 10 per cent night-time). In other studies, children with encopresis without constipation had extremely high rates of additional wetting problems (Van Ginkel et al 2000) – similar to those of children with encopresis and constipation (Gabel et al 1986, Loening-Baucke 2000).

The most important study is that of Loening-Baucke (1997), who examined 234 children aged 5 to 18 years (mean age 9 years) with chronic encopresis and constipation, prospectively. In total, 46 per cent of the children wetted, 34 per cent at night and 17 per cent only at night; 29 per cent wetted during the day, 12 per cent only during the day; 11 per cent had additional urinary tract infections, with a significant difference between girls (33 per cent) and boys (3 per cent). The constipation was treated intensively by regulating toilet habits and by prescribing laxatives; 52 per cent of all children were treated successfully after 12 months (success was defined as achieving more than three stools per week). Of this successful group, only 3 per cent wetted during the day (compared to 28 per cent initially) and 15 per cent at night (compared to 41 per cent initially). Even if only partial success (defined as fewer than three stools per week) was achieved, children still had a lower rate of wetting. Only 14 per cent wetted during the day (initially 36 per cent) and 26 per cent at night (initially 39 per cent). In other words, even if treatment does not lead to complete success, treating constipation alone can reduce coexisting wetting (Loening-Baucke 1997). This success does not depend on the type of laxative. In another study (Loening-Baucke 2002), 49 children with encopresis and constipation, aged 4–17 years, were treated with either polyethylene glycol (PEG) or milk of magnesia (MOM). After 12 months of treatment, day wetting was reduced from 29 to 9 per cent with PEG, and from 29 to 0 per cent with MOM. The rate of nocturnal enuresis dropped from 36 to 30 per cent with PEG and from 48 to 36 per cent with MOM. The similar effect of the two laxatives demonstrates that the treatment of constipation has a greater effect on reducing daytime wetting than it has on nocturnal enuresis.

Unfortunately, this question – i.e. how many children with enuresis and urinary incontinence also have encopresis – has not been addressed in epidemiological studies such as the famous longitudinal study of Fergusson et al (1986).

In early clinical studies, 4.3 per cent of children with nocturnal enuresis and 25 per cent of children with daytime wetting were also affected by encopresis (Berg et al 1977). Among child psychiatric patients, 4.4 per cent of all children with wetting problems also soiled (Steinhausen and Göbel 1989).

Finally, in a recent study, 12 per cent (20) of 167 consecutively presented wetting children had encopresis as an additional diagnosis (von Gontard and Hollmann 2004). Most of these 20 children with combined problems had encopresis with constipation; 24.6 per cent wetted during the day, 5.5 per cent during the night. The rate of encopresis differed greatly with regard to the type of wetting problem. Encopresis was most common in children with dysfunctional voiding (42.9 per cent), voiding postponement (25.0 per cent), urge incontinence (18.2 per cent) and primary, non-monosymptomatic nocturnal enuresis, i.e. night-time wetting with additional daytime micturition problems (15.6 per cent). Only one child with secondary and not a single child with primary monosymptomatic nocturnal enuresis had additional soiling problems. In other words, the comorbidity is highly associated with any type of bladder dysfunction and primarily affects children with day wetting or with non-monosymptomatic enuresis (see Figure 7.5 for a graphic representation of the prevalences of the different disorders and their overlap).

Children with combined voiding problems had more problems in relaxing the pelvic floor (30 per cent showed no relaxation on the EMG), and had a thicker bladder wall (von Gontard and Hollmann 2004). They showed an extremely high rate of comorbid behavioural disorders: 65 per cent had a CBCL total score, 50 per cent an externalizing score and 40 per cent an internalizing score, in the clinical range. Externalizing disorders (defined according to ICD-10), especially oppositional defiant disorder, were more common (45 per cent) than emotional disorders (25 per cent). These results mean that children with combined voiding disorders not only have higher rates of bladder dysfunction, but also show the highest rates of comorbid behavioural and emotional disorders – much higher than those of children with encopresis or wetting problems alone. This means that both disorders need to be addressed even more carefully in this group of children.

AETIOLOGY OF COMBINED ENCOPRESIS AND WETTING

Even though both local and central factors play a role in the association of wetting and encopresis, the local aetiology has been explored in more detail. Basically, four different, interacting local factors play a role:

1 Local stool masses compress the bladder retrovesically, leading to residual urine, vesico-ureteric reflux and/or hydronephrosis (Dohil et al 1994). Twenty-four children with chronic constipation had significant pelvicalyceal dilatation, which resolved completely after treatment of constipation (Dohil et al 1994). These changes can easily be seen on ultrasound.

2   The compression of stool masses can induce uninhibited contractions of the detrusor (O'Regan et al 1986). All patients with encopresis (most with constipation) who were examined urodynamically had signs of an overactive bladder. Treatment of constipation alone again led to a reduction of wetting in most children. It was hypothesized that stretch-receptors of the detrusor were activated by stool masses, leading to contractions (O'Regan and Yazbeck 1985).

3   The rectal and urethral sphincters represent a common physiological unit, so that contractions of the rectal and urethral sphincter are often associated. Dysfunctional voiding (detrusor–sphincter discoordination) and rectal discoordination, as well as encopresis, are often associated (Yazbeck et al 1987, von Gontard and Hollmann 2004).

4   Finally, all these factors increase the risk for urinary tract infection by inducing residual urine (O'Regan and Yazbeck 1985). As has been shown previously, urinary tract infections, in turn, can induce wetting and a vicious circle can follow.

These aetiological models are very plausible as explanations for the association of encopresis with constipation and daytime wetting. They do not, however, explain why children with encopresis without constipation have such high rates of wetting (Van Ginkel et al 2000), and why the treatment of constipation does not necessarily have an effect on night-time wetting (Loening-Baucke 1997). In these cases, central factors might be active, as several animal studies have shown. Thus increased pressures of both bladder and gut can activate the pontine micturition centre (Pavcovich et al 1998) and the locus coeruleus (Lechner et al 1997). These two centres are involved in the aetiology of nocturnal enuresis, which can be induced if the micturition reflex is not inhibited (pontine micturition centre) or if the full bladder does not lead to arousal (locus coeruleus). The locus coeruleus is seen as the link between visceral functions and affective behaviour. Thus, the stretching of bladder, rectum and even stomach could activate the noradrenergic neurons of the locus coeruleus without inducing a sympathetic activity (Elam et al 1986). In other words, the common association of wetting and encopresis might not just be due to local, mechanical factors associated with increased stool masses. It seems that both bowel and bladder function are regulated by the same pathways and neurons in the central nervous system.

SUMMARY AND CLINICAL GUIDELINES

Combined problems require an especially careful assessment addressing both organic and psychological aspects. The assessment should follow the guidelines that have been described – both for encopresis (see pages 231–238) and for wetting (see pages 139–141). Each separate sub-disorder should be diagnosed separately. Once a diagnosis has been reached, treatment should follow a clear sequence:

1   Encopresis/constipation should be treated first, since in many children the wetting problems will subside without any other treatment.

2   Any day-wetting problems (or micturition problems without daytime wetting) should be treated next, as these are associated with bladder dysfunction. If treated properly,

some children with concomitant nocturnal enuresis will stop wetting during the night without further treatment.

3   If nocturnal enuresis should persist despite successful treatment of encopresis/ constipation and daytime wetting, this should be addressed last.

Toilet refusal syndrome

Toilet refusal syndrome is defined by a typical behaviour: children use the toilet for micturition, but refuse to use it for defecation and insist on using a diaper (Christopherson and Edwards 1992). If this persists for longer than one month, the syndrome is diagnosed. It is a common condition, affecting one-fifth of all infants aged between 18 and 30 months (Taubman 1997).

AETIOLOGY

Four factors have been associated with toilet refusal syndrome (TRS):

1   Birth of a younger sibling
2   Behavioural problems
3   Late toilet training
4   Stool retention

In fact, stool retention actually precedes toilet refusal syndrome in almost half of the children. Therefore hard bowel movements and painful defecation are risk factors that contribute towards TRS (Blum et al 2004a).

In one study, it was hypothesized that parents were too relaxed, did not set limits adequately and that their demands were generally too low. There were no signs of coercive toilet training. Instead, late toilet training (after 42 months of age) was associated with higher rates of TRS and with constipation (Blum et al 2004b). Thus, toilet refusal syndrome is seen as a risk factor for later encopresis. Children with primary encopresis, who had previously shown toilet refusal syndrome, were especially difficult to treat (Taubman and Buzby 1997).

Children with TRS do not necessarily have more behavioural problems, but they show a trend towards a more difficult temperament (Blum et al 1997). In clinical practice, oppositional defiant disorder (ODD) is a common comorbidity, with ensuing interactional problems between parent and child. TRS has also been observed when mothers have psychiatric disorders such as depression; these mothers need not only treatment for their own problems but also guidance and counselling for their children.

Fortunately, TRS shows a high spontaneous remission rate of 73 per cent (Taubman 1997). TRS persists for longer than six months in 19 per cent of children.

Treatment is clear-cut and simple: parents are asked to give their child a diaper again. They are instructed to tell their child that underpants can only be worn when he/she passes stools and urinates in the potty or toilet. Then the parents are asked to make no effort to toilet-train the child (Taubman 1997). Although some of the parents are reluctant to do this, the success rate is high. A small group of children will require behaviour modification, mainly because of the stool retention. This simple approach is effective mainly in infancy: the children Taubman (1997) described were 18 to 30 months old.

Toilet refusal syndrome in an older child is usually a more chronic and severe condition. By this time, stool retention and constipation are common, and a more intensive regime, including disimpaction, laxatives and stool regulation, will be necessary. It can be helpful to adapt the toilet seat to the child's needs, as some children are actually afraid of sitting on the toilet. Sturdy children's toilet seats and foot-stools aid stability and make the children feel secure.

Z.P., 3-year-old girl
Diagnoses: Toilet refusal syndrome; chronic constipation

Z. had been chronically constipated from the age of 3 months, passing hard stools once every eight days. She had been treated with lactulose and paraffin oil from the age of 2 years. She preferred a low-fibre diet. A plain abdominal X-ray did not indicate an organic cause of the constipation.

Z. was referred because she obstinately refused to use the toilet for defecation. Instead she insisted on a diaper. There were no other signs of behavioural deviance. Her CBCL total scores were in the subclinical range. Ultrasound showed a markedly enlarged rectal diameter of 42 to 54 mm.

Z. was treated with polyethylene glycol (Movicol®). She was allowed to continue using a diaper until she was ready for further toilet training. In this case, chronic constipation preceded the toilet refusal syndrome, as recently described by Blum et al (2004a).

Toilet phobia
Toilet phobia is basically an isolated phobia, i.e. a circumscribed, object-bound phobia or anxiety. Some children are afraid to sit on the toilet. They fear that animals or monsters could emerge out of the toilet and attack them; they are afraid that they might fall into the toilet;

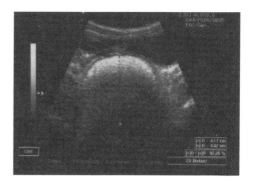

Fig. 9.3 Z.P: ultrasound: retrovesical impressions and enlarged rectum (diameter 42–54 mm) in a transversal view.

or they fear the flushing noises. These anxieties are generalized and the children avoid the toilet altogether. In contrast to toilet refusal syndrome, the toilet is avoided both for micturition and for bowel movements.

Toilet phobia can be associated with early toilet training (Bellman 1966). It is often overlooked and is seldom mentioned in the literature (Krisch 1985). The treatment is the same as for any other isolated phobia. Cognitive-behavioural techniques – usually some form of systematic desensitization – are most effective. If other emotional symptoms are present, further psychiatric and psychotherapeutic interventions may be necessary.

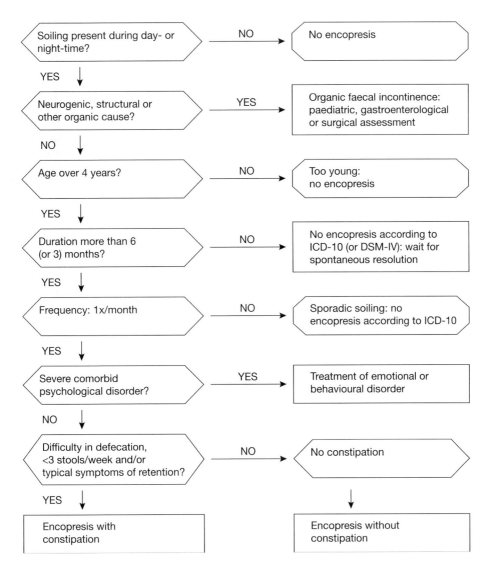

Chart 9.1 Diagnosis of functional faecal incontinence (encopresis).

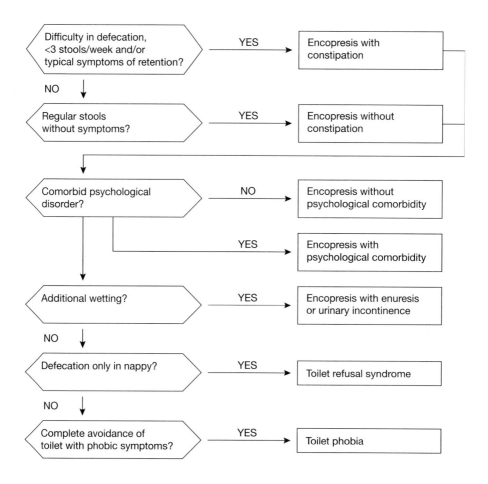

Chart 9.2 Differential diagnosis of functional faecal incontinence (encopresis).

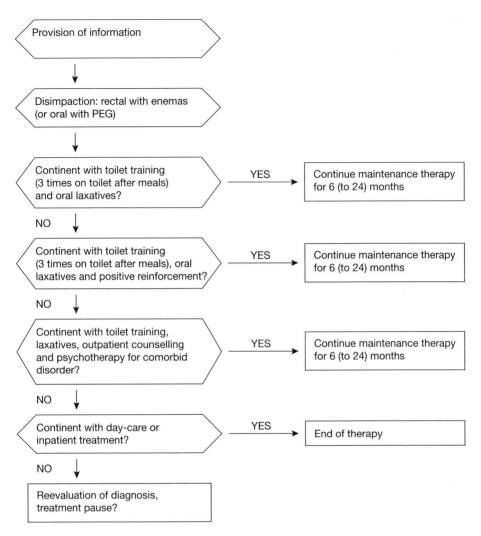

Chart 9.3 Therapy of functional faecal incontinence (encopresis) with constipation.

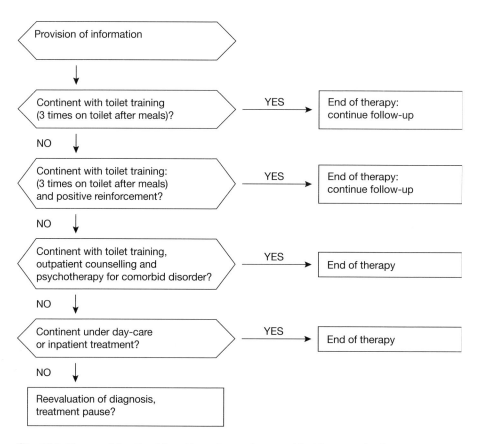

Chart 9.4 Therapy of functional faecal incontinence (encopresis) without constipation.

10
ORGANIC FAECAL INCONTINENCE

Structural faecal incontinence

CONGENITAL MALFORMATIONS

Congenital anorectal malformations *per se* do not cause faecal incontinence, with the exception of obvious cases such as cloacal malformations (Shaul and Harrison 1997). More commonly they result in obstructed faecal voiding. The typical cases are anal atresia of various degrees or the ectopic location of the anus in the perineum or vulva. Congenital rectovesical fistulas may cause meconium and faeces to have to force their way out through the urethra. But these cases present no differential diagnostic problem and are not the subject of this book.

The relevance of congenital anorectal malformations for this text is that these children commonly experience encopresis as a long-term postoperative complication (Ottolenghi et al 1994). Only around 50 per cent of children with corrected distal anorectal malformations have normal bowel function (Rintala et al 1997). Constipation is the most prevalent problem, and 25 per cent are faecally incontinent (Pena and Hong 2000).

POSTOPERATIVE FAECAL INCONTINENCE

Structural faecal incontinence is usually synonymous with postoperative faecal incontinence. The crucial causative factor is that the surgeon has been forced to damage, or has not been able to save, the internal anal sphincter (Lindsey et al 2004).

Children who have been operated on for Hirschsprung disease (see below) suffer a risk of approximately 50 per cent of becoming faecally incontinent (Catto-Smith et al 1995, Ludman et al 2002). The risk is highest if the usual endorectal pull-through operation has to be performed before 10 months of age (Foster et al 1990). The same operation carries the same risk for children with inflammatory bowel disease (Ceriati et al 2004).

EVALUATION AND TREATMENT

For in-depth guidelines on how to handle surgical faecal incontinence, the reader is advised to consult handbooks of paediatric surgery.

Children with postoperative faecal incontinence differ from those with functional constipation or encopresis in that invasive evaluation with anal EMG or anorectal manometry can often be useful and indicated (Hettiarachchi et al 2002, Abbasoglu et al 2004). Likewise, MRI is appropriate in these cases, since it gives excellent anatomical detail (Hettiarachchi et al 2002).

A majority of children with postoperative faecal incontinence can be successfully treated conservatively (Pena et al 1998) with laxatives, enemas, and – possibly – biofeedback (Hibi et al 2003). But treatment has to be long-term, since the underlying cause cannot be corrected, and in some cases surgical treatment, as outlined under neurogenic faecal incontinence below, has to be resorted to (Pena and Hong 2000).

Neurogenic faecal incontinence

AETIOLOGY AND PATHOGENESIS

The mechanisms behind neurogenic bowel disturbance are in many ways similar to those underlying the neurogenic bladder, and so are the causes. The reasons are obvious; the lowest part of the gastrointestinal canal, i.e. the anal sphincter, is innervated by the last part of the conus medullaris, and the more proximal large intestine receives innervation from neurons located slightly higher in the spinal medulla. Thus, neural damage above the conus medullaris results in slow faecal transport in most of the colon except in the rectosigmoid area, whereas damage to the conus or the cauda equina leads to a slowing of transport in the rectosigmoid colon (Krogh et al 2000). If the sacral roots S2–4 are damaged, the patient's ability to counter raised intra-abdominal or rectal pressure by raising his/her anal pressure is restricted, and the risk for faecal incontinence is increased (Agnarsson et al 1993).

The most prevalent cause is, not surprisingly, *spinal dysraphism*. It has been estimated that 80 per cent of children with myelomeningocele suffer from neurogenic bowel disturbance, and 40 per cent need to empty their bowels manually, usually with the assistance of a parent (Lie et al 1991). More than 50 per cent of these children have occasional faecal incontinence (Malone et al 1994). The presence of tethered-cord related neural damage further compromises bowel function (Levitt et al 1997). The situation for patients with spinal damage for other reasons – trauma, malignancy – is similar; a majority of these patients suffer from constipation and faecal incontinence (Glickman and Kamm 1996, De Looze et al 1998).

Most children with cerebral palsy of more than mild degree have clinically significant gastrointestinal problems. Many of these disturbances – such as vomiting, gastro-oesophageal reflux, swallowing difficulties – belong to the upper gastrointestinal tract, but colon transit time is often prolonged as well (Del Giudice et al 1999), and approximately half of these patients have some degree of faecal incontinence (Feldkamp et al 1976). The severity of the symptoms is not necessarily proportional to the damage visible on MRI or CT (Del Giudice et al 1999).

TREATMENT

First-line treatment of neurogenic faecal incontinence is similar to treatment of retentive encopresis. The children receive laxatives, enemas and bowel therapy, preferably under the supervision of a skilled anotherapist. Manual evacuation of the bowel is often necessary – a procedure that is rendered more difficult by the fact that many children with myelomeningocele have impaired manipulative skills or are obese.

In an increasing number of cases operative treatment is now performed, with the provision of a continent stoma by which enemas may be introduced directly into the proximal colon. The stoma is usually fashioned using the appendix, if present, but other parts of the intestine may also be used. This so-called Malone antegrade continence enema (MACE) procedure (Malone et al 1990) has proven safe and reliable in cases of severe neurogenic constipation and faecal incontinence (Yerkes et al 2003); success rates seem to depend more on motivation, age and habitus than on what tissue is used to fabricate the stoma (Clark et al 2002).

Treatment of the bowel problems of patients with multiple sclerosis or cerebrovascular insults is entirely empirical, and there is today no ground for treating them differently from other constipated or encopretic patients – although biofeedback has shown some promise in open studies (Wiesel et al 2000).

Other medical causes of faecal incontinence and constipation

Diarrhoea

Diarrhoea, for any cause, may if sufficiently severe cause faecal incontinence. This is not surprising. What is surprising is that most children do *not* become faecally incontinent when they have diarrhoea. The *inflammatory bowel diseases* ulcerative colitis and Crohn's disease, for instance, may force the child to go to the toilet more than a dozen times daily and regularly wake them up at night with a need to pass watery stools, but even so, patients seldom lose continence. And even perianal manifestations of Crohn's disease do not usually lead to faecal incontinence (Singh et al 2004). However, children with diarrhoea do sometimes soil their clothes. The usual case is faecal incontinence in a child with acute viral gastroenteritis.

Allergies and Food Intolerance

Cow's milk allergy or intolerance is a common condition, affecting a small percentage of the population (Moneret-Vautrin 1999). Both IgE- and non-IgE-mediated effects may be causative, and symptoms in children past infancy include various combinations of diarrhoea, constipation, vomiting and eczema. Most of these children have other allergies as well, and an atopic disposition is very common, as is a positive family history (Buisseret 1978).

Cow's milk allergy is not uncommon in children with chronic constipation with or without encopresis (Loening-Baucke 2000, Turunen et al 2004), but symptoms from other organs, such as the skin or lungs, are usually present as well.

Although skin prick testing or specific blood tests are often positive in IgE-mediated cases, the mainstay of diagnosis is elimination and provocation (Moneret-Vautrin 1999). Thus, if cow's milk intolerance (or, indeed, intolerance/allergy to any food component) is suspected, cow's milk should be eliminated for a week or two and then reintroduced. It is an important rule to remember: whenever elimination is tried, provocation should follow. The symptoms with and without cow's milk can then be evaluated. Cow's milk elimination and provocation should certainly be considered in children with chronic constipation of unclear aetiology, especially if they have an atopic predisposition or a family history of allergies (Daher et al 2001).

HIRSCHSPRUNG DISEASE AND RELATED DISORDERS

Although congenital aganglionosis of the colon, or Hirschsprung disease, is an important, albeit uncommon, cause of severe constipation in children, it does not usually lead to encopresis, and thus only deserves passing mention here (see Table 9.14). The severity of the constipation is proportional to the length of the distal colonic segment that is affected. Most cases will present during the first year of life. Diagnosis is made with anal manometry (one of the few indications for this procedure) and rectal biopsy. Treatment is surgical, usually a rectal pull-through anastomosis. As mentioned above, faecal incontinence is quite common among children who have been operated on because of this disease.

Intestinal neuronal dysplasia is a somewhat controversial condition which is distinguished from Hirschsprung disease by histological criteria (Kapur 2003, Puri 2003, Tomita et al 2004). The typical distinguishing feature is hyperplasia of the submucosal plexus (Hutson et al 2001). These children are reported to have earlier symptoms than those with functional constipation (Montedonico et al 2002). The condition can often be treated conservatively (Gillick et al 2001).

MYOPATHIES

Myopathies of various kinds, all exceedingly rare, may affect the bowel either exclusively (Fitzgibbons and Chandrasoma 1987, Jayachandar et al 1988) or in addition to striated muscle (Fuger et al 1995). These children may have stomach pains, abdominal distension, nausea, vomiting and alternating constipation and diarrhoea. Although constipation may be severe, with toxic megacolon or intestinal pseudo-obstruction as the end result in extreme cases, faecal incontinence is not typical (Mathias and Clench 1995). The evaluation of these children would typically include extensive metabolic screening, neurography and both rectal and muscle biopsy. Treatment of the bowel symptoms is empirical. In cases of megacolon, extensive surgery may be needed, and children with chronic intestinal pseudo-obstruction often become dependent on intravenous nutrition.

CYSTIC FIBROSIS

Cystic fibrosis is a recessively inherited multi-organ disease primarily affecting the lungs and the gastrointestinal tract. The children suffer from recurrent pulmonary infections, and malabsorption due to exocrine pancreatic insufficiency, and have varying degrees of constipation. Just as is the case with Hirschsprung disease, however, although constipation may be severe, the children are almost uniformly faecally continent (Littlewood 1992). Indeed, urinary incontinence is a more common voiding disorder in cystic fibrosis patients than encopresis (Nixon et al 2002).

A suspected diagnosis of cystic fibrosis is strengthened by measuring sodium chloride in sweat or elastase in faeces, and confirmed via genetic analysis. Treatment of the gastrointestinal complications is multifaceted, with pancreatic enzymes, vitamins, and specific barium enemas for the sometimes severe constipation. Surgical treatment of constipation should be avoided at all costs.

Faecal incontinence in chronic paediatric illness

IMMOBILIZATION

Any condition that immobilizes the child in bed may lead to faecal incontinence, usually via constipation. The child may be bedridden due to pain, in which case opioid side effects on bowel motility may aggravate constipation. Severely ill children may be too weak, and children with severe neuromuscular disability may not be mobile enough, to go to the toilet. Thus, in one study, nearly 30 per cent of children with spinal muscular atrophy had urinary incontinence – most of them were also affected by constipation and/or encopresis (von Gontard et al 2001b).

Treatment of faecal incontinence in these children obviously depends on why they are immobilized. In cases where the situation can be predicted, such as when a child has osteomyelitis and needs prolonged intravenous antibiotic treatment, and has skeletal pain when moving, it is advised that (1) laxatives be given before severe constipation develops; (2) complete pain relief is sought but preferably without IV morphine; (3) a physiotherapist is employed to improve mobility.

MENTAL RETARDATION

Soiling is more common in individuals with mental retardation than in the general population, but it is by no means universal. About 80 per cent of these individuals have attained full bowel control at the age of 20 years, even though 30 per cent are not fully continent yet at the age of 7 (von Wendt et al 1990).

Again, though burdensome for parents, encopresis has not been studied much in specific syndromes of mental retardation (behavioural phenotypes). In one study, 20 per cent of boys with fragile-X syndrome had encopresis (Backes et al 2000).

Treatment needs to be adapted according to intellectual abilities and associated behavioural problems. The outcome seems to be fairly encouraging according to a review of 21 studies (Lancioni et al 2001). The treatment of non-retentive encopresis relies mainly on behavioural technique packages. These include scheduled toileting, pants checks, positive and negative reinforcement, shaping and fading. Retentive encopresis (with constipation) requires additional medical components such as enemas, laxatives and dietary changes.

Specific programmes for adults rely on prompting, sitting on the toilet after meals, and immediate positive reinforcement – and omit all negative consequences (Smith 1996). In children with compulsive, repetitive and resistant behaviour, gradual transfer of stimulus control was effective. Children were allowed to defecate in their diaper and were rewarded immediately when this occurred. Next, they were asked to sit on a chair with a wooden toilet seat with their diaper on while being read to by their mother. Gradually, the chair was moved towards the toilet and the diaper size was reduced – until the toilet was accepted for defecation (Smith et al 2000). Long training times, ranging from two months to two years, were needed.

In summary, children with all degrees of mental retardation can achieve faecal continence by a combination of adapted behavioural techniques (and laxatives if constipated).

11
CONCLUSION

The aim of this book has been to provide a comprehensive overview of functional voiding disorders – a group of common disorders in children and adolescents. These disorders include different types of nocturnal enuresis, functional urinary incontinence and encopresis. Since the borderline between functional and organic disturbances is not always clear-cut, and the evaluation of the former requires some knowledge of the latter, we have also discussed organic causes for enuresis, incontinence and encopresis.

As both somatic and psychological factors are intertwined in the development as well as the treatment of these disorders, it was our explicit wish to present an interdisciplinary view of the approaches in paediatrics, child psychiatry and paediatric urology. We are convinced that an optimal treatment requires not only an interdisciplinary approach, i.e. the involvement of members of different professions, but actually more than that. Each person dealing with these children and families should have a basic understanding of the approaches of the other disciplines. Paediatricians and urologists need to know how to recognize and counsel children with child psychiatric disorders – and when to refer them. Conversely, child psychiatrists need to be aware of the enormous advances in non-invasive paediatric and urological diagnostics and treatments. We hope that we have been able to contribute towards such an all-encompassing approach to dealing with children and their families.

Our second aim was to provide a clinical handbook that could be used in everyday clinical practice. We have tried to present the current state of the art in a way that we hope can be implemented by many practitioners in diverse settings around the world. Wherever possible, the recommendations are evidence based. Due to the poor database for some disorders, views based on clinical experience are given in some cases and this is stated explicitly. We hope that future research will help to fill in the gaps of knowledge – to be condensed one day in another Mac Keith Press volume.

Finally, we hope that we have completed the task in the way that Kelm Hjälmås, our third co-author, would have wanted us to do it.

APPENDIX 1
HISTORY OF WETTING PROBLEM AND POSSIBLE COMORBID DISORDERS

Presenting symptom

General introduction:	Do you know why you and your parents are here today?
Time of wetting:	Is it because you wet the bed or because your pants are wet during the day?

Start with the most important symptom, i.e. night- or daytime problems

Nocturnal wetting

Frequency of wetting:	Do you wet the bed every night or are there dry nights? How many nights per week is your bed wet (or dry)?
Amount of wetting:	Is the bed damp or completely wet?
Depth of sleep:	How deeply does your child sleep? Is it easy or difficult to wake him/her? What do you have to do to wake your child? Does your child sometimes wake up at night to go to the toilet (nocturia)?
Dry intervals:	What is the longest time period that your child has been completely dry (days, weeks, months)? How old was your child then? Were there events at the time of the relapse which might have had some influence on your child starting wetting again?
Impact and distress:	How is it for you when your bed is wet? Are you sad, annoyed, angry, ashamed – or do you feel it does not matter? Do you want to get dry? Are you willing to do something about it and put some effort into the therapy?
Social consequences:	Have you been teased by somebody else about the wetting? Have you avoided sleeping over with friends or joining in on outings with your school class?

Daytime wetting and micturition problems during the day

Frequency of wetting:	Are your pants wet every day or do you also have dry days? How many days per week are your trousers wet? Does it happen that you wet during the day not once, but several times? How many times does it usually occur?
Amount of wetting:	Are your pants damp or really wet? Can the wet spot be seen through your clothing?
Timing during the day:	Do you usually wet during the morning or in the afternoons (evenings)?
Frequency of micturition:	How often does your child go to the toilet during the day (3, 5, 10 or 20 times? Normal range: 5 to 7 times per day)?
Voiding postponement:	Have you ever noticed that your child does not go to the toilet right away, but postpones going as long as possible? In which situations does this happen most often (for example, in school, coming home from school, while playing, while watching TV or during other activities)?
Holding manoeuvres:	How do you notice that your child needs to go to the toilet? Does he/she seem to be absent-minded? What exactly does your child do to postpone voiding? Have you ever noticed that he/she crosses his/her legs, jumps from one leg to the next, holds his/her tummy or genitals, squats or sits on his/her heels?
Urge symptoms:	Does it happen that your child feels a sudden and strong urge to go to the toilet (even though he/she goes to the toilet often)? For example, how long can you drive in the car or go shopping, before your child has to go to the toilet? Do you have enough time to wait for the next restroom or do you have to stop right away to let your child void?
Dry intervals during the day:	When did your child become dry during the day? Is he/she still wetting during the day? What is the longest time period your child has ever been dry (days, weeks, months)? How old was your child then? Were there events at the time of the relapse which might have had some influence on your child starting wetting again?
Problems with micturition:	Does your child have to strain at the beginning of micturition or does the urine come spontaneously? When voiding, is there one continuous stream or is the voiding interrupted? If it is interrupted, how many portions are there? And does your child have to strain to get it going again?
Urinary tract infections:	Does your child complain about pain during voiding? Does your child have to go to the toilet more often than usual? How many

urinary tract infections has your child had so far? When did the first infection occur? Has your child had infections with fever and pain in the kidney area? Have the infections been treated with antibiotics? Has your child had long-term antibiotic prophylaxis? Is he/she taking medication at the moment? Has your child had skin infections in the genital area (dermatitis)?

Medical complications: Have there been other medical complications such as reflux, operations, etc.?

Eating and drinking habits: Please describe the eating habits of your child. Does he/she prefer biscuits, white bread or other low-fibre food? How much and what does your child drink during the day?

Attributions: What do you think is the cause of your child's wetting problem? Do you have any idea how it happened? Have you ever felt guilty about it? Have you ever blamed yourself for it? Have you ever been blamed by others? Do you think your child is doing it on purpose? Who is more distressed about the wetting: you or your child? What do you think should change? What are your expectations? Are you and your child willing to cooperate actively?

Treatment trials

Previous therapy: What have you tried so far to get your child dry? (Ineffective forms of 'treatment': fluid restriction, waking, lifting, punishment, other measures? Effective forms of treatment: charts and calendars, rewards, alarm treatment, medication – which? Desmopressin, imipramine, others?) How were the treatment trials conducted? Please describe for how long and with what effects. Whom have you consulted about your child's wetting problem (paediatrician, urologist, psychologist, psychiatrist, child guidance centre, etc.)? Which investigations have been performed so far?

Encopresis

Soiling: Does your child sometimes soil his/her underwear? How many times per week does it happen? Is it large amounts or stool smearing? Does it happen only during the day or also at night? How does your child react when he/she soils? How old was your child when he/she became clean (i.e. stools in the toilet and not in the diaper)? Have there been any relapses in the past?

Toilet habits: How often does your child have bowel movements (per week)? Does it ever happen that your child does not have bowel movements for several days in a row? Is your child constipated regularly? Is the voiding of stool painful? Has there ever been blood on the stools? What have you done so far?

Child psychiatric history

The child psychiatric history is divided into the presenting symptom(s), the personal and developmental history and the family history. In most cases, parents and child are seen and questioned together – this way differing views can be assessed easily. In some cases, it is better to see the parents alone without the child (i.e. in cases of marital conflict, abuse, etc.). In others, it can be useful to see and talk to the child alone. Some children are more willing to talk about their problems when their parents are not present (less conflict of loyalty towards the parents).

Presenting symptom

At the end of the wetting history, it is useful to ask an open question regarding other problem areas.

Other behavioural problems:	Are there other areas of your child's behaviour that you are worried about? Please describe these in detail.

As in the history of the wetting problem, each presenting symptom should be dealt with in turn. The following points are useful to consider:

Presenting symptom:	Please describe the problem in your own words in as much detail as possible. How often does it occur? In which situations (at home, at school, with friends)? How does your child react? How do you react? When did it begin? How has it developed so far? Has it remained the same, got worse or diminished in intensity, frequency, etc.? What have you done about it so far? Has the child been presented, examined or treated for the problem? Where, by whom and with what effect? What are your main worries? What would you like to change? How do you think this could change? What do you expect from this visit?

It is also useful to ask a few general questions about possible problem domains that can occur in children and which might be missed by an open question. If parents answer positively, each of the problems should be explored in detail.

Other problem areas

Externalizing problems:	Is your child restless, constantly in movement, too active for their age? Is your child distracted easily? How long can he/she

concentrate on one thing? Are there certain situations in which it is especially difficult for them to sustain concentration – in school, for example? Does your child act impulsively, without thinking? Is he/she sometimes aggressive – verbally, towards objects or people? How does your child react to rules? Does he/she obey your rules? Or is he/she oppositional? How does he/she react if you set limits and say no? Are there any special problem areas: homework, coming home too late, lying, stealing, etc.?

Internalizing problems: Is your child sad, unhappy, withdrawn? Has your child lost interest in play, seeing other children? Does he/she find it difficult to get an activity going? Does your child worry? Are there problems with sleeping or eating? Are there fears and anxieties: towards certain objects or animals (phobias)? Towards strangers, groups of children (social anxiety)? When you go away (separation anxiety)? Or without apparent reason (generalized anxiety)? Has your child developed any peculiar habits, rituals or interests? Does he/she tend to repeat things in the same way?

Personal and developmental history

Pregnancy: Was the pregnancy planned (desired?) or unexpected? What were your feelings during pregnancy? Were there any medical complications? Were there any events that you found stressful?

Birth: Was the delivery at the expected date, too early, too late? Was it a spontaneous birth? Were there any complications during or after birth? What was the birthweight of your child?

Infancy: Was your child breastfed? For how long? If not, what were the reasons? Was your child a quiet, content or active baby (temperament)? Were there any problems with feeding, weight gain, sleeping, excessive crying?

Motor development: When did your child start sitting, standing, walking freely?

Speech and language: When did your child say their first words (and what were they)? When did your child say their first two-word sentences? Were there any problems with articulation, the way sentences were formed (expressive language), or with understanding (receptive language)?

Kindergarten: When did your child enter kindergarten? Did he/she show problems staying there (i.e. separation)? Were there any problems with other children or with the kindergarten teachers? If yes, please describe.

School:	When did your child enter school? Which grade is he/she in now? What type of school? Did he/she have to repeat a grade? Does your child like going to school? If yes or no, please describe. What are his/her favourite subjects? What are his/her grades in the different subjects? Does your child have special problems with the teachers, or with other children? Please describe.
Leisure time:	What does your child do in his/her free time? What are his/her favourite games and type of play (role playing, construction games, activity games, computer games, etc.)? Are there any planned activities? What are his/her interests and hobbies? Does he/she do any sports? Does your child have friends (how many and how intense)? Does your child spend his/her free time alone or with friends? What role does your child have in groups with other children of the same age?
Illnesses:	What illnesses, operations, hospital treatment, accidents, allergies has your child had so far?

Family history

Parents:	Age, occupation (school training), illnesses? Marital relationship? Did you wet as a child? How would you describe your relationship with your child?
Siblings:	Age, biological siblings? School grade, illnesses and wetting problems? How would you describe the relationship of the brothers and sisters with each other? Are there especially close bonds or rivalries?
Other relatives:	Other cases of wetting, other illnesses, especially psychiatric and nephrological?

Regarding the problem of enuresis and urinary incontinence (as well as nocturia and micturition problems such as urge) we have made it part of our routine to draw up a complete family history over three generations. Often, other relatives will be missed, unless one asks directly and explicitly if they have wetted in the past (or currently).

It is usually best to end the history by asking another open question, such as: is there anything else we might have missed or that you might feel to be of importance?

284

APPENDIX 2
FREQUENCY-VOLUME CHART

Instructions for parents

Dear parents,

In order to be able to assess and treat your child's wetting problem in the best possible way, we would be very grateful for your help and your observations.

Please fill out this chart on a day when there is no school or kindergarten (weekend or holiday). Please record whenever your child goes to the toilet or when he/she wets. This should start on one morning and continue through to the next morning. **If possible, please fill out two charts on two days in a row, as this is even more reliable.**

Please talk to your child about it beforehand. You should not send your child to the toilet. Instead, he/she should tell you when he/she wants to go to the toilet and he/she should empty the urine into a measuring cup. Please measure the amount of urine, and record it with the time of day on the chart. You do not have to keep the urine, but can discard it afterwards.

If your child needs to strain to start getting the micturition going, or if the stream is interrupted, please note this in the next column.

If your child wets his/her clothes, again please note the time and if they were wet or damp.

If your child feels a sudden urge to go to the toilet, please note this with the time in the next column.

If you observe that your child crosses his/her legs, squats or tries to hold back the urine in any other way, please note this (with the time) in the next column.

Finally, please measure and note the amount of fluids your child drinks during the day (with times).

Thank you very much for your help!

24- (48-) HOUR FREQUENCY-VOLUME CHART

Name _____ Date of birth _____

Date _____

Time	Urine volume (ml)	Straining/ interrupted stream	Wetting: damp/wet?	Urge	Comments/ observations	Drinking fluids (ml)

APPENDIX 3
PARENTAL QUESTIONNAIRE:
ENURESIS/URINARY INCONTINENCE

(Beetz et al 1994; translated and adapted by von Gontard, 2003)

Name _____ Date of birth _____

Date _____

	YES	NO
DAYTIME WETTING		
Does your child wet his/her clothes during the day?	❏	❏
Has your child ever been dry during the day?	❏	❏
If yes, for how long? _____ (weeks/months/years)		
And at what age? _____ (years)		
On how many days a week does your child wet during the daytime? _____ (days per week)		
How many times a day does your child wet? _____ (times per day)		
Is the clothing usually damp?	❏	❏
Is the clothing usually wet?	❏	❏
Does urine dribble constantly?	❏	❏
Does your child wet his/her clothes immediately after having gone to the toilet?	❏	❏
Does your child notice when he/she wets?	❏	❏

NIGHT-TIME WETTING	YES	NO
Does your child wet the bed (or diaper) during the night?	❏	❏
Has your child ever been dry during the night?	❏	❏
If yes, for how long? _____ (weeks/months/ years)		
And at what age? _____ (years)		
On how many nights a week does your child wet? _____ (nights per week)		
Is the bed usually damp?	❏	❏
Is the bed usually wet?	❏	❏
Does your child wake up to go to the toilet?	❏	❏
Does your child wake up after wetting the bed?	❏	❏
Is your child a deep sleeper, i.e. difficult to wake up?	❏	❏
Has any other member of your family wetted (day or night)?	❏	❏
If yes, who? _____		

TOILET HABITS	YES	NO
How many times a day does your child void (on average)? _____ (times/day)		
How long can your child manage without going to the toilet (during shopping, car trips, etc.)? _____ (hours)		
Does your child go to the toilet him/herself if he/she needs to?	❏	❏
Do you have to send your child to the toilet?	❏	❏
If your child wants to urinate, does he/she have to strain at the beginning or during voiding?	❏	❏
When your child voids, is the stream interrupted?	❏	❏
Does your child hurry and not take enough time for voiding?	❏	❏

OBSERVABLE REACTIONS	YES	NO
Does your child feel a sudden urge to go to the toilet?	❏	❏
When your child needs to void, does he/she have to rush to the toilet immediately?	❏	❏
Does your child cross his/her legs, squat, sit on the heels, etc. to prevent wetting?	❏	❏
Does your child postpone going to the toilet as long as possible? If yes, in which situations (school, play, TV, etc.)? Please specify _____	❏	❏

URINARY TRACT INFECTIONS	YES	NO
Has your child ever had a urinary tract infection? If yes, how many times? _____ (times)	❏	❏
Has your child had urinary tract infections with fever?	❏	❏
Has your child been treated for an illness of the urinary tract? If yes, please specify _____	❏	❏

STOOL HABITS	YES	NO
Does your child have daily bowel movements? If not, how many times/week? _____ (times/week)	❏	❏
Is your child regularly constipated?	❏	❏
Does your child soil his/her underwear (during the day)?	❏	❏
Does your child soil during sleep?	❏	❏
If yes, is it small amounts (smear)?	❏	❏
Or large amounts (stool)?	❏	❏
How often does your child soil? _____ (times/week) _____ (times/month)		
Has your child previously had complete bowel control? If yes, at what age? _____ (years) And for how long? _____ (months/years)	❏	❏
Does the soiling occur in special situations? If yes, please specify _____	❏	❏

BEHAVIOUR: WETTING	YES	NO
Is your child distressed by the wetting?	❏	❏
Are you distressed because of your child's wetting?	❏	❏
Has your child been teased because of the wetting?	❏	❏
Are there any things your child does not do (school outings, sleeping over with friends) because of the wetting?	❏	❏
Does your child wet more often during stressful times?	❏	❏
Is your child cooperative and motivated for treatment?	❏	❏
If your child was previously dry, can you think of any event that might be associated with the relapse? If yes, please specify _____	❏	❏

What in your opinion is the reason for the wetting?
Please specify_____
_____ _____

BEHAVIOUR: GENERAL	YES	NO
Does your child have difficulty in accepting rules?	❏	❏
Is your child restless, on the go, easily distracted?	❏	❏
Does your child have difficulty concentrating?	❏	❏
Is your child sometimes anxious?	❏	❏
Is your child sometimes sad, unhappy, withdrawn?	❏	❏
Does your child have problems at school? If yes, please specify _____	❏	❏
Does your child have problems in other areas? If yes, please specify_____	❏	❏

APPENDIX 4
ENCOPRESIS QUESTIONNAIRE – LONG VERSION

(von Gontard 2004)

Questions		Answers
Frequency of encopresis		
Does your child soil during the day?	❏	yes
	❏	no
How often does your child soil during the day?	_____	days per week
	_____	days per month
How often does your child soil per day?	_____	times per day
During what time of day does your child usually soil?	❏	morning
	❏	noon
	❏	afternoon
	❏	evening
Does your child soil during the night?	❏	yes
	❏	no
How often does your child soil during the night?	_____	nights per week
	_____	nights per month
Encopresis symptoms		
If your child soils, how large are the stool masses?	❏	only smearing
	❏	smearing and stool masses
	❏	only stool masses
What is the consistency of your child's stool?	❏	hard
	❏	soft
	❏	watery
In which situations does your child soil?	❏	no specific situation
	❏	at home
	❏	while quarrelling
	❏	during play
	❏	in school/kindergarten
	❏	in the car/travelling
	❏	other situations

Does your child soil in stressful situations?	❏	yes
	❏	no
Can your child postpone defecating if no toilet is available, e.g. while driving?	❏	yes
	❏	no
If yes, how long?	_____	hours

Relapses

Has your child ever had a period in their life without soiling?	❏	yes
	❏	no
If yes, what was the longest period?	_____	years, months

If yes, at what age did this occur?   from age of _____ years, months

to age of _____ years, months

Was there a reason for the relapse?	❏	yes
	❏	no
If yes, what was the reason?	❏	constipation
	❏	diarrhoea
	❏	pain when defecating
	❏	going to kindergarten
	❏	going to school
	❏	birth of a sibling
	❏	separation of parents
	❏	other life events
		_____

Toileting behaviour

Does your child wear a diaper?	❏	yes
	❏	no
If yes, when?	❏	daytime
	❏	night-time
	❏	both day- and night-time
On how many days per week does your child pass stools into the toilet?	_____	days per week
How many times per day does your child defecate?	_____	times per day
How large are the stool masses in the toilet?	❏	small
	❏	medium
	❏	large
What is the consistency of your child's stool in the toilet?	❏	hard
	❏	soft
	❏	watery
	❏	with blood

Do you have to send your child to the toilet?	❑	yes
	❑	no
If yes, how does he/she react?	❑	he/she complies
	❑	he/she gets angry
	❑	he/she refuses
Does your child take enough time for going to the toilet?	❑	yes
	❑	no
If yes, how long?	_____	minutes
Does your child play or read while sitting on the toilet?	❑	yes
	❑	no
Does your child go to the toilet regularly at certain times of the day?	❑	yes
	❑	no
If yes, when?	_____	
Does your child have difficulty passing stools?	❑	yes
	❑	no
Does he/she have to strain?	❑	yes
	❑	no
Is defecation painful for your child?	❑	yes
	❑	no
Does your child have stomach or abdominal pains?	❑	yes
	❑	no
How often does your child have abdominal pains?	_____	times per week
	_____	times per month
How strong are the abdominal pains?	❑	light
	❑	medium
	❑	severe
When does your child experience stomach pains?	❑	before meals
	❑	after meals
	❑	no specific time
Are the pains relieved after going to the toilet?	❑	yes
	❑	no
Does your child pass wind?	❑	yes
	❑	no

Perceptions and reactions after soiling

Does your child notice when he/she has soiled?	❑	yes
	❑	no
Do you notice when your child has soiled?	❑	yes
	❑	no
How do you notice it?	❑	seems absent-minded
	❑	complains of pains
	❑	other _____

Does your child tell you when he/she has soiled?	❏	yes
	❏	no
If no, does your child try to conceal it?	❏	yes
	❏	no
Does your child hide his/her underpants?	❏	yes
	❏	no
How does your child react when he/she has soiled?	❏	indifferent
	❏	no reaction
	❏	sad
	❏	anxious
	❏	disappointed
	❏	ashamed
	❏	desperate
	❏	angry
	❏	other reactions
Who removes the stools from the clothing (or the bed)?	❏	parents
	❏	child
	❏	both
Does your child suffer emotionally due to the soiling?	❏	yes
	❏	no
If yes, how intensely?	❏	a little
	❏	a lot
	❏	very much
If yes, how does this distress show?	_____	
Is your child motivated for treatment?	❏	yes
	❏	no

Reaction of parents and others

How do you react when your child has soiled?	❏	understanding
	❏	soothing
	❏	neutral
	❏	angry
	❏	scolding
	❏	punishing
	❏	other _____
Are you distressed by your child's soiling?	❏	yes
	❏	no
If yes, how intensely?	❏	a bit
	❏	a lot
	❏	very much
Have you punished your child because of his/her soiling?	❏	yes
	❏	no
Do you think that your child soils on purpose?	❏	yes
	❏	no

Who knows that your child soils?	❏	mother/father/siblings
	❏	other relatives
	❏	teachers
	❏	friends
	❏	others
Has your child been rejected because of his/her soiling?	❏	yes
	❏	no
If yes, how?	❏	he/she is teased
	❏	he/she is excluded from activities
	❏	he/she is made fun of
	❏	other ways _____
How often does this occur?	❏	seldom
	❏	often
Who teases your child?	_____	
Has your child not been able to take part in activities because of his/her soiling?	❏	yes
	❏	no
If yes, which activities?	❏	school outings
	❏	swimming
	❏	others _____
Does your child engage in sports?	❏	yes
	❏	no
If yes, what types of sports?	_____	

Wetting

How often does your child go to the toilet to urinate?	_____	times per day
Does your child wet during the day?	❏	yes
	❏	no
If yes, how often?	_____	days per week
Does your child wet at night?	❏	yes
	❏	no
If yes, how often?	_____	days per week
Does your child show a sudden urge to go to the toilet?	❏	yes
	❏	no
Does your child postpone going to the toilet?	❏	yes
	❏	no
If your child postpones going to the toilet, how do you notice it?	❏	pressing legs together
	❏	moving back and forth
	❏	sitting on heels
		other _____

Eating and drinking habits

How much fluid does your child drink per day?	_____	litres per day
Does your child prefer to eat low-fibre foods?	❏	yes
	❏	no
If yes, which foods?	_____	
Does your child prefer to eat other specific types of foods?	❏	yes
	❏	no
If yes, which foods?	_____	

Previous forms of treatment

Does your child take laxatives?	❏	yes
	❏	no
If yes, which?	_____	
If yes, how often?	_____	times per week
If yes, for how long?	_____	weeks/months
Has your child been investigated because of his/her soiling?	❏	yes
	❏	no
If yes, where and when?	_____	
Has your child been operated on because of his/her soiling?	❏	yes
	❏	no
If yes, where and when?	_____	
What have you personally done to treat the soiling?	_____	

Family history

Has anyone else in your family soiled?	❏	yes
	❏	no
If yes, who?	_____	
Has any member of your family been affected by constipation?	❏	yes
	❏	no
If yes, who?	_____	
Has anyone in your family had wetting problems?	❏	yes
	❏	no
If yes, who?	_____	

APPENDIX 5
ENCOPRESIS QUESTIONNAIRE – SCREENING VERSION

(von Gontard 2004)

Questions	Answers	
Frequency of encopresis		
Does your child soil during the day?	❑	yes
	❑	no
How often does your child soil during the day?	_____	days per week
	_____	days per month
How often does your child soil per day?	_____	times per day
Does your child soil during the night?	❑	yes
	❑	no
How often does your child soil during the night?	_____	nights per week
	_____	nights per month
Encopresis symptoms		
If your child soils, how large are the stool masses?	❑	only smearing
	❑	smearing and stool masses
	❑	only stool masses
What is the consistency of your child's stool?	❑	hard
	❑	soft
	❑	watery
Relapses		
Has your child ever had a period in his/her life without soiling?	❑	yes
	❑	no
If yes, at what age did this occur?	from age of _____ years, months	
	to age of _____ years, months	

Toileting behaviour

On how many days per week does your child pass stools into the toilet?	_____	days per week
How many times per day does your child defecate?	_____	times per day
How large are the stool masses in the toilet?	❏	small
	❏	medium
	❏	large
What is the consistency of your child's stool in the toilet?	❏	hard
	❏	soft
	❏	watery
	❏	with blood
Is defecation painful for your child?	❏	yes
	❏	no
Does your child have stomach or abdominal pains?	❏	yes
	❏	no

Perceptions and reactions after soiling

Does your child suffer emotionally due to the soiling?	❏	yes
	❏	no
Is your child motivated for treatment?	❏	yes
	❏	no
Have you punished your child because of his/her soiling?	❏	yes
	❏	no

Wetting

How often does your child go to the toilet to urinate?	_____	times per day
Does your child wet during the day?	❏	yes
	❏	no
If yes, how often?	_____	days per week
Does your child wet at night?	❏	yes
	❏	no
If yes, how often?	_____	days per week
How much fluid does your child drink per day?	_____	litres per day

APPENDIX 6
VOIDING DIARY

One-week voiding diary

Date							
Time	Monday	Tuesday	Wednesday	Thursday	Friday	Saturday	Sunday
6.00							
7.00							
8.00							
9.00							
10.00							
11.00							
12.00							
13.00							
14.00							
15.00							
16.00							
17.00							
18.00							
19.00							
20.00							
21.00							
22.00							
23.00							
24.00							
night							

X = urinating without leakage
V = urinating with some leakage (underpants damp)
W = urinating with more leakage (underpants wet)

APPENDIX 7
TITRATION CHART FOR
DESMOPRESSIN (INTRANASAL)

Weeks 1 and 2: Desmopressin intranasal spray: 20 µg in the evening

Date	Dry	Amount of urine: reduced	Amount of urine: same as before	Remarks

If dry or marked reduction of wet nights → continue with this dose (20 µg)
If not effective → increase to 30 µg

Week 3: Desmopressin intranasal spray: 30µg in the evening

Date	Dry	Amount of urine: reduced	Amount of urine: same as before	Remarks

If dry or marked reduction of wet nights → continue with this dose (30µg)
If not effective → increase to 40µg

Week 4: Desmopressin intranasal spray: 40µg in the evening

Date	Dry	Amount of urine: reduced	Amount of urine: same as before	Remarks

If dry or marked reduction of wet nights → continue with this dose (40µg)
If not effective → discontinue (desmopressin non-responder)

APPENDIX 8
TITRATION CHART FOR
DESMOPRESSIN (ORAL)

Weeks 1 and 2: Desmopressin tablets: 0.2 mg (200 μg) in the evening (one tablet)

Date	Dry	Amount of urine: reduced	Amount of urine: same as before	Remarks

If dry or marked reduction of wet nights → continue with this dose (0.2 mg – one tablet)
If not effective → increase to 0.4 mg (two tablets)

Weeks 3 and 4: Desmopressin tablets: 0.4 mg (400 µg) in the evening (two tablets)

Date	Dry	Amount of urine: reduced	Amount of urine: same as before	Remarks

If dry or marked reduction of wet nights → continue with this dose (0.4 mg – two tablets)

If not effective → discontinue (desmopressin non-responder)

APPENDIX 9
DOCUMENTATION OF
ALARM TREATMENT

(modified from Butler 1987)

If dry			If wet					
Date	Dry	Got up and went to toilet without alarm	Time of alarm	Child awoke by him/herself		Amount of urine in bed (diaper) L = large M = medium	Passed urine in toilet	
				Yes	No	S = small	Yes	No

APPENDIX 10
NOCTURNAL ENURESIS
BASELINE CHART

This chart belongs to: _____

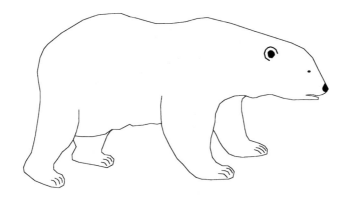

(Dry nights registered as 'suns', wet ones as 'clouds' – or any other symbol)

	Monday	Tuesday	Wednesday	Thursday	Friday	Saturday	Sunday
1							
2							
3							
4							

APPENDIX 11
CHART FOR TREATMENT OF URGE INCONTINENCE/OVERACTIVE BLADDER

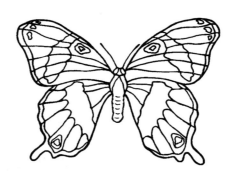

This chart belongs to: _____

My sign for 'wet': [ ]   **My sign for 'dry':** [ ]

	Dry or wet going to toilet
Monday	
Tuesday	
Wednesday	
Thursday	
Friday	
Saturday	
Sunday	

APPENDIX 12
CHART FOR TREATMENT OF
VOIDING POSTPONEMENT

This chart belongs to: _____

My sign for 'wet':

My sign for 'dry':

	1	2	3	4	5	6	7
Monday							
Tuesday							
Wednesday							
Thursday							
Friday							
Saturday							
Sunday							

APPENDIX 13
72-HOUR FREQUENCY-VOLUME CHART

Day					Day					Day				
Time	Urinating How much?	Dry/wet	Drinks How much?	Stool	Time	Urinating How much?	Dry/wet	Drinks How much?	Stool	Time	Urinating How much?	Dry/wet	Drinks How much?	Stool
Night					Night					Night				
05.00					05.00					05.00				
06.00					06.00					06.00				
07.00					07.00					07.00				
08.00					08.00					08.00				
09.00					09.00					09.00				
10.00					10.00					10.00				
11.00					11.00					11.00				
12.00					12.00					12.00				
13.00					13.00					13.00				
14.00					14.00					14.00				
15.00					15.00					15.00				
16.00					16.00					16.00				
17.00					17.00					17.00				
18.00					18.00					18.00				
19.00					19.00					19.00				
20.00					20.00					20.00				
21.00					21.00					21.00				
22.00					22.00					22.00				
23.00					23.00					23.00				

APPENDIX 14

DOCUMENTATION OF TOILET TRAINING (ENCOPRESIS CHART)

Date	Monday	Tuesday	Wednesday	Thursday	Friday	Saturday	Sunday
Morning							
Sent to toilet (→) Went alone (!)							
Pants: dry (D) wet (W) stools small (S) stools large (L)							
Toilet: urine (U) stools (S)							
Midday							
Sent to toilet (→) Went alone (!)							
Pants: dry (D) wet (W) stools small (S) stools large (L)							
Toilet: urine (U) stools (S)							
Evening							
Sent to toilet (→) Went alone (!)							
Pants: dry (D) wet (W) stools small (S) stools large (L)							
Toilet: urine (U) stools (S)							

REFERENCES

AACP (2002) Practice parameters for the use of stimulant medications in the treatment of children, adolescents and adults. *J Am Acad Child Adolesc Psychiatry* 41: 26S–49S.

AACP (2004) Practice parameter for the assessment and treatment of children and adolescents with enuresis. *J Am Acad Child Adolesc Psychiatry* 43: 1540–1550.

Ab E, Schoemaker M, van Empelen R. (2002) Paradoxical movement of the pelvic floor in dysfunctional voiding and the results of biofeedback training. *BJU Int* 89 Suppl 2: 48.

Abbasoglu L, Tansu Salman F, Baslo B, Isler S, Gun F. (2004) Electromyographic studies on the external anal sphincter in children with operated anorectal malformations. *Eur J Pediatr Surg* 14: 103–107.

Abe K, Oda N, Hatta H. (1984) Behavioural genetics of early childhood: fears, restlessness, motion sickness and enuresis. *Acta Genet Med Gemellol* 33: 303–306.

Abrahamsson K, Hansson E, Sillén U, Hermansson G, Hjälmås K. (1998) Bladder dysfunction: an integral part of the ectopic ureterocele complex. *J Urol* 160: 1468–1470.

Abrahamsson K, Hansson S, Larsson P, Jodal U. (2002) Antibiotic treatment for five days is effective in children with acute cystitis. *Acta Paediatr* 91: 55–58.

Abrams P. (1997) *Urodynamics*. London: Springer.

Abrams P, Klevmark B. (1996) Frequency volume charts: an indispensable part of lower urinary tract assessment. *Scand J Urol Nephrol* 179: 47–53.

Abrams P, Cardozo L, Fall M, Griffiths D, Rosier P, Ulmsten U, Van Kerrebroeck P, Victor A, Wein A. (2002) The standardisation of terminology in lower urinary tract function. *Neurourol Urodyn* 21: 167–178.

Aceto G, Penza R, Coccioli MS, Palumbo F, Cresta L, Cimador M, Chiozza ML, Caione P. (2003) Enuresis subtypes based on nocturnal hypercalciuria: a multicenter study. *J Urol* 170: 1670–1673.

Achenbach TM. (1991) *Manual for the Child Behavior Checklist/4–18 and 1991 Profile*. Burlington: University of Vermont.

Agersø H, Seiding Larsen L, Riis A, Lövgren U, Karlsson MO, Senderovitz T. (2004) Pharmacokinetics and renal excretion of desmopressin after intravenous administration to healthy subjects and renally impaired patients. *Br J Clin Pharmacol* 58: 352–358.

Agnarsson U, Warde C, McCarthy G, Clayden GS, Evans N. (1993) Anorectal problems in patients with neurological problems. I: Spina bifida. *Dev Med Child Neurol* 35: 893–902.

Aikawa T, Kasahara T, Uchiyama M. (1998) The arginine-vasopressin secretion profile of children with primary nocturnal enuresis. *Eur Urol* 33 Suppl 3: 41–44.

Akbal C, Ekici S, Erkan I, Tekgul S. (2004) Intermittent oral desmopressin therapy for monosymptomatic primary nocturnal enuresis. *J Urol* 171: 2603–2606.

Alhano JP, Shannon SG, Alem NM, Mason KT. (1996) Injury risk for research subjects with spina bifida occulta in a repeated impact study: a case review. *Aviat Space Environ Med* 67: 767–769.

Alhasso A, Glazener CM, Pickard R, N'Dow J. (2003) Adrenergic drugs for urinary incontinence in adults. *Cochrane Database Syst Rev* 2: CD001842.

Allen TD. (1972) Psychogenic urinary retention. *South Med J* 65: 302–304.

Allen TD. (1977) The non-neurogenic neurogenic bladder. *J Urol* 117: 232–238.

Allen TD, Bright TC. (1978) Urodynamic patterns in children with dysfunctional voiding problems. *J Urol* 119: 247–249.

Alon U, Woodward CP, Howard CP. (1992) Urine volume, age and nocturnal enuresis: a prospective study on newly diagnosed children with diabetes mellitus. *Children's Hospital Quarterly* 4: 157–160.

Al-Waili NS. (2000) Carbamazepine to treat primary nocturnal enuresis: double-blind study. *Eur J Med Res* 5: 40–44.

Amarenco G, Ismael SS, Even-Schneider A, Raibaut P, Demaille-Wlodyka S, Parratte B, Kerdraon J. (2003) Urodynamic effect of acute transcutaneous posterior tibial nerve stimulation in overactive bladder. *J Urol* 169: 2210–2215.

Åmark P, Beck O. (1992) Effect of phenylpropanolamine on incontinence in children with neurogenic bladders. A double-blind crossover study. *Acta Paediatr* 81: 345–350.

American Psychiatric Association. (1994) *Diagnostic and Statistical Manual of Mental Disorders (DSM-IV)*. Washington, DC: APA.

Anderson LT, David R, Bonnet K, Dancis J. (1979) Passive avoidance learning in Lesch–Nyhan disease: effect of 1-desamino-8-D-arginine vasopressin. *Life Sci* 24: 905–910.

Andersson G, Johansson JE, Garpenholt O, Nilsson K. (2004) Urinary incontinence – prevalence, impact on daily living and desire for treatment: a population-based study. *Scand J Urol Nephrol* 38: 125–130.

Andersson KE. (2003) Storage and voiding symptoms: pathophysiologic aspects. *Urology* 62 Suppl 2: 3–10.

Andersson KE, Hedlund P. (2002) Pharmacologic perspective on the physiology of the lower urinary tract. *Urology* 60 Suppl 1: 13–21.

Andersson KE, Pehrson R. (2003) CNS involvement in overactive bladder. Pathophysiology and opportunities for pharmacological intervention. *Drugs* 63: 2595–2611.

Ang VTY, Jenkins JS. (1982) Blood–cerebrospinal fluid barrier to arginine-vasopressin, desmopressin and desglycinamide arginine-vasopressin in the dog. *J Endocrinol* 93: 319–325.

Angold A, Erkanli A, Egger H, Costello J. (2000) Stimulant treatment for children: a community perspective *J Am Acad Child Adolesc Psychiatry* 39: 975–983.

Anthony E, Bene E. (1957) A technique for the objective assessment of the child's family relationships. *J Ment Sci* 103: 541–555.

Araki I, de Groat WC. (1997) Developmental synaptic depression underlying reorganization of visceral reflex pathways in the spinal cord. *J Neurosci* 17: 8402–8407.

Argenti D, Ireland D, Heald DL. (2001) A pharmacokinetic and pharmacodynamic comparison of desmopressin administered as whole, chewed and crushed tablets, and as an oral solution. *J Urol* 165: 1446–1451.

Arhan P, Devroede G, Jehannin B, Faverding C, Revillon Y, Lefevre D, Pellerin D. (1983) Idiopathic disorders of fecal continence in children. *Paediatrics* 71: 744–779.

Arhan P, Devroede G, Jehannin B, et al. (1989) Determination of total and segmental colonic transit time in constipated patients: results in 91 patients with a new simplified method. *Dig Dis Sci* 34: 1168–1172.

Arnell H, Hjälmås M, Jägervall G, et al. (1997) The genetics of primary nocturnal enuresis: inheritance and suggestion of a second major gene on chromosome 12q. *J Med Genet* 34: 360–365

Aronson AS, Andersson KE, Bergstrand CG, Mulder JL. (1973) Treatment of diabetes insipidus in children with DDAVP, a synthetic analogue of vasopressin. *Acta Pædiatr Scand* 62: 133–140.

Artibani W. (1997) Diagnosis and significance of idiopathic overactive bladder. *Urology* 50 Suppl 6A: 25–32.

Aruffo RN, Ibarra S, Strupp KR. (2000) Encopresis and anal masturbation. *J Am Psychoanal Assoc* 48: 1327–1354.

Arya LA, Myers DL, Jackson ND. (2000) Dietary caffeine intake and the risk for detrusor instability: a case-control study. *Obstet Gynecol* 96: 85–89.

Austin PF, Homsy YL, Masel JL, Cain MP, Casale AJ, Rink RC. (1999) Alpha-adrenergic blockade in children with neuropathic and nonneuropathic voiding dysfunction. *J Urol* 162: 1064–1067.

Awad SA, Gajewski JB, Sogbein SK, Murray TJ, Field CA. (1984) Relationship between neurological and urological status in patients with multiple sclerosis. *J Urol* 132: 499–502.

Axline V. (1947) *Play Therapy. The Inner Dynamics of Childhood*. Boston: Houghton Mifflin.

Azrin NH, Sneed TJ, Foxx RM. (1974) Dry-bed training: rapid elimination of childhood enuresis. *Behav Res Ther* 12: 147–156.

Backes M, Genc B, Doerfler W, Schreck J, Lehmkuhl G, von Gontard A. (2000) Cognitive and behavioral profile of Fragile X boys – correlations to molecular data. *Am J Med Genet* 95: 150–156.

Baeyens D. (2005) The relationship between attention-deficit/hyperactivity disorder (ADHD) and enuresis in children. PhD thesis, Gent, Belgium.

Baeyens D, Van Hoecke E, Van Laecke E, Raes A, Hoebecke P, Vande Walle J. (2001) Behavioural and emotional problems in children with voiding problems. *Br J Urol Int* 87 Suppl 1: 56.

Baeyens D, Roeyers H, Hoebecke P, Verte S, Van Hoecke E, Vande Walle J. (2004) Attention deficit/ hyperactivity disorder in children with nocturnal enuresis. *J Urol* 171: 2576–2579.

Bailey JN, Ornitz EM, Gehricke JG, Gabikian P, Russell AT, Smalley SL. (1999) Transmission of primary nocturnal enuresis and attention deficit hyperactivity disorder. *Acta Paediatr* 88: 1364–1368.

Baker SS, Liptak GS, Colletti RB, Croffie JM, DiLorenzo C, Ector W, Nurko S. (1999) Constipation in infants and children: evaluation and treatment. *J Pediatr Gastroenterol Nutr* 29: 612–626.

Bakker E, van Gool JD, Wyndaele JJ. (2001) Results of a questionnaire evaluating different aspects of personal and familial situation, and the methods of potty-training in two groups of children with a different outcome of bladder control. *Scand J Urol Nephrol* 35: 35.

Bakker E, van Sprundel M, van der Auwera JC, van Gool JD, Wyndaele JJ. (2002) Voiding habits and wetting in a population of 4,332 Belgian schoolchildren aged between 10 and 14 years. *Scand J Urol Nephrol* 36: 354–362.

Bakker E, van Gool JD, van Sprundel M, van der Auwera JC, Wyndaele JJ. (2004) Risk factors for recurrent urinary tract infection in 4,332 Belgian schoolchildren aged between 10 and 14 years. *Eur J Pediatr* 163: 234–238

Bakwin H. (1961) Enuresis in children. *J Pediatr* 58: 806–819.

Bakwin H. (1971) Enuresis in twins. *Am J Dis Child* 121: 222–225.

Bakwin H. (1973) The genetics of enuresis. In: Kolvin I, MacKeith RC, Meadow SR, editors. *Bladder Control and Enuresis*. London: William Heinemann Medical Books, pp 73–77.

Bakwin H, Davidson MD. (1971) Constipation in twins. *Am J Dis Child* 121: 179–181.

Ballauff A, Kersting M, Manz F. (1988) Do children have an adequate fluid intake? Water balance studies carried out at home. *Ann Nutr Metab* 32: 332–339.

Barr RG, Levine MD, Wilkinson RH, Mulvihill D. (1979) Chronic and occult stool retention: a clinical tool for its evaluation in school-aged children. *Clin Pediatr* 18: 674–686.

Barrington FJF. (1921) The relation of hindbrain to micturition. *Brain* 44: 23–53.

Barrington FJF. (1925) The effect of lesions of the hind- and midbrain on micturition in the cat. *Quart J Exp Physiol* 15: 81–102.

Bass A. (1994) Aspects of urethrality in women. *Psychoanal Q* 63: 491–517.

Batislam E, Nohoglu B, Peskircioglu L, Emir L, Uygur C, Germiyanoglu C, Erol D. (1995) A prostaglandin synthesis inhibitor, diclofenac sodium in the treatment of primary nocturnal enuresis. *Acta Urol Belg* 63: 35–38.

Bauer SB, Retik AB, Colodny AH, Hallett M, Khoshbin S, Dyro FM. (1980) The unstable bladder of childhood. *Urol Clin North Am* 7: 321–336.

Baumann FW, Hinman F. (1974) Treatment of incontinent boys with non-obstructive disease. *J Urol* 111: 114–116.

Bayliss M, Wu C, Newgreen D, Mundy AR, Fry CH. (1999) A quantitative study of atropine-resistant contractile responses in human detrusor smooth muscle, from stable, unstable and obstructed bladders. *J Urol* 162: 1833–1839.

Beach PS, Beach RE, Smith LR. (1992) Hyponatremic seizures in a child treated with desmopressin to control enuresis. A rational approach to fluid intake. *Clin Pediatr* 31: 566–569.

Becker P, Schaller S, Schmidtke A. (1980) *Coloured Progressive Matrices – Manual*, 2nd edition. Weinheim: Beltz Test Gesellschaft.

Beckwith BE, Petros TV, Bergloff PJ, Staebler RJ. (1987) Vasopressin analog (DDAVP) facilitates recall of narrative prose. *Behav Neurosci* 101: 429–432.

Beetz R. (1993) Funktionelle Aspekte der Enuresis im Kindesalter – Bedeutung für Diagnostik und Therapie. *Akt Urol* 24: 241–250.

Bellman M. (1966) Studies on encopresis. *Acta Paediatr Scand* 170 Suppl: 1–151.

Benninga MA, Buller HA, Heymans HS, Tygat GN, Taminiau JA. (1994) Is encopresis always the result of constipation? *Arch Dis Child* 71: 186–193.

Benninga MA, Voskuijl WP, Akkerhuis GW, Taminiau JA, Buller HA. (2004) Colonic transit times and behaviour profiles in children with defecation disorders. *Arch Dis Child* 89: 13–16.

Berg I, Fielding D, Meadow R. (1977) Psychiatric disturbance, urgency, and bacteriuria in children with day and night wetting. *Arch Dis Child* 52: 651–657.

Berg I, Ellis M, Forsythe I, McGuire R. (1981) The relationship between the Rutter A Questionnaire and an interview with mother in assessing child psychiatric disturbance among enuretic children. *Psychol Med* 11: 647–650.

Bergman A, Koonings PP, Ballard CA. (1989) Detrusor instability. Is the bladder the cause or the effect? *J Reprod Med* 34: 834–838.

Bernard-Bonnin AC, Haliy N, Belanger S, Nadeau D. (1993) Parental and patient perceptions about encopresis and its treatment. *J Dev Behav Pediatr* 14(6): 397–400.

Bernstein SA, Williford SL. (1997) Intranasal desmopressin-associated hyponatremia: a case report and literature review. *J Fam Pract* 44: 203–208.

Biederman J, Santagelo SL, Faraone SV, Kiely K, Guite J, Mick E, Reed ED, Kraus I, Jellinek M, Perrin J. (1995) Clinical correlates of enuresis and ADHD and non-ADHD children. *J Child Psychol Psychiatry* 36: 865–877.

Bird JR. (1980) Psychogenic urinary retention. *Psychother Psychosom* 34: 45–51.

Bird HR. (1996) Epidemiology of childhood disorders in a cross-cultural context. *J Child Psychol Psychiatry* 37: 35–49

Birkasova M, Birkas O, Flynn MJ, Cort JH. (1978) Desmopressin in the management of nocturnal enuresis in children: a double-blind study. *Pediatrics* 62: 970–974.

Bishop WP. (2001) Miracle laxative? *J Pediatr Gastroenterol Nutr* 32: 514–515.

Björkström G, Hellström A-L, Andersson S. (2000) Electro-acupuncture in the treatment of children with monosymptomatic nocturnal enuresis. *Scand J Urol Nephrol* 34: 21–26.

Blaivas JG. (1982) The neurophysiology of micturition: a clinical study of 550 patients. *J Urol* 127: 958–963.

Blaivas JG, Labib KB, Michalik J, Zayed AAH. (1980) Cystometric response to propantheline in detrusor hyperreflexia: therapeutic implications. *J Urol* 124: 259–262.

Blethyn AJ, Verrier Jones K, Newcombe R, Roberts GM, Jenkins HR. (1995) Radiological assessment of constipation. *Arch Dis Child* 73: 532–533.

Blok BF, Holstege G. (1998) The central nervous system control of micturition in cats and humans. *Behav Brain Res* 92: 119–125.

Blok BF, Willemsen ATM, Holstege G. (1997a) A PET study on the brain control of micturition in humans. *Brain* 120: 111–121

Blok BF, de Weerd H, Holstege G. (1997b) The pontine micturition center projects to sacral cord GABA immunoreactive neurons in the cat. *Neurosci Lett* 233: 109–112.

Blok BF, Sturms LM, Holstege G. (1998) Brain activation during micturition in women. *Brain* 121: 2033–2042.

Bloom DA, Seeley WW, Ritchey ML, McGuire EJ. (1993) Toilet habits and incontinence in children: an opportunity sampling in search of normal parameters. *J Urol* 149: 1087–1090.

Blum NJ, Taubman B, Osborne ML. (1997) Behavioral characteristics of children with stool toileting refusal. *Pediatrics* 99: 50–53.

Blum NJ, Taubman B, Nemeth N. (2003) Relationship between age at initiation of toilet training and duration of training: a prospective study. *Pediatrics* 111: 810–814.

Blum NJ, Taubman B, Nemeth N. (2004a) During toilet training, constipation occurs before stool toileting refusal. *Pediatrics* 113: e520–e522.

Blum NJ, Taubman B, Nemeth N. (2004b) Why is toilet training occurring at older ages? A study of factors associated with later training. *J Pediatr* 145: 107–111.

Bonde HV, Andersen JP, Rosenkilde P. (1994) Nocturnal enuresis: change of nocturnal voiding pattern during alarm treatment. *Scand J Urol Nephrol* 28: 349–352.

Bonnet MH, Johnson LC. (1978) Relationship of arousal threshold to sleep stage distribution and subjective estimates of depth and quality of sleep. *Sleep* 1: 161–168.

Boon F. (1991) Encopresis and sexual assault. *J Am Acad Child Adolesc Psychiatry* 30(3): 509–510.

Borowitz SM, Sutphen J, Ling W, Cox DJ. (1996) Lack of correlation of anorectal manometry with symptoms of chronic childhood constipation and encopresis. *Dis Colon Rectum* 39: 400–405

Borowitz SM, Cox DJ, Kovatchev B, Ritterband LM, Sheen J, Sutphen JL. (2005) Treatment of childhood constipation by primary care physicians: efficacy and predictors of outcome. *Pediatrics* 115: 873–877.

Bosch R. (1990) Instability of the bladder: pathophysiology unknown? A synopsis of clinical points of interest. *Neurourol Urodyn* 9: 563–565.

Bouchoucha M, Thomas SR. (2000) Error analysis of classic colonic transit time estimates. *Am J Physiol Gastrointest Liver Physiol* 279: G520–G527.

Bowden DM, German DC, Poynter WD. (1978) An autoradiographic, semistereotaxic mapping of major projections from locus coeruleus and adjacent nuclei in Macaca mulatta. *Brain Res* 145: 257–276.

Bower WF, Yeung CK. (2004) A review of non-invasive electro neuromodulation as an intervention for non-neurogenic bladder dysfunction in children. *Neurourol Urodyn* 23: 63–67.

Bower WF, Moore KH, Shepherd RB, Adams RD. (1996) The epidemiology of childhood enuresis in Australia. *Br J Urol* 78: 602–606.

Bower WF, Moore KH, Adams RD. (2001) A pilot study of the home application of transcutaneous neuro-modulation in children with urgency or urge incontinence. *J Urol* 166: 2420–2422.

Bower WF, Sit FK, Yeung CK. (2004) What children tell us about the effect of incontinence on their quality of life. Gent: ICCS meeting. Abstract 35, pp 55–56.

Bradbury M, Meadow SR. (1995) Combined treatment with enuresis alarm and desmopressin for nocturnal enuresis. *Acta Paediatr* 84: 1014–1018.

Brading AF. (1997) A myogenic basis for the overactive bladder. *Urology* 50 Suppl 6A: 57–67.

Brading AP, Turner WH. (1994) The unstable bladder: towards a common mechanism. *Br J Urol* 73: 3–8.

Bradley WE. (1980) Cerebro-cortical innervation of the urinary bladder. *Tohoku J Exp Med* 131: 7–13.

Bradley WE, Timm GW, Scott FB. (1974) Innervation of the detrusor muscle and urethra. *Urol Clin North Am* 1: 3–27.

Brazelli M, Griffiths P. (2002) Behavioural and cognitive interventions with or without other treatments for defaecation disorders in children. In: The Cochrane Library, Issue 2. Oxford: Update Software.

Brem-Gräser L. (1995) *Familie in Tieren: Die Familiensituation im Spiegel der Kinderzeichnung.* München, Basel: Ernst Reinhhardt Verlag

Brierly RD, Hindley RG, McLarty E, Harding DM, Thomas PJ. (2003) A prospective controlled quantitative study of ultrastructural changes in the underactive detrusor. *J Urol* 169: 1374–1378.

Brocklebank JT, Meadow SR. (1981) Cure of giggle micturition. *Arch Dis Child* 56: 232–234.

Brooks LJ, Topol HI. (2003) Enuresis in children with sleep apnea. *J Pediatr* 142: 515–518.

Brooks RS, Copen RM, Cox DJ, Morris J, Borowitz S, Sutphen J. (2000) The treatment literature for encopresis, constipation, and stool-toileting refusal. *Ann Behav Med* 22: 260–267.

Brosen K, Gram LF, Klysner R, et al. (1986) Steady-state levels of imipramine and its metabolites: significance of dose-dependent kinetics. *Eur J Clin Pharmacol* 30: 43–49.

Broughton RJ. (1968) Sleep disorders: disorders of arousal? Enuresis, somnambulism, and nightmares in confusional states of arousal, not in 'dreaming sleep'. *Science* 159: 1070–1078.

Buderus S. (2002) Rationale Diagnostik der chronischen Obstipation. *Monatsschr Kinderheilkd* 150: 587–593.

Buisseret PD. (1978) Common manifestations of cow's milk allergy in children. *Lancet* 1(8059): 304–305.

Bulmer P, Abrams P. (2004) The unstable detrusor. *Urol Int* 72: 1–12.

Busby K, Pivik RT. (1983) Failure of high intensity auditory stimuli to affect behavioral arousal in children during the first sleep cycle. *Pediatr Res* 17: 802–805.

Busby KA, Mercier L, Pivik RT. (1994) Ontogenic variations in auditory arousal threshold during sleep. *Psychophysiology* 31: 182–188.

Butler RJ. (1986) Maternal attributions and tolerance for nocturnal enuresis. *Behav Res Ther* 24: 307–312.

Butler RJ. (1987) *Nocturnal Enuresis: Psychological Perspectives.* Bristol: John Wright.

Butler RJ. (1991) Etablishment of working definitions in nocturnal enuresis. *Arch Dis Child* 66: 267–271.

Butler RJ. (1994) Nocturnal enuresis – the child's experience. Oxford: Butterworth-Heinemann.

Butler RJ. (1998) Annotation: night wetting in children: psychological perspectives. *J Child Psychol Psychiatry* 39: 453–463.

Butler RJ. (2001) Impact of nocturnal enuresis on children and young people. *Scand J Urol Nephrol* 35: 169–176.

Butler RJ, Robinson JC. (2002) Alarm treatment of childhood nocturnal enuresis: an investigation of within-treatment variables. *Scand J Urol Nephrol* 36: 268–272.

Butler RJ, Robinson JC, Holland P, Doherty-Williams D. (2004a) Investigating the three systems approach to complex childhood nocturnal enuresis. *Scand J Urol Nephrol* 38: 117–121.

Butler RJ, Robinson JC, Holland P, Doherty-Williams D. (2004b) An exploration of outcome criteria in nocturnal enuresis treatment. *Scand J Urol Nephrol* 38: 196–206.

Buttarazzi PJ. (1977) Oxybutynin chloride (Ditropan) in enuresis. *J Urol* 118: 46.

Buttross S. (1999) Encopresis in the child with a behavioral disorder: when the initial treatment does not work. *Pediatr Ann* 28(5): 317–321.

Byrd RS, Weitzmann M, Lamphear N, Auinger P. (1996) Bed-wetting in US children: epidemiology and related behavior problems. *Pediatrics* 98: 414–419.

Cadman D, Boyle M, Offord D. (1988) The Ontario Child Health study: social adjustment and mental health of siblings of children with chronic health problems. *J Dev Behav Pediatr* 9: 117–121.

Cain MP, Wu SD, Austin PF, Herndon CD, Rink RC. (2003) Alpha blocker therapy for children with dysfunctional voiding and urinary retention. *J Urol* 170: 1514–1515.

Caione P, Arena F, Biraghi M, Cigna RM, Chendi D, Chiozza ML, De Lisa A, De Grazia E, Fano M, Formica P, Garofalo S, Gramenzi R, von Heland M, Lanza P, Lanza T, Maffei S, Manieri C, Merlini E, Miano L,

Nappo S, Pagliarulo A, Paolini Paoletti F, Pau AC, Porru D, Riccipetitoni G, Scarpa RM, Artibani W. (1997) Nocturnal enuresis and daytime wetting: a multicentric trial with oxybutynin and desmopressin. *Eur Urol* 31: 459–463.

Can G, Topbas M, Okten A, Kizil M. (2004) Child abuse as a result of enuresis. *Pediatr Int* 46: 64–66.

Cardozo LD. (2000) Biofeedback in overactive bladder. *Urology* 55 Suppl 5A: 24–28.

Cardozo LD, Stanton SL. (1980) Genuine stress incontinence and detrusor instability: a review of 200 patients. *Br J Obstet Gynaecol* 87: 184–190.

Cardozo LD, Chapple CR, Tooz-Hobson P, et al. (2000) Efficacy of trospium chloride in patients with detrusor instability: a placebo-controlled, randomized, double-blind, multicenter clinical trial. *BJU Int* 85: 659–664.

Caress JB, Kothari MJ, Bauer SB, Shefner JM. (1996) Urinary dysfunction in Duchenne muscular dystrophy. *Muscle Nerve* 19: 819–822.

Carey MP, De Jong S, Friedhuber A, Moran PA, Dwyer PL, Scurry J. (2000) A prospective evaluation of the pathogenesis of detrusor instability in women, using electron microscopy and immunohistochemistry. *BJU Int* 86: 970–976.

Carruthers SG. (1994) Adverse effects of alpha 1-adrenergic blocking drugs. *Drug Saf* 11: 12–20.

Castleden CM, George CF, Renwick AG, Asher MJ. (1981) Imipramine – a possible alternative to current therapy for urinary incontinence in the elderly. *J Urol* 125: 318–320.

Catell RB, Weiss RH, Osterland J. (1997) *Grundintelligenz Skala 1 (CFT 1)*, 5th edition. Göttingen: Hogrefe.

Catto-Smith AG, Coffey CM, Nolan TM, Hutson JM. (1995) Fecal incontinence after the surgical treatment of Hirschsprung disease. *J Pediatr* 127: 954–957.

Cayan S, Doruk E, Bozlu M, Duce MN, Ulusoy E, Akbay E. (2001) The assessment of constipation in monosymptomatic primary nocturnal enuresis. *Int Urol Nephrol* 33: 513–516.

Ceriati E, Deganello F, De Peppo F, Ciprandi G, Silveri M, Marchetti P, Rava L, Rivosecchi M. (2004) Surgery for ulcerative colitis in pediatric patients: functional results of 10-year follow-up with straight endorectal pull-through. *Pediatr Surg Int* 20: 573–578.

Chambless DL, Hollon SD. (1998) Defining empirically supported therapies. *J Consult Clin Psychol* 66: 7–18.

Chan YL, Chan KW, Yeung CK, Roebuck DJ, Chu WC, Lee KH, Metreweli C. (1999) Potential utility of MRI in the evaluation of children at risk of renal scarring. *Pediatr Radiol* 29: 856–862.

Chandra M, Saharia R, Shi QS, Hill V. (2002) Giggle incontinence in children: a manifestation of detrusor instability. *J Urol* 168: 2184–2187.

Chang G, Warner V, Weissman MM. (1988) Physician's recognition of psychiatric disorders in children and adolescents. *Am J Dis Child* 142: 736–739.

Chang SS, Ng CFN, Wong SN. (2002) Behavioural problems in children and parenting stress associated with primary nocturnal enuresis in Hong Kong. *Acta Paediatr* 91: 475–479.

Chase JH, Homsy Y, Siggard S, Bower W. (2004) Functional constipation in children. *J Urol* 171: 2641–2643.

Cher TW, Lin GJ, Hsu KH. (2002) Prevalence of nocturnal enuresis and associated familial factors in primary school children in Taiwan. *J Urol* 168: 1142–1146.

Christophersen ER, Edwards K. (1992) Treatment of elimination disorders: state of the art 1991. *Appl Prev Psychol* 1: 15–22.

Chugh DK, Weaver TE, Dinges DF. (1996) Neurobehavioral consequences of arousals. *Sleep* 19 Suppl 10: S198–S201.

Cinar U, Vural C, Cakir B, Topuz E, Karaman MI, Turgut S. (2001) Nocturnal enuresis and upper airway obstruction. *Int J Pediatr Otorhinolaryngol* 59: 115–118.

Cisternino A, Passerini-Glazel G. (1995) Bladder dysfunction in children. *Scand J Urol Nephrol* Suppl 173: 25–29.

Clark T, Pope JC 4th, Adams C, Wells N, Brock JW 3rd. (2002) Factors that influence outcomes of the Mitrofanoff and Malone antegrade continence enema reconstructive procedures in children. *J Urol* 168: 1537–1540.

Close CE, Carr MC, Burns MW, Miller JL, Bavendam TG, Mayo ME, Mitchell ME. (1996) Interstitial cystitis in children. *J Urol* 156: 860–862.

Cook BJ, Lim E, Cook D, Chow CW, Stanton MP, Southwell BR, Hutson JM. (2002) Radionuclear transit to assess sites of delay in large bowel transit in chronic idiopathic constipation in children. ICCS meeting, Hong Kong.

Costello CH, Cook CK. (2004) Intravenous urography and imaging of the urinary tract. *Hosp Med* 65: 426–430.

Cox DJ, Sutphen J, Ling W, Quillian W, Borowitz S. (1996) Additive benefits of laxative, toilet training, and biofeedback therapies in the treatment of pediatric encopresis. *J Pediatr Psychol* 21: 659–670.

315

Cox DJ, Sutphen JL, Borowitz SM, Korvatchev B, Ling W. (1998) Contribution of behavior therapy and biofeedback to laxative therapy in the treatment of pediatric encopresis. *Ann Behav Med* 20: 70–76.

Cox DJ, Morris JB, Borowitz SM, Sutphen JL. (2002) Psychological differences between children with and without chronic encopresis. *J Pediatr Psychol* 27: 585–591.

Cox DJ, Ritterband LM, Quillian W, Kovatchev B, Morris JB, Sutphen JL, Borowitz SM. (2003) Assessment of behavioural mechanisms maintaining encopresis: Virginia Encopresis-Constipation Apperception Test. *J Pediatr Psychol* 28: 375–382.

Crimmins CR, Rathburn SR, Husman DA. (2003) Management of urinary incontinence and nocturnal enuresis in attention-deficit hyperactivity disorder. *J Urol* 170: 1347–1350.

Cunningham C, Taylor HG, Minich AM, Hack M. (2001) Constipation in very-low-birth-weight children at 10 to 14 years of age. *J Pediatr Gastroenterol Nutr* 33: 23–27.

Curran MJ, Kaefer M, Peters C, Logigian E, Bauer SB. (2000) The overactive bladder in childhood: long-term results with conservative management. *J Urol* 163: 574–577.

Cvitkovic-Kuzmic A, Brkljacic B, Ivankovic D, Grga A. (2002) Ultrasound assessment of detrusor muscle thickness in children with non-neuropathic bladder/sphincter dysfunction. *Eur Urol* 41: 214–219.

Czernichow P, Pomarede R, Basmaciogullari A, Rappaport R. (1979) Diabetes insipidus in children: I. Arginine-vasopressin determination in plasma during short dehydration test. *Acta Paediatr Scand* Suppl 277: 64–67.

d'Agay-Abensour L, Fjellestad-Paulsen A, Höglund P, Ngô Y, Paulsen O, Rambaud JC. (1993) Absolute bioavailability of an aqueous solution of 1-deamino-8-D-arginine vasopressin from different regions of the gastrointestinal tract in man. *Eur J Clin Pharmacol* 44: 473–476.

Daher S, Tahan S, Sole D, Naspitz CK, Da Silva Patricio FR, Neto UF, De Morais MB. (2001) Cow's milk protein intolerance and chronic constipation in children. *Pediatr Allergy Immunol* 12: 339–342.

Dauvilliers Y, Baumann CR, Carlander B, Bishof M, Blatter T, Lecendreux M, Maly F, Besset A, Touchon J, Billiard M, Tafti M, Basetti CL. (2003) CSF hypocretin-1 levels in narcolepsy, Kleine–Levin syndrome, and other hypersomnias and neurological conditions. *J Neurol Neurosurg Psychiatry* 74: 1667–1673.

Dauvilliers Y, Bouin J-L, Neidhart E, Carlander B, Eliaou J-F, Antonarakis SE, Billiard M, Tafti M. (2004) A narcolepsy susceptibility locus maps to a 5Mb region of chromosome 21q. *Ann Neurol* 56: 383–388.

Dawson PM, Griffith K, Boeke KM. (1990) Combined medical and psychological treatment of hospitalized children with encopresis. *Child Psychiatry Hum Dev* 20: 181–190.

de Gatta MF, Garcia MJ, Acosta A, Rey F, Gutierrez JR, Dominguez-Gil A. (1984) Monitoring of serum levels of imipramine and desipramine and individualization of dose in enuretic children. *Ther Drug Monit* 6: 438–443.

de Gennaro M, Capitanucci ML, Mastracci P, Silveri M, Gatti C, Mosiello G. (2004) Percutaneous tibial nerve neuromodulation is well tolerated in children and effective for treating refractory vesical dysfunction. *J Urol* 171: 1911–1913.

de Groat WC. (1975) Nervous control of the urinary bladder in the cat. *Brain Res* 87: 201–211.

de Groat WC. (1993) Anatomy and physiology of the lower urinary tract. *Urol Clin North Am* 20: 383–401.

de Groat WC. (2002) Influence of central serotonergic mechanisms on lower urinary tract function. *Urology* 59(5 Suppl 1): 30–36.

de Groat WC, Booth AM. (1980) Physiology of the urinary bladder and urethra. *Ann Intern Med* 92: 312–315.

de Groat WC, Lalley PM. (1972) Reflex firing in the lumbar sympathetic outflow to activation of vesical afferent fibers. *J Physiol* 226: 289–309.

de Groat WC, Downie JW, Levin RM, et al. (1999) Basic neurophysiology and neuropharmacology. In: Abrams P, Khoury S, Wein A, editors. *Incontinence: 1st International Consultation on Incontinence*. Plymouth: Plymbridge Distributors Ltd, pp 105–154.

De Looze D, Van Laere M, Muynck D, Beke R, Elewaut A. (1998) Constipation and other chronic gastrointestinal problems in spinal cord injury patients. *Spinal Cord* 36: 63–66.

de Lorijn F, van Wijk MP, Reitsma JB, van Ginkel R, Taminiau JA, Benninga MA. (2004) Prognosis of constipation: clinical factors and colonic transit time. *Arch Dis Child* 89: 723–727.

de Luca FG, Swenson O, Fisher JH, Loutfi AH. (1962) The dysfunctional 'lazy' bladder syndrome in children. *Arch Dis Child* 37: 117–121.

de Paepe H, Renson C, Van Laecke E, Raes A, Vande Walle J, Hoebeke P. (2000) Pelvic-floor therapy and toilet training in young children with dysfunctional voiding and obstipation. *BJU Int* 85: 889–893.

Decter RM, Bauer SB, Khoshbin S, Dyro FM, Krarup C, Colodny AH, Retik AB. (1987) Urodynamic assessment of children with cerebral palsy. *J Urol* 138: 1110–1112.

Deen PM, Knoers NV. (1998) Vasopressin type-2 receptor and aquaporin-2 water channel mutants in nephrogenic diabetes insipidus. *Am J Med Sci* 316: 300–309.

Del Giudice E, Staiano A, Capano G, et al. (1999) Gastrointestinal manifestations in children with cerebral palsy. *Brain Dev* 21: 307–311.

Dell RB, Hein K, Ramakrishnan R, et al. (1990) Model for the kinetics of imipramine and its metabolites in adolescents. *Ther Drug Monit* 12: 450–459.

Deutsche Gesellschaft für Ernährung. (1989) *Empfehlungen zur Nährstoffzufuhr*. Frankfurt am Main: Umschau Verlag, pp 23–25.

DeVane CL, Walker RD 3rd, Sawyer WP, Wilson JA. (1984) Concentrations of imipramine and its metabolites during enuresis therapy. *Pediatr Pharmacol* 4: 245–251.

Devlin JB. (1991) Prevalence and risk factors for childhood nocturnal enuresis. *Ir Med J* 84: 118–120.

Devlin JB, O'Cathain C. (1990) Predicting treatment outcome in nocturnal enuresis. *Arch Dis Child* 65: 1158–1161.

Di Lorenzo C, Benninga MA. (2004) Pathophysiology of pediatric fecal incontinence. *Gastroenterology* 126: S33–S40.

Dimson SB. (1977) Desmopressin as a treatment for enuresis. *Lancet* 1: 1260.

Djurhuus JC, Matthiesen TB, Rittig S. (1999) Similarities and dissimilarities between nocturnal enuresis in childhood and nocturia in adults. *BJU Int* 84 Suppl 1: 9–12.

Dmochowski RR. (1999) Female voiding dysfunction and movement disorders. *Int Urogynecol J Pelvic Floor Dysfunct* 10: 144–151.

Dmochowski RR, Davila GW, Zinner NR, et al. (2002) Efficacy and safety of transdermal oxybutynin in patients with urge and mixed urinary incontinence. *J Urol* 168: 580–586.

Dobson W. (1968) Another treatment for nocturnal enuresis. *Practitioner* 200: 568–570.

Dohil R, Roberts E, Verrier Jones K, Jenkins HR. (1994) Constipation and reversible urinary tract abnormalities. *Arch Dis Child* 70: 56–57.

Döpfner M, Berner W, Flechtner H, Lehmkuhl G, Steinhausen HC. (1999) *Psychopathologische Befund-Dokumentation für Kinder und Jugendliche (CASCAP-D): Befundbogen, Glossar und Explorationsleitfaden*. Göttingen: Hogrefe.

Duel BP, Steinberg-Epstein R, Hill M, Lerner M. (2003) A survey of voiding dysfunction in children with attention deficit-hyperactivity disorder. *J Urol* 170: 1521–1524.

Duker PC, Averink M, Melein L. (2001) Response restriction as a method to establish diurnal bladder control. *Am J Ment Retard* 106: 209–215.

Dundas I. (1994) The Family Adaptability and Cohesion Scale III in a Norwegian sample. *Fam Process* 33: 191–202.

Dunger DB, Seckl JR, Grant DB, Yeoman L, Lightman SL. (1988) A short water deprivation test incorporating urinary arginine vasopressin estimations for the investigation of posterior pituitary function in children. *Acta Endocrinol* 117: 13–18.

Dupont C, Ammar F, Leluyer B, Mathiex-Fortunet H, Garnier P. (2000) Polyethylene glycol (PEG) 4000 in constipated children (6 months – 15 years): a dose determination study. *Gastroenterology* 118 Suppl. Abstract 4437.

Dwyer PL, Teele JS. (1992) Prazosin: a neglected cause of genuine stress incontinence. *Obstet Gynecol* 79: 117–121.

Ebenezer IS. (1994) The effects of subcutaneous administration of arginine-8-vasopressin on the electroencephalogram of conscious rats are mediated by peripheral vasopressin V1 receptors. *Methods Find Exp Clin Pharmacol* 16: 315–321.

Edwards CRW, Kitau MJ, Chard T, Besser GM. (1973) Vasopressin analogue DDAVP in diabetes insipidus: clinical and laboratory studies. *BMJ* 3: 375–378.

Eggert P, Kühn B. (1995) Antidiuretic hormone regulation in patients with primary nocturnal enuresis. *Arch Dis Child* 73: 508–511.

Eiberg H. (1998) Total genome scan analysis in a single extended family for primary nocturnal enuresis (PNE). Evidence for a new locus (ENUR 3) for PNE on chromosome 22q.11. *Eur J Urol* 33 Suppl 3: 34–36.

Eiberg H, Berendt I, Mohr J. (1995) Assignment of dominant inherited nocturnal enuresis (ENUR 1) to chromosome 13q. *Nat Genet* 10: 354–356.

Eiberg H, Schaumburg HL, von Gontard A, Rittig S. (2001) Linkage study in a large Danish four generation family with urge incontinence and nocturnal enuresis. *J Urol* 166: 2401–2403.

Eiser C. (1990) Psychological effects of chronic disease. *J Child Psychol Psychiatry* 31: 85–98.

317

Eiser C, Morse R. (2001) Quality-of-life measures in chronic diseases in childhood. *Health Technol Assess* 5(4): 1–147.

Elam M, Thoren P, Svensson TH. (1986) Locus coeruleus neurons and sympathetic nerves: activation by visceral afferents. *Brain Res* 375: 117–125.

El-Badawi A, Schenk EA. (1966) Dual innervation of the mammalian urinary bladder. A histochemical study of the distribution of cholinergic and adrenergic nerves. *Am J Anat* 119: 405–416.

El-Badawi A, Yalla SV, Resnick NM. (1993) Structural basis of geriatric voiding dysfunction. 3. Detrusor overactivity. *J Urol* 150: 1668–1680.

Eliasson K, Larsson T, Mattsson E. (2002) Prevalence of stress incontinence in nulliparous elite trampolinists. *Scand J Med Sci Sports* 12: 106–110.

Eller DA, Homsy YL, Austin PF, Tanguay S, Cantor A. (1997) Spot urine osmolality, age and bladder capacity as predictors of response to desmopressin in nocturnal enuresis. *Scand J Urol Nephrol* 31 Suppl 183: 41–45.

Eller DA, Austin PF, Tanguay S, Homsy YL. (1998) Daytime functional bladder capacity as a predictor of response to desmopressin in monosymptomatic nocturnal enuresis. *Eur Urol* 33 Suppl 3: 25–29.

Ellinas PA, Rosner F, Jaume JC. (1993) Symptomatic hyponatremia associated with psychosis, medications, and smoking. *J Natl Med Assoc* 85: 135–141.

El-Sadr A, Sabry AA, Abdel-Rahman M, El-Barnachawy R, Koraitim M. (1990) Treatment of primary nocturnal enuresis by oral androgen mesterolone. A clinical and cystometric study. *Urology* 36: 331–335.

Elsherif I, Kareemullah C. (1999) Tonsil and adenoid surgery for upper airway obstruction in children. *Ear Nose Throat J* 78: 617–620.

Elzinga-Plomp A, Boemers TML, Messer AP, Vijverberg MAW, de Jong TPVM, van Gool JD. (1995) Treatment of enuresis risoria in children by self-administered electric and imaginary shock. *Br J Urol* 76: 775–778.

Ertunc D, Tok EC, Pata O, Dilek U, Ozdemir G, Dilek S. (2004) Is stress urinary incontinence a familial condition? *Acta Obstet Gynecol Scand* 83: 912–916.

Esperanca M, Gerrard JW. (1969) Nocturnal enuresis: studies in bladder function in normal children and enuretics. *Can Med Assoc J* 101: 324–327.

Everaert K, Pevernagie D, Oosterlinck W. (1995) Nocturnal enuresis provoked by an obstructive sleep apnea syndrome. *J Urol* 153: 1236.

Feber J, Cochat P, Hadj-Aissa A, Dubourg L, Wright C, Pozet N. (1993) Renal concentrating capacity test by desmopressin in children: intranasal or intravenous route? *Am J Nephrol* 13: 129–131.

Feehan CJ. (1995) Enuresis secondary to sexual assault. *J Am Acad Child Adolesc Psychiatry* 34: 1404.

Feehan M, McGee R, Stanton W, Silva PA. (1990) A 6-year follow-up of childhood enuresis: prevalence in adolescence and consequences for mental health. *J Paediatr Child Health* 26: 75–79.

Fehlow P. (1991) Zur Bedeutung der Elektroenzephalographie bei der körperlichen Untersuchung von Kindern mit Enkopresis. *Kinderärztl Praxis* 59: 262–265.

Feldkamp M, Bartmann D, Sureth H, Steinhausen D. (1976) Vegetative Störungen bei zerebralparetischen Kindern Ergebnisse einer Elternbefragung. *Monatsschr Kinderheilkd* 124: 583–589.

Feldman W. (1983) Nocturnal enuresis. *Can Med Assoc J* 128: 114–116.

Felt B, Wise CG, Olsen A, Kochhar P, Marcus S, Coran A. (1999) Guideline for the management of pediatric idiopathic constipation and soiling. *Arch Pediatr Adolesc Med* 153: 380–385.

Fennig S, Fennig S. (1999) Management of encopresis in early adolescence in a medical-psychiatric unit. *Gen Hosp Psychiatry* 21: 360–367.

Fergusson DM, Horwood LJ. (1994) Nocturnal enuresis and behavioral problems in adolescence: a 15-year longitudinal study. *Pediatrics* 94: 662–668.

Fergusson DM, Horwood LJ, Shannon FT. (1986) Factors related to the age of attainment of nocturnal bladder control. *Pediatrics* 78: 884–890.

Fergusson DM, Horwood LJ, Shannon FT. (1990) Secondary enuresis in a birth cohort of New Zealand children. *Paediatr Perinat Epidemiol* 4: 53–63.

Fiedorek S, Pumphrey CL, Casteel HB. (1990) Breath methane production in children with constipation and encopresis. *J Pediatr Gastroenterol Nutr* 10: 473–477.

Fielding D. (1980) The response of day and night wetting children and children who wet only at night to retention control training and the enuresis alarm. *Behav Res Ther* 18: 305–317.

Fishman L, Rappaport L, Schonwald A, Nurko S. (2003) Trends in referral to a single encopresis clinic over 20 years. *Pediatrics* 111: 604–607.

Fitzgibbons PL, Chandrasoma PT. (1987) Familial visceral myopathy. Evidence of diffuse involvement of intestinal smooth muscle. *Am J Surg Pathol* 11: 846–854.

Fjellestad A, Czernichow P. (1986) Central diabetes insipidus in children. Oral treatment with a vasopressin hormone analogue (DDAVP). *Acta Paediatr Scand* 75: 605–610.

Fjellestad-Paulsen A, Wille S, Harris AS. (1987a) Comparison of intranasal and oral desmopressin for nocturnal enuresis. *Arch Dis Child* 62: 674–677.

Fjellestad-Paulsen A, Tubiana-Rufi N, Harris AS, Czernichow P. (1987b) Central diabetes insipidus in children. Antidiuretic effect and pharmacokinetics of intranasal and peroral 1-deamino-8-D-arginine vasopressin. *Acta Endocrinol* 115: 307–312.

Fjellestad-Paulsen A, Höglund P, Lundin S, Paulsen O. (1993a) Pharmacokinetics of 1-deamino-8-D-arginine vasopressin after various routes of administration in healthy volunteers. *Clin Endocrinol* 38: 177–182.

Fjellestad-Paulsen A, Laborde K, Kindermans C, Czernichow P. (1993b) Water-balance hormones during long-term follow-up of oral DDAVP treatment in diabetes insipidus. *Acta Paediatr* 82: 752–757.

Flämig J, Wörner U. (1977) Standardisierung einer deutschen Fassung des Family Relations Test (FRT) an Kindern von 6 bis 11 Jahren. *Prax Kinderpsychol Kinderpsychiatr* 26: 5–11, 38–46.

Foldspang A, Mommsen S. (1994) Adult female urinary incontinence and childhood bedwetting. *J Urol* 152: 85–88.

Foote SL, Bloom FE, Aston-Jones G. (1983) Nucleus locus coeruleus: new evidence of anatomical and physiological specificity. *Physiol Rev* 63: 844–914.

Fordham KE, Meadow SR. (1989) Controlled trial of standard pad and bell alarm against mini alarm for nocturnal enuresis. *Arch Dis Child* 64: 651–656.

Foreman DM, Thambirajah MS. (1996) Conduct disorder, enuresis and specific developmentel delays in two types of encopresis: a case-note study of 63 boys. *Eur J Child Adolesc Psychiatry* 5: 33–37.

Forsythe WI, Redmond A. (1974) Enuresis and spontaneous cure rate: study of 1129 enuretics. *Arch Dis Child* 49: 259–263.

Foster P, Cowan G, Wrenn ELJ. (1990) Twenty-five years' experience with Hirschsprung's disease. *J Pediatr Surg* 25: 531–534.

Fotter R. (1998) Imaging of constipation in infants and children. *Pediatr Radiol* 8: 248–258.

Foxman B, Valdez B, Brook RH. (1986) Childhood enuresis: prevalence, perceived impact, and prescribed treatment. *Pediatrics* 77: 482–487.

Fraser AM, Taylor DC. (1986) Childhood encopresis extending into adult life. *Br J Psychiatry* 149: 370–371.

Freeman RM, McPherson FM, Baxby K. (1985) Psychological features of women with idiopathic detrusor instability. *Urol Int* 40: 257–259.

Freitag CM, Röhling D, Seifen S, Pukrop R, von Gontard A. (2006) Neurophysiology of nocturnal enuresis: evoked potentials and prepulse inhibition of the startle reflex. *Dev Med Child Neurol*, in print.

Freunek K. (1993) Störung der analen Sphinkterfunktion bei Kindern mit Enkopresis. Universität Würzburg: Medical doctoral thesis.

Frieling T. (1993) Interaktion zwischen enterischem und zerebralem Nervensystem. *Z Gastroenterol* 31 Suppl 3: 21–25.

Fritz GK, Rockney RM, Yeung AS. (1994) Plasma levels and efficacy of imipramine treatment for enuresis. *J Am Acad Child Adolesc Psychiatry* 33: 60–64.

Fry CH, Ikeda Y, Harvey R, Wu C, Sui GP. (2004a) Control of bladder function by peripheral nerves: avenues for novel drug targets. *Urology* 63(3 Suppl 1): 24–31.

Fry CH, Sui GP, Severs NJ, Wu C. (2004b) Spontaneous activity and electrical coupling in human detrusor smooth muscle: implications for detrusor overactivity? *Urology* 63(3 Suppl 1): 3–10.

Fuger K, Barnert J, Hopfner W, Wienbeck M. (1995) Intestinal pseudoobstruction as a feature of myotonic muscular dystrophy. *Z Gastroenterol* 33: 534–538.

Fujiwara J, Kimura S, Tsukayama H, Nakahara S, Haibara S, Fujita M, Isobe N, Tamura K. (2001) Evaluation of the autonomic nervous system function in children with primary monosymptomatic nocturnal enuresis – power spectrum analysis of heart rate variability using 24-hour Holter electrocardiograms. *Scand J Urol Nephrol* 35: 350–356.

Furlanut M, Montanari G, Benetello P, Bonin P, Schiaulini P, Pellegrino PA. (1989) Steady-state serum concentrations of imipramine, its main metabolites and clinical response in primary enuresis. *Pharmacol Res* 21: 561–566.

Fusch C, Hungerland E, Scharrer B, Moeller H. (1993) Water turnover of healthy children measured by deuterated water elimination. *Eur J Pediatr* 152: 110–114.

Gabel S, Hegedus AM, Wald A, Chandra R, Chiponis D. (1986) Prevalence of behavior problems and mental health utilization among encopretic children: implications for behavioral pediatrics. *J Dev Behav Pediatr* 7: 293–297.

Gastaut H, Orfanos A, Lob H, Poiré R. (1964) Polygraphic study of enuresis during grand mal attacks. *Electroenceph Clin Neurophysiol* 16: 626–627.

Gattuso JM, Kamm MA. (1997) Clinical features of idiopathic megarectum and idiopathic megacolon. *Gut* 41: 93–99.

Gattuso JM, Kamm MA, Talbot IC. (1997) Pathology of idiopathic megarectum and megacolon. *Gut* 41: 252–257.

Geirsson G, Lindström S, Fall M. (1999) The bladder cooling reflex and the use of cooling as stimulus to the lower urinary tract. *J Urol* 162: 1890–1896.

Gepertz S, Nevéus T. (2004) Imipramine for therapy resistant enuresis: a retrospective evaluation. *J Urol* 171: 2607–2610.

Gerlach M, Warnke A, Wewetzer C, editors. (2004) *Neuro-Psychopharmaka im Kindes- und Jugendalter.* Vienna, New York: Springer.

Gibb S, Nolan T, South M, Noad L, Bates G, Vidmar S. (2004) Evidence against a synergistic effect of desmopressin with conditioning in the treatment of nocturnal enuresis. *J Pediatr* 144: 351–357.

Gillick J, Tazawa H, Puri P. (2001) Intestinal neuronal dysplasia: results of treatment in 33 patients. *J Pediatr Surg* 36: 777–779.

Gladh G, Mattsson S, Lindström S. (2001) Anogenital electrical stimulation as treatment of urge incontinence in children. *BJU Int* 87: 366–371.

Gladh G, Mattsson S, Lindström S. (2004) Outcome of the bladder cooling test in children with nonneurogenic bladder problems. *J Urol* 172: 1095–1098.

Glahn BE. (1979) Giggle incontinence (enuresis risoria). A study and an aetiological hypothesis. *Br J Urol* 51: 363–366.

Glazener CM, Evans JH. (2000) Tricyclic and related drugs for nocturnal enuresis in children. *Cochrane Database Syst Rev* 2: CD002117.

Glazener CMA, Evans JHC. (2002a) Simple behavioural and physical interventions for nocturnal enuresis in children (Cochrane Review). In: The Cochrane Library, Issue 2. Oxford: Update Software.

Glazener CMA, Evans JHC. (2002b) Alarm interventions for nocturnal enuresis in children (Cochrane Review). In: The Cochrane Library, Issue 2. Oxford: Update Software.

Glazener CM, Evans JH. (2002c) Desmopressin for nocturnal enuresis. *Cochrane Database Syst Rev* 3: CD002112.

Glazener CMA, Evans JH, Peto RE. (2004) Complex behavioural and educational interventions for nocturnal enuresis in children (Cochrane Review). *Cochrane Database Syst Rev* 1: CD004668.

Glicklich LB. (1951) An historical account of enuresis. *Pediatrics* 8: 859–876.

Glickman S, Kamm MA. (1996) Bowel dysfunction in spinal-cord-injury patients. *Lancet* 347: 1651–1653.

Goldman M, Bistritzer T, Horne T, Zoareft I, Aladjem M. (2000a) The etiology of renal scars in infants with pyelonephritis and vesicoureteral reflux. *Pediatr Nephrol* 14: 385–388.

Goldman M, Lahat E, Strauss S, Reisler G, Livne A, Gordin L, Aladjem M. (2000b) Imaging after urinary tract infection in male neonates. *Pediatrics* 105: 1232–1235.

Green RG, Harris RN, Forte JA, Robinson M. (1991) Evaluating FACES III and the Circumplex Model: 2440 families. *Fam Process* 30: 55–73.

Greiff L, Andersson M, Svensson J, Wollmer P, Lundin S, Persson CGA. (2002) Absorption across the nasal airway mucosa in house dust mite perennial allergic rhinitis. *Clin Physiol Func Im* 22: 55–57.

Griffiths DJ, Scholtmeijer RJ. (1983) Detrusor sphincter dyssynergia in neurologically normal children. *Neurourol Urodyn* 2: 27–37.

Griffiths DJ, Scholtmeijer RJ. (1987) Vesicoureteral reflux and lower urinary tract dysfunction: evidence for 2 different reflux/dysfunction complexes. *J Urol* 137: 240–244.

Guay DRP. (2003) Clinical pharmacokinetics of drugs used to treat urge incontinence. *Clin Pharmacokinet* 42: 1243–1285.

Guillaud R, Amram S, Lememme F, Lesbros D. (1993) Desmopressine et intoxication par l'eau. A propos d'un cas traité pour enuresie. *Pediatrie* 48: 697–699.

Guilleminault C, Pelayo R, Leger D, Clerk A, Bocian RBZ. (1996) Recognition of sleep-disordered breathing in children. *Pediatrics* 98: 871–882.

320

Gümüs B, Vurgun N, Lekili M, Iscan A, Müezzinoglu T, Büyüksu C. (1999) Prevalence of nocturnal enuresis and accompanying factors in children aged 7–11 years in Turkey. *Acta Paediatr* 88: 1369–1372.

Gur E, Turhan P, Can G, Akkus S, Sever L, Guzeloz S, Cifcili S, Arvas A. (2004) Enuresis: prevalence, risk factors and urinary pathology among school children in Istanbul, Turkey. *Pediatr Int* 46: 58–63.

Gutierrez Segura C. (1997) Urine flow in childhood: a study of flow chart parameters based on 1,361 uroflowmetry tests. *J Urol* 157: 1426–1428.

Haab F, Stewart L, Dwyer P. (2004) Darifenacin, an M3 selective receptor antagonist, is an effective and well-tolerated once-daily treatment for overactive bladder. *Eur Urol* 45: 420–429.

Hägglöf B, Andren O, Bergström E, Marklund L, Wendelius M. (1997) Self-esteem before and after treatment in children with nocturnal enuresis and urinary incontinence. *Scand J Urol Nephrol* Suppl 183: 79–82.

Halaska M, Ralph G, Wiedemann A, Primus G, Ballering-Bruhl B, Hofner K, Jonas U. (2003) Controlled, double-blind, multicentre clinical trial to investigate long-term tolerability and efficacy of trospium chloride in patients with detrusor instability. *World J Urol* 20: 392–399.

Hallgren B. (1957) Enuresis: a clinical and genetic study. *Acta Psychiatr Neurol Scand* Suppl 114.

Hallgren B. (1960) Nocturnal enuresis in twins. *Acta Psychiatr Neurol Scand* 35: 73–90.

Halliday S, Meadow SR, Berg I. (1987) Successful management of daytime enuresis using alarm procedures: a randomly controlled trial. *Arch Dis Child* 62: 132–137.

Hamed M, Mitchell H, Clow DJ. (1993) Hyponatremic convulsion associated with desmopressin and imipramine treatment. *BMJ* 306(6886): 1169.

Hammer M, Vilhardt H. (1985) Peroral treatment of diabetes insipidus with a polypeptide hormone analog, desmopressin. *J Pharmacol Exp Ther* 234: 754–760.

Hansen AF, Jorgensen TM. (1997) Alarm treatment: influence on functional bladder capacity. *Scand J Urol Nephrol* 31 Suppl 183: 59–60.

Hansen A, Hansen B, Dahm TL. (1997) Urinary tract infection, day wetting and other voiding symptoms in seven- to eight-year-old Danish children. *Acta Paediatr* 86: 1345–1349.

Hanson E, Hellström A-L, Hjälmås K. (1987) Non-neurogenic discoordinated voiding in children. The longterm effect of bladder retraining. *Z Kinderchir* 42: 109–111.

Hanson E, Hanson M, Hellström A-L, Hjälmås K, Holmdahl G, Jansson U-B, Sillén U. (1995) Four-hour voiding observation in infants. Third International Children's Continence Symposium, Sydney, Australia.

Hansson S, Jodal U, Lincoln K, Svanborg-Edén C. (1989) Untreated asymptomatic bacteriuria in girls. II. Effect of phenoxymethylpenicillin and erythromycin given for intercurrent infections. *BMJ* 298: 856–859.

Hansson S, Hjälmås K, Jodal U, Sixt R. (1990) Lower urinary tract dysfunction in girls with untreated asymptomatic or covert bacteriuria. *J Urol* 143: 333–335.

Haque M, Ellerstein NS, Gundy JH, Shelov SP, Weiss JC, McIntire MS, Olness KN, Jones DJ, Heagarty MC, Starfield BH. (1981) Parental perceptions of enuresis. *Am J Dis Child* 135: 809–811.

Harper PS. (1982) *Practical Genetic Counseling*. Bristol: John Wright.

Harrington L, Schuh S. (1997) Complications of Fleet enema administration and suggested guidelines for use in the pediatric emergency department. *Pediatr Emerg Care* 13: 225–226.

Harrison SC, Hunnam GR, Farman P, Ferguson DR, Doyle PT. (1987) Bladder instability and denervation in patients with bladder outflow obstruction. *Br J Urol* 60: 519–522.

Haruno A, Yamasaki Y, Miyoshi K, et al. (1989) Effects of propiverine hydrochloride and its metabolites on isolated guinea pig urinary bladder. *Folia Pharmacol Jpn* 94: 145–150.

Hatch TF. (1988) Encopresis and constipation in children. *Pediatr Clin North Am* 35: 257–280.

Hellerstein S, Linebarger JS. (2003) Voiding dysfunction in pediatric patients. *Clin Pediatr* 42: 43–49.

Hellström A-L, Hjälmås K, Jodal U. (1987) Rehabilitation of the dysfunctional bladder in children: method and 3-year follow-up. *J Urol* 138: 847–849.

Hellström A-L, Hjälmås K, Jodal U. (1989) Terodiline in the treatment of children with unstable bladders. *Br J Urol* 63: 358–362.

Hellström A-L, Hansson E, Hansson S, Hjälmås K, Jodal U. (1990) Incontinence and micturition habits in 7-year-old Swedish school entrants. *Eur J Pediatr* 149: 434–437.

Hellström A-L, Hanson E, Hansson S, Hjälmås K, Jodal U. (1995) Micturition habits and incontinence at age 17 – reinvestigation of a cohort studied at age 7. *Br J Urol* 76: 231–234.

Heslington K, Hilton P. (1996) Ambulatory monitoring and conventional cystometry in asymptomatic female volunteers. *Br J Obstet Gynaecol* 103: 211–214.

Hettiarachchi M, Garcea G, DeSouza NM, Williams AD, Clayden GS, Ward HC. (2002) Evaluation of dysfunction following reconstruction of an anorectal anomaly. *Pediatr Surg Int* 18: 405–409.

321

Hibi M, Iwai N, Kimura O, Sasaki Y, Tsuda T. (2003) Results of biofeedback therapy for fecal incontinence in children with encopresis and following surgery for anorectal malformations. *Dis Colon Rectum* 46 (10 Suppl): S54–S58.

Hinchliffe SA, Sargent PH, Howard CV, et al. (1991) Human intra-uterine renal growth expressed in absolute number of glomeruli assessed by 'disector' method and Cavalieri principle. *Lab Invest* 54: 777–784.

Hindmarsh JR, Byrne PO. (1980) Adult enuresis – a symptomatic and urodynamic assessment. *Br J Urol* 52: 88–91.

Hinds JP, Eidelmann BH, Wald A. (1990) Prevalence of bowel dysfunction in multiple sclerosis. A population study. *Gastroenterology* 98: 1538–1542.

Hinman F. (1974) Urinary tract damage in children who wet. *Pediatrics* 54: 142–150.

Hinman F. (1986) Non-neurogenic neurogenic bladder (the Hinman Syndrome) – 15 years later. *J Urol* 136: 769–777.

Hinman F, Baumann FW. (1973) Vesical and ureteral damage from voiding dysfunction in boys without neurologic or obstructive disease. *J Urol* 109: 727–732.

Hinman, F, Baumann FW. (1976) Complications of vesicoureteral operations from incoordination of micturition. *J Urol* 116: 638–642.

Hirasing RA, van Leerdam FJ, Bolk-Bennink L, Janknegt RA. (1997a) Enuresis nocturna in adults. *Scand J Urol Nephrol* 31: 533–536.

Hirasing RA, van Leerdam FJM, Bolk-Bennink LB, Bosch JD. (1997b) Bedwetting and behavioural and/or emotional problems. *Acta Paediatr* 86: 1131–1134.

Hirasing RA, van Leerdam FJM, Bolk-Bennink LB, Koor HM. (2002) Effect of dry bed training on behavioural problems in enuretic children. *Acta Paediatr* 91: 960–964.

Hjälmås K. (1976) Micturition in infants and children with normal lower urinary tract. *Scand J Urol Nephrol* Suppl 37: 1–106.

Hjälmås K. (1988) Urodynamics in normal infants and children. *Scand J Urol Nephrol* Suppl 114: 20–27.

Hjälmås K. (1992) Vesicoureteral reflux in infants and children: a disorder of the bladder. *Curr Opin Urol* 4: 321–326.

Hjälmås K. (1995a) Is dyscoordinated voiding in children an hereditary disorder? *Scand J Urol Nephrol* Suppl 173: 31–35.

Hjälmås K. (1995b) The Swedish Enuresis Trial (SWEET): long-term use of desmopressin in primary monosymptomatic nocturnal enuresis. Preliminary results. Third International Children's Continence Symposium, Sydney, Australia.

Hjälmås K, Bengtsson B. (1993) Efficacy, safety, and dosing of desmopressin for nocturnal enuresis in Europe. *Clin Pediatr* (spec no.): 19–24.

Hjälmås K, Hanson E, Hellström A-L, Kruse S, Sillén U. (1998) Long-term treatment with desmopressin in children with primary monosymptomatic nocturnal enuresis: an open multicentre study. Swedish Enuresis Trial (SWEET) Group. *Br J Urol* 82: 704–709.

Hjälmås K, Hellström A-L, Mogren K, Läckgren G, Stenberg A. (2001) The overactive bladder: a potential future indication for tolterodine. *Br J Urol Int* 87: 569–574.

Hjälmås K, Arnold T, Bower W, Caione P, Chiozza LM, von Gontard A, Han SW, Husman DA, Kawauchi A, Läckgren G, Lottmann H, Mark S, Rittig S, Robson L, Vande Walle J, Yeung CK. (2004) Nocturnal enuresis: an international evidence-based management strategy. *J Urol* 171: 2545–2561.

Hoang-Böhm J, Jünemann KP, Köhrmann KU, Zendler S, Alken P. (1999) Kindgerechtes Biofeedback-Training bei einnässenden Kindern mit Detrusor-Sphinkter-Dyskoordination. *Akt Urol* 30: 118–122.

Hoang-Böhm J, Lusch A, Sha W, Alken P. (2004) Biofeedback bei kindlichen Blasenfunktionsstörungen. *Urologe* (A) 43: 813–819.

Hoberman A, Wald ER, Reynolds EA, Penchansky L, Charron M. (1994) Pyuria and bacteriuria in urine specimens obtained by catheter from young children with fever. *J Pediatr* 124: 513–519.

Hoebeke P, van Laecke E, Van Camp C, Raes A, Vande Walle J. (2001) One thousand video-urodynamic studies in children with non-neurogenic bladder sphincter dysfunction. *BJU Int* 87: 575–580.

Hoebeke P, Van Laecke E, Renson C, Raes A, Dehoorne J, Vermeiren P, Vande Walle J. (2004) Pelvic floor spasms in children: an unknown condition responding well to pelvic floor therapy. *Eur Urol* 46: 651–654.

Hoefnagels WA, Padberg GW, Overweg J, van der Velde EA, Roos RA. (1991) Transient loss of consciousness: the value of the history for distinguishing seizure from syncope. *J Neurol* 238: 39–43.

322

Hoekx L, Wyndaele JJ, Vermandel A. (1998) The role of bladder biofeedback in the treatment of children with refractory nocturnal enuresis associated with idiopathic detrusor instability and small bladder capacity. *J Urol* 160: 858–860.

Holland AJ, King PA, Chauvel PJ, O'Neill MK, McKnight DL, Barker AP. (1997) Intravesical therapy for the treatment of neurogenic bladder in children. *Aust NZ J Surg* 67: 731–733.

Holliday JM, Segar C. (1957) The maintenance need for water in parenteral fluid therapy. *Pediatrics* 19: 823–832.

Holmdahl G. (1997) Bladder dysfunction in boys with posterior urethral valves. *Scand J Urol Nephrol* 188(Suppl): 1–36.

Holmdahl G, Sillén U, Bachelard M, Hansson E, Hermansson G, Hjälmås K. (1995) The changing urodynamic pattern in valve bladders during infancy. *J Urol* 153: 463–467.

Holmdahl G, Hanson E, Hanson M, Hellström A-L, Hjälmås K, Sillén U. (1996) Four-hour voiding observation in healthy infants. *J Urol* 156: 1809–1812.

Holmdahl G, Sillén U, Bertilsson M, Hermansson G, Hjälmås K. (1997) Natural filling cystometry in small boys with posterior urethral valves: unstable valve bladders become stable during sleep. *J Urol* 158: 1017–1021.

Holme E, Greter J, Jacobson CE, Lindstedt S, Nordin I, Kristiansson B, Jodal U. (1989) Carnitine deficiency induced by pivampicillin and pivmecillinam therapy. *Lancet* 2(8661): 469–473.

Holmes WC, Slap GB. (1998) Sexual abuse of boys: definition, prevalence, correlates, sequelae, and management. *JAMA* 280: 1855–1862.

Holstege G, Griffiths D, De Wall H, Dalm E. (1986) Anatomical and physiological observations on supraspinal control of bladder and urethral sphincter muscles in the cat. *J Comp Neurol* 250: 449–461.

Homsy YL, Nsouli I, Hamberger B, Laberge I, Schuck E. (1985) Effects of oxybutinin on vesico-ureteral reflux in children. *J Urol* 134: 1168–1171.

Horner RL. (1996) Autonomic consequences of arousal from sleep: mechanisms and implications. *Sleep* 19(10 Suppl): S193–S195.

Hourihane J, Salisbury AJ. (1993) Use caution in prescribing desmopressin for nocturnal enuresis. *BMJ* 306(6891): 1545.

Houts AC, Berman JS, Abramson H. (1994) Effectiveness of psychological and pharmacological treatments for nocturnal enuresis. *J Consult Clin Psychol* 62: 737–745.

Hoyle CH. (1994) Non-adrenergic, non-cholinergic control of the urinary bladder. *World J Urol* 12: 233–244.

Hublin C, Kaprio J, Partinen M, Koskenvuo M. (1998) Nocturnal enuresis in a nationwide twin cohort. *Sleep* 21: 579–585.

Hunsballe JM, Hansen TK, Rittig S, Nørgaard JP, Pedersen EB, Djurhuus JC. (1995) Polyuric and non-polyuric bedwetting – pathogenetic differences in nocturnal enuresis. *Scand J Urol Nephrol* S173: 77–79.

Hunsballe JM, Rittig S, Pedersen EB, Olesen OV, Djurhuus JC. (1997) Single dose imipramine reduces nocturnal urine output in patients with nocturnal enuresis and nocturnal polyuria. *J Urol* 158: 830–836.

Hunsballe JM, Hansen TK, Rittig S, Pedersen EB, Djurhuus JC. (1998) The efficacy of DDAVP is related to the circadian rhythm of urine output in patients with persisting nocturnal enuresis. *Clin Endocrinol* 49: 793–801.

Hutson JM, McNamara J, Gibb S, Shin YM. (2001) Slow transit constipation in children. *J Paediatr Child Health* 37: 426–430.

Hutson JM, Catto-Smith T, Gibb S, Chase J, Shin Y-M, Stanton M, King S, Sutcliffe J, Ong SY, Djaja P, Southwell B. (2004) Chronic constipation: no longer stuck! Characterization of colonic dismotility as a new disorder in children. *J Pediatr Surg* 39: 795–799.

Hvistendahl GM, Kamperis K, Rawashdeh F, Rittig S, Djurhuus JC. (2004) The effect of alarm treatment on the functional bladder capacity in children with monosymptomatic nocturnal enuresis. *J Urol* 171: 2611–2614.

Hyams G, McCoull K, Smith PS, Tyrer SP. (1992) Behavioural continence training in mental handicap: a 10-year follow-up study. *J Int Disabil Res* 36: 551–558.

Hyman PE, Fleisher DR. (1994) A classification of disorders of defecation in infants and children. *Semin Gastrointest Dis* 5: 20–23.

Ichioka M, Hirata Y, Inase N, Tojo N, Yoshizawa M, Chida M, et al. (1992) Changes in circulating atrial natriuretic peptide and antidiuretic hormone in obstructive sleep apnea syndrome. *Respiration* 59: 164–168.

Illowsky BP, Kirch DG. (1988) Polydipsia and hyponatremia in psychiatric patients. *Am J Psychiatry* 145: 675.

Ishigooka M, Hashimoto T, Sasagawa I, Izumiya K, Nakada T. (1992) Terodiline in the treatment of nocturnal enuresis in children. *Int Urol Nephrol* 24: 509–513.

Issenman RM, Filmer RB, Gorski PA. (1999) A review of bowel and bladder control development in children: how gastrointestinal and urologic conditions relate to problems in toilet training. *Pediatrics* 103: 1346–1352.

Iwata G, Iwai N, Nagashima M, Fukata R. (1995) New biofeedback therapy in children with encopresis. *Eur J Pediatr Surg* 142: 231–234.

Jabs CFI, Stanton SL. (2001) Urge incontinence and detrusor instability. *Int Urogynecol J* 12: 58–68.

Jakobsson I. (1985) Unusual presentation of adverse reactions to cow's milk proteins. *Klin Pädiatr* 197: 360–362.

Jakobsson B, Berg U, Svensson L. (1994) Renal scarring after acute pyelonephritis. *Arch Dis Child* 70: 111–115.

Jameson JS, Scott AD. (1997) Medical causes of faecal incontinence. *Eur J Gastroenterol Hepatol* 9: 428–430.

Janknegt RA, Zweers HM, Delaere KP, Kloet AG, Khoe SG, Arendsen HJ. (1997) Oral desmopressin as a new treatment modality for primary nocturnal enuresis in adolescents and adults: a double-blind, randomized, multicenter study. Dutch Enuresis Study Group. *J Urol* 157: 513–517.

Järvelin MR, Vikeväinen-Tervonen L, Moilanen I, Huttunen N-P. (1988) Enuresis in seven-year-old children. *Acta Paediatr Scand* 77: 148–153.

Järvelin MR, Moilanen I, Vikeväinen-Tervonen L, Huttunen N-P. (1990a) Life changes and protective capacities in enuretic and non-enuretic children *J Child Psychol Psychiatry* 31: 763–774.

Järvelin MR, Huttunen NP, Seppänen J, Seppänen U, Moilanen I. (1990b) Screening for urinary tract abnormalities among day and night wetting children. *Scand J Urol Nephrol* 24: 181–189.

Jayachandar J, Frank JL, Jonas MM. (1988) Isolated intestinal myopathy resembling progressive systemic sclerosis in a child. *Gastroenterology* 95: 1114–1118.

Jensen P, Kettle L, Roper M, et al. (1999) Are stimulants overprescribed? Treatment of ADHD in four communities. *J Am Acad Child Adolesc Psychiatry* 38: 797–804.

Jodal U. (2000) Selective approach to diagnostic imaging of children after urinary tract infection. *Acta Paediatr* 89: 767–768.

Jodal U, Koskimies O, Hansson E, Löhr G, Olbing H, Smellie J, Tamminen-Möbius T. (1992) Infection pattern in children with vesicoureteral reflux randomly allocated to operation or long-term antibacterial prophylaxis. *J Urol* 148: 1650–1652.

Johanson JF, Lafferty J. (1996) Epidemiology of fecal incontinence: the silent affliction. *Am J Gastroenterol* 91: 33–36.

Johnston BD, Wright JA. (1993) Attentional dysfunction in children with encopresis. *J Dev Behav Pediatr* 14: 381–385.

Jonas U, Tanagho EA. (1975) Studies on vesicourethral reflexes. I. Urethral sphincteric responses to detrusor stretch. *Invest Urol* 12: 357–373.

Jonat S, Santer R, Schneppenheim R, Obser T, Eggert P. (1999) Effect of DDAVP on nocturnal enuresis in a patient with nephrogenic diabetes insipidus. *Arch Dis Child* 81: 57–59.

Jonge GG. (1969) *Children with Enuresis*. Assen: Van Gorcum.

Jonville AP, Dutertre JP, Autret E, Barbellion M. (1992) Effets indesirables du chlorure d'oxybutynine (Ditropan). Bilan de l'enquête officielle des Centres Regionaux de Pharmacovigilance. *Thérapie* 47: 389–392.

Jørgensen OS, Lober M, Christiansen J, Gram LF. (1980) Plasma concentration and clinical effect in imipramine treatment of childhood enuresis. *Clin Pharmacokinet* 5: 386–393.

Jost W, Marsalek P. (2004) Duloxetine: mechanism of action at the lower urinary tract and Onuf's nucleus. *Clin Auton Res* 14: 220–227.

Jung SY, Fraser MO, Ozawa H, Yokohama O, Yoshiyama M, De Groat WC, Chancellor MB. (1999) Urethral afferent nerve activity affects the micturition reflex; implication for the relationship between stress incontinence and detrusor instability. *J Urol* 162: 204–212.

Jurzak M, Schmidt HA. (1998) Vasopressin and sensory circumventricular organs. *Prog Brain Res* 119: 221–245.

Jurzak M, Muller AR, Gerstberger R. (1995) Characterization of vasopressin receptors in cultured cells derived from the region of rat brain circumventricular organs. *Neuroscience* 65: 1145–1159.

Kajiwara M, Inoue K, Usui A, Kurihara M, Usui T. (2004) The micturition habits and prevalence of daytime urinary incontinence in Japanese primary school children. *J Urol* 171: 403–407.

Kakizaki H, Nonomura K, Asano Y, Shinno Y, Ameda K, Koyanagi T. (1994) Preexisting neurogenic voiding dysfunction in children with imperforate anus: problems in management. *J Urol* 151: 1041–1044.

Kallio J, Rautava P, Huupponen R, Korvenranta H. (1993) Severe hyponatremia caused by intranasal desmopressin for nocturnal enuresis. *Acta Paediatr* 82: 881–882.

Kalo BB, Bella H. (1996) Enuresis: prevalence and associated factors among primary school children in Saudi Arabia. *Acta Paediatr* 85: 1217–1222.

Kamperis K, Rittig S, Schaumburg HL, Hansen MN, Djurhuus JC. (2001) Predictors of response to DDAVP in monosymptomatic nocturnal enuresis. The role of bladder capacity (abstract). *Pediatr Nephrol* 16(Suppl): C109.

Kanie S, Yokoyama O, Komatsu K, et al. (2000) GABAergic contribution to rat bladder hyperactivity after middle cerebral artery occlusion. *Am J Physiol Regul Integr Comp Physiol* 279: R1230–R1238.

Kaplan GW, Wallace WW, Orgel HA, Miller JR. (1977) Serum immunoglobulin E and incidence of allergy in group of enuretic children. *Urology* 10: 428–430.

Kapoor VK, Saksena PN. (1969) Methylamphetamine hydrochloride (methedrine) in enuresis. *Ind J Pediatr* 36: 169–170.

Kapur RP. (2003) Neuronal dysplasia: a controversial pathological correlate of intestinal pseudo-obstruction. *Am J Med Genet* 122A(4): 287–293.

Kardash S, Hillman ES, Werry J. (1968) Efficacy of imipramine in childhood enuresis: a double-blind control study with placebo. *Can Med Assoc J* 99: 263–266.

Kaufman JJ. (1957) A new recording uroflowmeter: a simple automatic device for measuring voiding velocity. *J Urol* 78: 97–99.

Kaufman AS, Kaufman NL. (1983) *K-ABC: Kaufman Assessment Battery for Children*. Circle Pines, Minn.: American Guidance Service.

Kazdin A. (2000) *Psychotherapy for Children and Adolescents – Directions for Research and Practice*. New York, Oxford: Oxford University Press.

Keefe FB, Johnson LC, Hunter EJ. (1971) EEG and autonomic response pattern during waking and sleep stages. *Psychophysiology* 8: 198–212.

Keller K-M. (2002) Evidenz-basierte Therapie der chronischen Obstipation und Enkopresis bei Kindern. *Monatsschr Kinderheilkd* 150: 594–601.

Keren R, Chan E. (2002) A meta-analysis of randomized, controlled trials comparing short- and long-course antibiotic therapy for urinary tract infections in children. *Pediatrics* 109: E70–0.

Kessler R, Constantinou CE. (1986) Internal urethrotomy in girls and its impact on the urethral intrinsic and extrinsic continence mechanisms. *J Urol* 136: 1248–1253.

Khaled SM, Elhilali M. (2003) Role of 5-HT receptors in treatment of overactive bladder. *Drugs Today* 39: 599–607.

Kimura Y, Sasaki Y, Hamada K, Fukui H, Ukai Y, Yoshikuni Y, Kimura K, Sugaya K, Nishizawa O. (1996) Mechanisms of the suppression of the bladder activity by flavoxate. *Int J Urol* 3: 218–227.

Kjolseth D, Knudsen LM, Madsen B, Norgaard JP, Djurhuus JC. (1993) Urodynamic biofeedback training for children with bladder-sphincter-dyscoordination during voiding. *Neurourol Urodyn* 12: 211–221.

Klackenberg G. (1981) Nocturnal enuresis in a longitudinal perspective. *Acta Paediatr Scand* 70: 453–457.

Klarskov P. (1987) Enkephalin inhibits presynaptically the contractility of urinary tract smooth muscle. *Eur Urol* 59: 31–35.

Kleran JL, De Jong AR. (1990) Urinary tract symptoms and urinary tract infection following sexual abuse. *Am J Dis Child* 144: 242–244.

Knudsen UB, Rittig S, Nørgaard JP, Lundemose JB, Pedersen EB, Djurhuus JC. (1991) Long-term treatment of nocturnal enuresis with desmopressin. A follow-up study. *Urol Res* 19: 237–240.

Kodman-Jones C, Hawkins L, Schulman SL. (2001) Behavioral characteristics of children with daytime wetting. *J Urol* 166: 2392–2395.

Koff SA. (1983) Estimating bladder capacity in children. *Urology* 21: 248.

Koff SA. (1996) Cure of nocturnal enuresis: why isn't desmopressin very effective? *Pediatr Nephrol* 10: 667–670.

Koff SA, Byard MA. (1988) The daytime urinary frequency syndrome of childhood. *J Urol* 140: 1280–1281.

Koff SA, Murtagh DS. (1983) The uninhibited bladder in children: effect of treatment on recurrence of urinary infection and on vesicoureteral reflux resolution. *J Urol* 130: 1138–1141.

Koff SA, Wagner TT, Jayanthi VR. (1998) The relationship among dysfunctional elimination syndromes, primary vesicoureteral reflux and urinary tract infections in children. *J Urol* 160: 1019–1022.

Koletzko S. (2002) Intestinale Motilitätsstörungen. *Monatsschr Kinderheilkd* 150: 574–586.

Kolvin I, MacKeith RC, Meadow SR, editors. (1973) *Bladder Control and Enuresis*. London: William Heinemann.

Kontiokari T, Laitinen J, Jarvi L, Pokka T, Sundqvist K, Uhari M. (2003) Dietary factors protecting women from urinary tract infection. *Am J Clin Nutr* 77: 600–604.

Kontiokari T, Nuutinen M, Uhari M. (2004) Dietary factors affecting susceptibility to urinary tract infection. *Pediatr Nephrol* 19: 378–383.

Koonings PP, Bergman A. (1991) Urethral pressure changes in women with detrusor instability. Bladder or urethral pathologic process? *Urology* 37: 540–542.

Korczyn AD, Kish I. (1979) The mechanism of imipramine in enuresis nocturna. *Clin Exp Pharmacol Physiol* 6: 31–35.

Kosar A, Arikan N, Dincel C. (1999) Effectiveness of oxybutynin hydrochloride in the treatment of enuresis nocturna. *Scand J Urol Nephrol* 33: 115–118.

Kramer NR, Bonitati AE, Millman RP. (1998) Enuresis and obstructive sleep apnea in adults. *Chest* 114: 634–637.

Krieger J, Follenius M, Sforza E, Brandenberger G, Peter JD. (1991) Effects of treatment with nasal continuous positive airway pressure on atrial natriuretic peptide and arginine vasopressin release during sleep in patients with obstructive sleep apnoea. *Clin Sci Colch* 80: 443–449.

Krisch K. (1985) *Enkopresis: Ursachen und Behandlung des Einkotens*. Bern: Hans Huber Verlag.

Kristensen G, Jensen IN. (2003) Meta-analyses of results of alarm treatment for nocturnal enuresis. *Scand J Urol Nephrol* 37: 232–238.

Krogh K, Mosdal C, Laurberg S. (2000) Gastrointestinal and segmental colonic transit times in patients with acute and chronic spinal cord lesions. *Spinal Cord* 38: 615–621.

Kruse S, Hellström A-L, Hjälmås K. (1999) Daytime bladder dysfuncion in therapy-resistant nocturnal enuresis: a pilot study in urotherapy. *Scand J Urol Nephrol* 33: 49–52.

Kubota M, Suita S, Kamimura T. (1997) Abnormalities in visceral evoked potentials from the anal canal in children with chronic constipation. *Surg Today* 27: 632–637.

Kuh D, Cardozo L, Hardy R. (1999) Urinary incontinence in middle aged women: childhood enuresis and other lifetime risk factors in a British prospective cohort. *J Epidemiol Community Health* 53: 453–458.

Kumar V, Templeman L, Chapple CR, Chess-Williams R. (2003) Recent developments in the management of detrusor overactivity. *Curr Opin Urol* 13: 285–291.

Kunin CM. (1970) A ten-year study of bacteriuria in schoolgirls: final report of bacteriologic, urologic and epidemiologic findings. *J Infect Dis* 122: 382–393.

Kuo HC. (2004) Urodynamic evidence of effectiveness of botulinum A toxin injection in treatment of detrusor overactivity refractory to anticholinergic agents. *Urology* 63: 868–872.

Kurol J, Modin H, Bjerkhoel A. (1998) Orthodontic maxillary expansion and its effect on nocturnal enuresis. *Angle Orthod* 68: 225–232.

Kuru M. (1965) Nervous control of micturition. *Physiol Rev* 45: 425–494.

Kusek JW, Nyberg LM. (2001) The epidemiology of interstitial cystitis: is it time to expand our definition? *Urology* 57 (6 Suppl 1): 95–99.

Laberge L, Denesle R, Tremblay R, Montplaisir J. (1996) Parasomnias in 2000 children aged 11. *J Sleep Res* 5(Suppl 1): 114.

Läckgren G, Nevéus T, Stenberg A. (1997) Diurnal plasma vasopressin and urinary output in adolescents with monosymptomatic nocturnal enuresis. *Acta Paediatr* 86: 385–390.

Läckgren G, Hjälmås K, van Gool J, von Gontard A, de Gennaro M, Lottmann H, Terho P. (1999) Nocturnal enuresis – a suggestion for a European treatment strategy. *Acta Paediatr* 88: 679–690.

Läckgren G, Wåhlin N, Sköldenberg E, Stenberg A. (2001) Long-term follow-up of children treated with dextranomer/hyaluronic acid copolymer for vesicoureteric reflux. *J Urol* 166: 1887–1892.

Lal R, Bhatnagar V, Mitra DK. (1999) Long-term prognosis of renal function in boys treated for posterior urethral valves. *Eur J Pediatr Surg* 9: 307–311.

Lancioni GE, O'Reilly MF, Basili G. (2001). Treating encopresis in people with intellectual disabilities: a literature review. *J Appl Res Int Disabil* 14: 47–63.

Landgraf JM, Abidari J, Cilento BC, Cooper CS, Schulman SL, Ortenberg J. (2004) Coping, commitment, and attitude: quantifying the everyday burden of enuresis on children and their families. *Pediatrics* 113: 334–344.

326

Landman GB, Rappaport L, Fenton T, Levine M. (1986) Locus of control and self-esteem in children with encopresis. *J Dev Behav Pediatr* 7: 111–113.

Langtry HD, McTavish D. (1990) Terodiline. A review of its pharmacological properties, and therapeutic use in the treatment of urinary incontinence. *Drugs* 40: 748–761.

Lantz RJ, Gillespie TA, Rash TJ, Kuo F, Skinner M, Kuan HY, Knadler MP. (2003) Metabolism, excretion, and pharmacokinetics of duloxetine in healthy human subjects. *Drug Metab Dispos* 31: 1142–1150.

Lapides J, Diokno AC, Silber SJ, Lowe BS. (1971) Clean, intermittent self-catheterization in the treatment of urinary tract disease. *Trans Am Assoc Genitourin Surg* 63: 92–96.

Largo RH, Stützle W. (1977) A longitudinal study of bowel and bladder control by day and by night in the first six years of life: the interrelations between bowel and bladder control. *Dev Med Child Neurol* 19: 598–606.

Largo R, Gianciaruso M, Prader A. (1978) Die Entwicklung der Darm- und Blasenkontrolle von der Geburt bis zum 18. Lebensjahr. *Schw med Wschr* 108: 155–160.

Largo RH, Molinari L, von Siebenthal K, Wolfensberger U. (1996) Does a profound change in toilet training affect development of bowel and bladder control? *Dev Med Child Neurol* 38: 1106–1116.

Largo RH, Molinari L, von Siebenthal K, Wolfensberger U. (1999) Development of bladder control: significance of prematurity, perinatal risk factors, psychomotor development and gender. *Eur J Pediatr* 158: 115–122.

Largo RH, Caflisch JA, Hug F, Muggli K, Molnar K, Molinari L, Sheehy A, Gasser T. (2001a) Neuromotor development from 5 to 18 years. Part 1: timed performance. *Dev Med Child Neurol* 42: 436–443.

Largo RH, Caflisch JA, Hug F, Muggli K, Molnar K, Molinari L. (2001b) Neuromotor development from 5 to 18 years. Part 2: associated movements. *Dev Med Child Neurol* 42: 444–453.

Larsson G, Hallen B, Nilvebrant L. (1999) Tolterodine in the treatment of overactive bladder: analysis of the pooled phase II efficacy and safety data. *Urology* 53: 990–998.

Laurenti C, de Dominicis C, dal Forno S, Iori F, Franco G, Bellino M. (1987) Il trattamento medico dell'enuresi essenziale con ossibutinina HCl e imipramina. *Minerva Urol Nefrol* 39: 195–200.

Lawrence D. (2002) Intranasal delivery could be used to administer drugs directly to the brain. *Lancet* 359(931B): 1674.

Lechner SM, Curtis AL, Brons R, Valentino RJ. (1997) Locus coeruleus activation by colon distention: role of corticotropin-releasing factor and excitatory amino acids. *Brain Res* 756: 114–124.

Lee B, Bhuta T, Craig J, Simpson J. (2002) Methenamine hippurate for preventing urinary tract infections. *Cochrane Database Syst Rev* 1: CD003265.

Leebeek-Groenewegen A, Blom J, Sukhai R, van der Heijden B. (2001) Efficacy of desmopressin combined with alarm therapy for monosymptomatic nocturnal enuresis. *J Urol* 166: 2456–2458.

Leech SC, McHugh K, Sullivan PB. (1999) Evaluation of a method of assessing faecal loading on plain abdominal radiographs in children. *Pediatr Radiol* 29: 255–258.

Leippold T, Reitz A, Schurch B. (2003) Botulinum toxin as a new therapy option for voiding disorders: current state of the art. *Eur Urol* 44: 165–174.

Lettgen B, von Gontard A, Olbing H, Heiken-Lowenau C, Gaebel E, Schmitz I. (2002) Urge incontinence and voiding postponement in children: somatic and psychosocial factors. *Acta Paediatr* 91: 978–986.

Levine MD. (1991) Encopresis. In: Levine MD, Carey WB, Crocker AC, editors. *Developmental–Behavioral Pediatrics*, 2nd edition. Philadelphia: Saunders, pp 389–397.

Levitt MA, Patel M, Rodriguez G, Gaylin DS, Pena A. (1997) The tethered spinal cord in patients with anorectal malformations. *J Pediatr Surg* 32: 462–468.

Lie HR, Lagergren J, Rasmussen F, Lagerkvist B, Hagelsteen J, Börjeson MC, Muttilainen M, Taudorf K. (1991) Bowel and bladder control of children with myelomeningocele: a Nordic study. *Dev Med Child Neurol* 33: 1053–1061.

Lightman SL, Todd K, Everitt BJ. (1984) Ascending noradrenergic projections from the brainstem: evidence for a major role in the regulation of blood pressure and vasopressin secretion. *Exp Brain Res* 55: 145–151.

Lindsey I, Jones OM, Smilgin-Humphreys MM, Cunningham C, Mortensen NJ. (2004) Patterns of fecal incontinence after anal surgery. *Dis Colon Rectum* 47: 1643–1649.

Linsenmeyer TA, Harrison B, Oakley A, Kirshblum S, Stock JA, Millis SR. (2004) Evaluation of cranberry supplement for reduction of urinary tract infections in individuals with neurogenic bladders secondary to spinal cord injury. A prospective, double-blind, placebo-controlled, crossover study. *J Spinal Cord Med* 27: 29–34.

Lister-Sharp D, O'Meara S, Bradley M, Sheldon TA. (1997) A systematic review of the effectiveness of interventions for managing childhood nocturnal enuresis. York: NHS Centre for Reviews and Dissemination, University of York.

Littlewood JM. (1992) Cystic fibrosis: gastrointestinal complications. *Br Med Bull* 48: 847–859.

Liu X, Sun Z, Uchiyama M, Li Y, Okawa M. (2000) Attaining nocturnal urinary control, nocturnal enuresis, and behavioral problems in Chinese children aged 6 through 16 years. *J Am Acad Child Adolesc Psychiatry* 39: 1557–1564.

Loening-Baucke V. (1990) Modulation of abnormal defecation dynamics by biofeedback treatment in chronically constipated children with encopresis. *J Pediatr* 116: 214–222.

Loening-Baucke V. (1994) Management of chronic constipation in infants and toddlers. *Am Fam Physician* 49: 397–406.

Loening-Baucke V. (1995) Biofeedback treatment for chronic constipation and encopresis in childhood: long-term outcome. *Pediatrics* 96: 105–110.

Loening-Baucke V. (1996) Biofeedback training in children with functional constipation: a critical review. *Dig Dis Sci* 41: 65–71.

Loening-Baucke V. (1997) Urinary incontinence and urinary tract infection and their resolution with treatment of chronic constipation of childhood. *Pediatrics* 100: 228–232.

Loening-Baucke V. (2000) Clinical approach to fecal soiling in children. *Clin Pediatr* 39: 603–607.

Loening-Baucke V. (2002) Polyethylene glycol without electrolytes for children with constipation and encopresis. *J Pediatr Gastroenterol Nutr* 34: 372–377.

Loening-Baucke V. (2004) Functional fecal retention with encopresis in childhood. *J Pediatr Gastroenterol Nutr* 38: 79–84.

Loening-Baucke VA, Cruikshank BM. (1986) Abnormal defecation dynamics in chronically constipated children with encopresis. *J Pediatr* 108: 562–566.

Loening-Baucke V, Yamada T. (1995) Is the afferent pathway from the rectum impaired in children with chronic constipation and encopresis? *Gastroenterology* 109: 397–403.

Loening-Baucke VA, Cruikshank B, Savage C. (1987) Defecation dynamics and behavior profiles in encopretic children. *Pediatrics* 80: 672–679.

Loening-Baucke VA, Miele E, Staiano A. (2004) Fiber (Glucomannan) is beneficial in the treatment of childhood constipation. *Pediatrics* 113: 259–264.

Loeys B, Hoebeke P, Raes A, Messiaen L, de Pape A, Vande Walle J. (2002) Does monosymptomatic enuresis exist? A molecular genetic exploration of 32 families with enuresis/incontinence. *BJU Int* 90: 76–83.

Longstaffe S, Moffat M, Whalen J. (2000) Behavioral and self-concept changes after six months of enuresis treatment: a randomized, controlled trial. *Pediatrics* 105: 935–940.

Lopez F, Siva R, Pestreich L, Munitz R. (2003) Comparative efficacy of two once daily methylphenidate formulations (Ritalin LA and Concerta) and placebo in children with attention deficit hyperactivity disorder across the school day. *Pediatr Drugs* 5: 545–555.

Lose G, Jorgensen L, Thunedborg P. (1989) Doxepin in the treatment of female detrusor overactivity: a randomised double-blind cross-over study. *J Urol* 142: 1024–1027.

Lovering JS, Tallett SE, McKendry BI. (1988) Oxybutynin efficacy in the treatment of primary enuresis. *Pediatrics* 82: 104–106.

Low JA. (1977) Urethral behavior during the involuntary detrusor contraction. *Am J Obstet Gynecol* 128: 32–42.

Ludman L, Spitz L, Tsuji H, Pierro A. (2002) Hirschsprung's disease: functional and psychological follow up comparing total colonic and rectosigmoid aganglionosis. *Arch Dis Child* 86: 348–351.

McClung HJ, Boyne LH, Linsheid T, Heitlinger LA, Murray RD, Fyda J, Li BU. (1993) Is combination therapy for encopresis nutritionally safe? *Pediatrics* 91(3): 591–594.

McCormack PL, Keating GM. (2004) Duloxetine: in stress urinary incontinence. *Drugs* 64: 2567–2573.

McCormack M, Infante-Rivard C, Schick E. (1992) Agreement between clinical methods of measurement of urinary frequency and functional bladder capacity. *Br J Urol* 69: 17–21.

McGee R, Makinson T, Williams S, Simpson A, Silva PA. (1984) A longitudinal study of enuresis from five to nine years. *Aust Paediatr J* 20: 39–42.

McGrath ML, Mellon MW, Murphy L. (2000) Empirically supported treatments in pediatric psychology: constipation and encopresis. *J Pediatr Psychol* 25: 225–254.

MacKeith RC. (1959) Micturition induced by giggling. Cataplexy. *Arch Dis Child* 34: 358.

MacKinnon AE, Roberts JP, Searles J. (2000) Day-care ultrasound avoids urodynamics. *Eur J Pediatr Surg* 10 Suppl 1: 24–25.

McLennan MT, Melick C, Bent AE. (2001) Urethral instability: clinical and urodynamic characteristics. *Neurourol Urodyn* 20: 653–660.

MacLeod M, Kelly R, Robb SA, Borzyskowski M. (2003) Bladder dysfunction in Duchenne muscular dystrophy. *Arch Dis Child* 88: 347–349.

Madersbacher H, Jilg G. (1991) Control of detrusor hyperreflexia by the intravesical instillation of oxybutynin hydrochloride. *Paraplegia* 29: 84–90.

Madersbacher H, Stohrer M, Richter R, Burgdorfer H, Hachen HJ, Murtz G. (1995) Trospium chloride versus oxybutynin: a randomized, double-blind, multicentre trial in the treatment of detrusor hyper-reflexia. *Br J Urol* 75: 452–456.

Maghnie M, Cosi G, Genovese E, Manca-Bitti ML, Cohen A, Zecca S, Tinelli C, Gallucci M, Bernasconi S, Boscherini B, Severi F, Arico M. (2000) Central diabetes insipidus in children and young adults. *N Engl J Med* 343: 998–1007.

Malinovsky JM, Le Normand L, Lepage JY, et al. (1998) The urodynamic effects of intravenous opioids and ketoprofen in humans. *Anesth Analg* 87: 456–461.

Malone PS, Ransley PG, Kiely EM. (1990) Preliminary report: the antegrade continence enema. *Lancet* 336(8725): 1217–1218.

Malone PS, Wheeler RA, Williams JE. (1994) Continence in patients with spina bifida: long term results. *Arch Dis Child* 70: 107–110.

Malone-Lee J, Lubel D, Szonyi G. (1992) Low dose oxybutynin for the unstable bladder. *BMJ* 304(6833): 1053.

Marinkovic S, Bedlani G. (2001) Voiding and sexual dysfunction after cerebrovascular accidents. *J Urol* 165: 359–370.

Marshall HJ, Beevers DG. (1996) Alpha-adrenoceptor blocking drugs and female urinary incontinence: prevalence and reversibility. *Br J Clin Pharmacol* 42: 507–509.

Martin IG. (1971) Imipramine pamoate in the treatment of childhood enuresis. *Am J Dis Child* 122: 42–47.

Marugan de Miguelsanz JM, Lapena Lopez de Armentia S, Rodriguez Fernandez LM, Palau Benavides MT, Torres Hinojal MC, Menau Martin G, Gutierrez Fernandez M, Alvaro Iglesias E. (1996) Analisis epidemiologico de la secuencia de control vesical y prevalencia de enuresis nocturna en ninos de la provincia de Leon. *An Esp Pediatr* 44: 561–567.

Massey JA, Abrams P. (1986) Dose titration in clinical trials: an example using emepronium carrageenate in detrusor instability. *Br J Urol* 58: 125–128.

Mathias JR, Clench MH. (1995) Neuromuscular diseases of the gastrointestinal tract. Specific disorders that often get a nonspecific diagnosis. *Postgrad Med J* 97: 101–102, 105–108.

Matthiesen TB, Rittig S, Djurhuus JC, Nørgaard JP. (1994) A dose titration, and an open 6-week efficacy and safety study of desmopressin tablets in the management of nocturnal enuresis. *J Urol* 151: 460–463.

Mattsson S. (1994a) Urinary incontinence and nocturia in healthy schoolchildren. *Acta Paediatr* 83: 950–954.

Mattsson S. (1994b) Voiding frequency, volumes and intervals in healthy schoolchildren. *Scand J Urol Nephrol* 28: 1–11.

Mattsson S, Gladh G. (2003) Urethrovaginal reflux – a common cause of daytime incontinence in girls. *Pediatrics* 111: 136–139.

Mattsson S, Lindström S. (1994) Diuresis and voiding pattern in healthy schoolchildren. *Br J Urol* 76: 783–789.

Mattsson S, Gladh G, Lindström S. (2003) Relative filling of the bladder at daytime voids in healthy school children. *J Urol* 170: 1343–1346.

Matza LS, Swensen AR, Flood EM, Secnik K, Leidy NK. (2004) Assessment of health-related quality of life in children: a review of conceptual, methodological, and regulatory issues. *Value in Health* 7: 79–92.

Mayo ME. (1992) Lower urinary tract dysfunction in cerebral palsy. *J Urol* 147: 419–420.

Mayo ME, Burns MW. (1990) Urodynamic studies in children who wet. *Br J Urol* 65: 641–645.

Mazur D, Wehnert J, Dorschner W, et al. (1995) Clinical and urodynamic effects of propiverine in patients suffering from urgency and urge incontinence. *Scand J Urol Nephrol* 29: 289–294.

Mazzola BL, von Vigier RO, Marchand S, Tonz M, Bianchetti MG. (2003) Behavioral and functional abnormalities linked with recurrent urinary tract infections in girls. *J Nephrol* 16: 133–138.

Meadow SR. (1990) Day wetting. *Pediatr Nephrol* 4: 178–184.

Mehler-Wex C, Scheuerpflug P, Peschke N, Roth M, Reitzle K, Warnke A. (2005) Enkopresis: Prognosefaktoren und Langzeitverlauf. *Z Kinder-Jugendpsychiatr* 33: 285–293.

Meierkord H, Will B, Fish D, Shorvon S. (1991) The clinical features and prognosis of pseudoseizures diagnosed using video-EEG telemetry. *Neurology* 41: 1643–1646.

Mellon MW, McGrath ML. (2000) Empirically supported treatments in pediatric psychology: nocturnal enuresis. *J Pediatr Psychol* 25: 193–214.

329

Mevorach RA, Kogan BA. (1995) Fetal lower urinary tract physiology: in vivo studies. *Adv Exp Med Biol* 385: 385–391.

Michelson D, Faries D, Wernicke J, Kelsey D, Kendrick K, Sallee FR, Spencer T, and the Atomoxetine Study Group. (2001) *Pediatrics* 108: e83.

Miller P, Champelli J, Dinello F. (1968) Imipramine in the treatment of enuretic school children. A double-blind study. *Am J Dis Child* 115: 17–20.

Miller M, Dalakos T, Moses AM, Fellerman H, Streeten DHP. (1970) Recognition of partial defects in antidiuretic hormone secretion. *Ann Intern Med* 73: 721–729.

Miller K, Goldberg S, Atkin B. (1989) Nocturnal enuresis: experience with long-term use of intranasally administered desmopressin. *J Pediatr* 114: 723.

Moffat MEK. (1997) Nocturnal enuresis: a review of the efficacy of treatments and practical advice for clinicians. *J Dev Behav Pediatr* 18: 49–56.

Moffat MEK, Kato C, Pless IB. (1987) Improvements in self-concept after treatment of nocturnal enuresis: randomized controlled trial. *J Pediatr* 110: 647–652.

Moffatt ME, Harlos S, Kirshen AJ, Burd L. (1993) Desmopressin acetate and nocturnal enuresis: how much do we know? *Pediatrics* 92: 420–425.

Moilanen I, Järvelin M, Vikeväinen-Torvonen L, Huttunen N-P. (1987) Personality and family characteristics of enuretic children. *Psychiatr Fenn* 18: 53–61.

Moltke H, Verder H. (1979) Enuresis nocturna. A double-blind study with furosemide, imipramine and placebo (Danish). *Ugeskr Laeger* 141: 1399–1401.

Monda JM, Husmann DA. (1995) Primary nocturnal enuresis: a comparison among observation, imipramine, desmopressin acetate and bed-wetting alarm systems. *J Urol* 154: 745–758.

Moneret-Vautrin DA. (1999) Cow's milk allergy. *Allerg Immunol* 31: 201–210.

Montague DK, Jones LR. (1979) Psychogenic urinary retention. *Urology* 13: 30–35.

Montedonico S, Acevedo S, Fadda B. (2002) Clinical aspects of intestinal neuronal dysplasia. *J Pediatr Surg* 37: 1772–1774.

Moore KL. (1980) *Embryologie – Lehrbuch der Entwicklungsgeschichte des Menschen.* Stuttgart, New York: Schattauer Verlag.

Moore KH. (2000) Conservative management for urinary incontinence. *Baillieres Best Pract Res Clin Obstet Gynaecol* 14: 251–289.

Moore KH, Gilpin SA, Dixon JS, Richmond DH, Sutherst JR. (1992a) Increase in presumptive sensory nerves of the urinary bladder in idiopathic detrusor instability. *Br J Urol* 70: 370–372.

Moore KH, Nickson P, Richmond DH, Sutherst JR, Manasse PR, Helliwell TR. (1992b) Detrusor mast cells in refractory idiopathic instability. *Br J Urol* 70: 17–21.

Moore KH, Simons A, Mukerjee C, Lynch W. (2000) The relative incidence of detrusor instability and bacterial cystitis detected on the urodynamic-test day. *BJU Int* 85: 786–792.

Moore KH, Ray FR, Barden JA. (2001) Loss of purinergic P2X$_3$ and P2X$_5$ receptor innervation in human detrusor from adults with urge incontinence. *J Neurosci* 21: 1–6.

Morgan RTT. (1978) Relapse and therapeutic response in the conditioning treatment of enuresis: a review of recent findings on intermittent reinforcement, overlearning and stimulus intensity. *Behav Res Ther* 16: 273–279.

Morison MJ, Tappin D, Staines H. (2000) 'You feel helpless, that's exactly it': parents' and young people's beliefs about bed-wetting and the implications for practice. *J Adv Nurs* 31: 1216–1227.

Morrow J, Yeager CA, Lewis DO. (1996) Encopresis and sexual abuse in a sample of boys in residential treatment. *Child Abuse Negl* 21: 11–18.

Moruzzi G, Magoun HW. (1949) Brain stem reticular formation and activation of the EEG. *Electroenceph Clin Neurophysiol* 1: 455–473.

Mowrer OH. (1980) Enuresis: the beginning work – what really happened. *J Hist Behav Sci* 16: 25–30.

Mowrer OH, Mowrer WM. (1938) Enuresis: a method for its study and treatment. *Am J Orthopsychiatry* 8: 436–459.

MTA Cooperative Group. (1999) A 14-month randomized clinical trial of treatement strategies for attention-deficit/hyperactivity disorder. *Arch Gen Psychiatry* 56: 1073–1086.

MTA Cooperative Group. (2004) National Institute of Mental Health multimodal treatment study of ADHD follow-up: changes in effectiveness and growth after the end of treatment. *Pediatrics* 113: 762–769.

Muller D, Marr N, Ankermann T, Eggert P, Deen PM. (2002) Desmopressin for nocturnal enuresis in nephrogenic diabetes insipidus. *Lancet* 359(9305): 495–497.

Mundy L, Merlin TL, Maddern GJ, Hiller JE. (2004) Systematic review of safety and effectiveness of an artificial bowel sphincter for faecal incontinence. *Br J Surg* 91: 665–672.

Murray KH, Feneley RC. (1982) Endorphins: a role in lower urinary tract function? The effect of opioid blockade on the detrusor and urethral sphincter mechanisms. *Br J Urol* 54: 638–640.

Murray K, Nurse D, Borzyskowski M, Mundy AR. (1987) The 'congenital' wide bladder neck anomaly: a common cause of incontinence in children. *Br J Urol* 59: 533–535.

Nagy F, Hamvas A, Frang D. (1990) Idiopathic bladder hyperactivity treated with Ditropan (oxybutynin chloride). *Int Urol Nephrol* 22: 519–524.

Natochin YV, Kuznetsova AA. (2000) Nocturnal enuresis: correction of renal function by desmopressin and diclofenac. *Pediatr Nephrol* 14: 42–47.

Nergårdh A, Boréus LO. (1972) Autonomic receptor function in the lower urinary tract of man and cat. *Scand J Urol Nephrol* 6: 32–36.

Nevéus T. (1999) The bladder and the brain. Studies on the pathogenesis and treatment of nocturnal enuresis. Dept of Women's and Children's Health, Uppsala University, Uppsala: 59.

Nevéus T. (2001) Oxybutynin, desmopressin and enuresis. *J Urol* 166: 2459–2462.

Nevéus T. (2006) Reboxetine in therapy-resistant enuresis – results and pathogenetic implications. *Scand J Urol Nephrol* 40: 31–34.

Nevéus T, Hetta J, Cnattingius S, Tuvemo T, Läckgren G, Olsson U, Stenberg A. (1999a) Depth of sleep and sleep habits among enuretic and incontinent children. *Acta Paediatr* 88: 748–752.

Nevéus T, Läckgren G, Tuvemo T, Stenberg A. (1999b) Osmoregulation and desmopressin pharmacokinetics in enuretic children. *Pediatrics* 103: 65–70.

Nevéus T, Läckgren G, Tuvemo T, Olsson U, Stenberg A. (1999c) Desmopressin-resistant enuresis: pathogenetic and therapeutic considerations. *J Urol* 162: 2136–2140.

Nevéus T, Läckgren G, Tuvemo T, Hetta J, Hjälmås K, Stenberg A. (2000) Enuresis – background and treatment. *Scand J Urol Nephrol* 202 Suppl 206: 1–44.

Nevéus T, Cnattingius S, Olsson U, Hetta J. (2001a) Sleep habits and sleep problems among a community sample of school children. *Acta Paediatr* 90: 1450–1455.

Nevéus T, Tuvemo T, Läckgren G, Stenberg A. (2001b) Bladder capacity and renal concentrating ability in enuresis – pathogenic implications. *J Urol* 165: 2022–2025.

Nevéus T, Hansell P, Stenberg A. (2002) Vasopressin and hypercalciuria in enuresis: a reappraisal. *BJU Int* 90: 725–729.

Nevéus T, Johansson E, Hansson S. (2004) Diuretic treatment of nocturnal enuresis: preliminary results of an open pilot study. *J Urol* 171: 2584–2585.

Nevéus T, von Gontard A, Hoebeke P, Hjälmås K, Bauer S, Bower W, Jørgensen TM, Rittig S, Vande Walle J, Yeung CK, Djurhuus JC. (2006) The standardisation of terminology of lower urinary tract function in children and adolescents: report from the standardisation committee of the International Children's Continence Society (ICCS). *J Urol* 176: 314–324.

Ng CF, Wong S, Hong Kong Childhood Enuresis Study Group. (2005) Comparing alarms, desmopressin, and combined treatment in Chinese enuretic children. *Pediatr Nephrol* 20: 163–169.

Nilsson CG, Lukkari E, Haarala M, et al. (1997) Comparison of a 10 mg controlled release oxybutynin tablet with a 5 mg oxybutynin tablet in urge incontinent patients. *Neurourol Urodyn* 16: 533–542.

Nixon GM, Glazner JA, Martin JM, Sawyer SM. (2002) Urinary incontinence in female adolescents with cystic fibrosis. *Pediatrics* 110: e22.

Nolan T, Debelle G, Oberklaid F, Coffey C. (1991) Randomised trial of laxatives in treatment of childhood encopresis. *Lancet* 338: 523–527.

Nolan T, Catto-Smith T, Coffey C, Wells J. (1998) Randomised controlled trial of biofeedback training in persistent encopresis with anismus. *Arch Dis Child* 79: 131–135.

Nørgaard JP, Pedersen EB, Djurhuus JC. (1985) Diurnal anti-diuretic hormone levels in enuretics. *J Urol* 134: 1029–1031.

Nørgaard JP, Jonler M, Rittig S, Djurhuus JC. (1995) A pharmacodynamic study of desmopressin in patients with nocturnal enuresis. *J Urol* 153: 1984–1986.

Nørgaard JP, van Gool JD, Hjälmås K, Djurhuus JC, Hellström A-L. (1998) Standardization and definitions in lower urinary tract dysfunction in children. *Br J Urol* 81 Suppl 3: 1–16.

Norton PA, Zinner NR, Yalcin I, et al. (2002) Duloxetine versus placebo in the treatment of stress urinary incontinence. *Am J Obstet Gynecol* 187: 40–48.

331

Noto H, Roppolo JR, Steers WD, de Groat WC. (1989) Excitatory and inhibitory influences on bladder activity elicited by electrical stimulation in the pontine micturition center in the rat. *Brain Res* 17: 99–115.

Nuutinen M, Uhari M. (2001) Recurrence and follow-up after urinary tract infection under the age of one year. *Pediatr Nephrol* 16: 69–72.

Ochoa B. (2004) Can a congenital dysfunctional bladder be diagnosed from a smile? The Ochoa syndrome updated. *Pediatr Nephrol* 19: 6–12.

Ochoa B, Gorlin RJ. (1987) Urofacial (Ochoa) syndrome. *Am J Med Genet* 27: 661–667.

Oei HD, Pelikan-Filipek M, Pelikan Z, van Vliet AC. (1989) Enuresis and encopresis as a reaction to food (Dutch). *Ned Tijdschr Geneeskd* 133: 1555–1557.

Ohel G, Haddad S, Samueloff A. (1995) Fetal urine production and micturition and fetal behavioral state. *Am J Perinatol* 12: 91–92.

Olbing H, editor. (1993) *Enuresis und Harninkontinenz bei Kindern.* München: Hans Marseille Verlag.

Oldani A, Zucconi M, Asselta R, Modugno M, Bonati MT, Dalpra L, Malcovati M, Tenchini ML, Smirne S, Ferini-Strambi L. (1998) Autosomal dominant nocturnal frontal lobe epilepsy. A video-polysomnographic and genetic appraisal of 40 patients and delineation of the epileptic syndrome. *Brain* 121: 205–223.

Olfson M, Gameroff MJ, Marcus SC, Jensen PS. (2003) National trends in the treatment of attention deficit hyperactivity disorder. *Am J Psychiatry* 160: 1071–1077.

Olson DH, Portner J, Lavee Y. (1985) *Faces-III.* University of Minnesota: Family Social Science.

Oredson AF, Jorgensen TM. (1998) Changes in nocturnal bladder capacity during treatment with the bell and pad for monosymptomatic nocturnal enuresis. *J Urol* 160: 166–169.

O'Regan S, Yazbeck S. (1985) Constipation: a cause of enuresis, urinary tract infection and vesicoureteral reflux in children. *Mel Hypotheses* 17: 409–413.

O'Regan S, Yazbeck S, Hamberger B, Schick E. (1986) Constipation – a commonly unrecognized cause of enuresis. *Am J Dis Child* 140: 260–261.

O'Reilly BA, Kosaka AH, Knight GF, Chang TK, Ford AP, Rymer JM, Popert R, Burnstock G, McMahon SB. (2002) P2X receptors and their role in female idiopathic detrusor instability. *J Urol* 167: 157–164.

Ornitz EM, Russell AT, Hanna G, Gabikian P, Gehricke J-G, Song D, Guthrie D. (1999) Prepulse inhibition of startle and the neurobiology of primary nocturnal enuresis. *Biol Psychiatry* 45: 1455–1466.

Osungbade KO, Oshiname FO. (2003) Prevalence and perception of nocturnal enuresis in children of a rural community in southwestern Nigeria. *Trop Doct* 33: 234–236.

Ottolenghi A, Sulpasso M, Bianchi S, Bettili G, Salloum A, Liber H. (1994) Ectopic anus in childhood. *Eur J Pediatr Surg* 4: 145–150.

Ottolini MC, Shaer CM, Rushton HG, Majd M, Gonzales EC, Patel KM. (1995) Relationship of asymptomatic bacteriuria and renal scarring in children with neuropathic bladders who are practicing clean intermittent catheterization. *J Pediatr* 127: 368–372.

Ouedraogo A, Kere M, Ouedraogo TL, Jesu F. (1997) Epidemiology of enuresis in children and adolescents aged 5–16 years in Ouagadougou (Burkina Faso) (French). *Archives de Pediatrie* 4: 947–951.

Overdeem S, Taal W, Gezici EÖ, Lammers GJ, van Dijk JG. (2004) Is motor inhibition during laughter due to emotional or respiratory influences? *Psychophysiology* 41: 254–258.

Owen GO, Canter RJ, Robinson A. (1996) Snoring, apnoea and ENT symptoms in the paediatric community. *Clin Otolaryngol* 21: 130–134.

PACCT Group. (2005) The Paris consensus on childhood constipation terminology (PACCT) group. *J Pediatr Gastroenterol Nutr* 40: 273–275.

Page ME, Akaoka H, Aston-Jones G, Valentino RJ. (1992) Bladder distension activates noradrenergic locus coeruleus neurons by an excitatory amino acid mechanism. *Neuroscience* 51: 555–563.

Palm L, Nielsen OH. (1967) Evaluation of bladder function in children. *J Pediatr Surg* 2: 529–531.

Palnaes Hansen C, Klarskov P. (1998) The accuracy of the frequency-volume chart: comparison of self-reported and measured volumes. *Br J Urol* 81: 709–711.

Papadopoulou A, Clayden GS, Booth IW. (1994) The clinical value of solid marker transit studies in childhood constipation and soiling. *Eur J Pediatr* 153: 560–564.

Partin JC, Hamill SK, Fischel JE, Partin JS. (1992) Painful defecation and fecal soiling in children. *Pediatrics* 89: 1007–1009.

Pashankar DS, Bishop WP. (2001) Efficacy and optimal dose of daily polyethylene glycol 3350 for treatment of constipation and encopresis in children. *J Pediatr* 139: 428–432.

Pashankar DS, Bishop WP, Loening-Baucke V. (2003a) Long-term efficacy of polyethylene glycol 3350 for the treatment of chronic constipation in children with and without encopresis. *Clin Pediatr (Phil)* 42: 815–819.

Pashankar DS, Loening-Baucke V, Bishop WP. (2003b) Safety of polyethylene glycol 3350 for the treatment of chronic constipation in children. *Arch Pediatr Adolesc Med* 157: 661–664.

Pavcovich LA, Yang M, Miselis RR, Valentino RJ. (1998) Novel role for the pontine micturition center, Barrington's nucleus: evidence for coordinaion of colonic and forebrain activity. *Brain Res* 784: 355–361.

Pedersen E. (1977) Studies on the effect and mode of action of flavoxate in human urinary bladder and sphincter. *Urol Int* 32: 202–208.

Pehrson R, Andersson KE. (2003) Tramadol inhibits detrusor overactivity due to dopamine receptor stimulation. *J Urol* 170: 272–275.

Pena A, Hong A. (2000) Advances in the management of anorectal malformations. *Am J Surg* 180: 370–376.

Pena A, Guardino K, Tovilla JM, Levitt MA, Rodriguez GRT. (1998) Bowel management for fecal incontinence in patients with anorectal malformations. *J Pediatr Surg* 33: 133–137.

Penders L, de Leval J, Petit R. (1984) Enuresis and urethral instability. *Eur Urol* 10: 317–322.

Persson J, Wolner-Hanssen P, Rydhstroem H. (2000) Obstetric risk factors for stress urinary incontinence: a population-based study. *Obstet Gynecol* 96: 440–445.

Persson-Jünemann CH, Seemann O, Kohrmann KU, Junemann KP, Alken P. (1993) Comparison of urodynamic findings and response to oxybutynin in nocturnal enuresis. *Eur Urol* 24: 92–96.

Petersen S. (1978) Long-term prophylaxis with methenamine hippurate in girls with recurrent urinary tract infections. *Acta Paediatr Scand* 67: 597–599.

Petersen T, Chandiramani V, Fowler CJ. (1997) The ice-water test in detrusor hyper-reflexia and bladder instability. *Br J Urol* 79: 163–167.

Philip T, Shah PJR, Worth PHL. (1988) Acupuncture in the treatment of bladder instability. *Br J Urol* 61: 490–496.

Piaget J. (1975) *Gesammelte Werke (Studienausgabe)*. Stuttgart: Ernst Klett Verlag.

Piers EV. (1984) *Piers–Harris Children's Self-concept Scale – Revised manual 1984*. Los Angeles: Western Psychological Services.

Pippi Salle JL, Capolicchio G, Houle AM, Vernet O, Jednak R, O'Gorman AM, Montes JL, Farmer JP. (1998) Magnetic resonance imaging in children with voiding dysfunction: is it indicated? *J Urol* 160: 1080–1083.

Porena M, Constantini E, Rociola W, Mearini E. (2000) Biofeedback successfully cures detrusor-sphincter dyssynergia in pediatric patients. *J Urol* 163: 1927–1931.

Potter WZ, Calil HM, Sutfin TA, Zavadil AP, Jusko WJ, Rapoport J, Goodwin FK. (1982) Active metabolites of imipramine and desipramine in man. *Clin Pharmacol Ther* 31: 393–401.

Poussaint FA, Ditman SK. (1965) A controlled study of imipramine (Tofranil) in the treatment of childhood enuresis. *J Pediatr* 67: 283–290.

Powell PH, Shepherd AM, Lewis P, Fenely RCL. (1980) The accuracy of clinical diagnosis assessed urodynamically. First joint meeting ICS and UDS, Los Angeles.

Power C, Manor O. (1995) Asthma, enuresis, and chronic illness: long term impact on height. *Arch Dis Child* 73: 298–304.

Preskorn SH, Bupp SJ, Weller EB, Weller RA. (1989) Plasma levels of imipramine and metabolites in sixty-eight hospitalized children. *J Am Acad Child Adolesc Psychiatry* 28: 373–375.

Pretlow RA. (1999) Treatment of nocturnal enuresis with an ultrasound bladder volume controlled alarm device. *J Urol* 162: 1224–1228.

Price KJ, Elliott TM. (2002) Stimulant laxatives and soiling in children (Cochrane Review). In: The Cochrane Library, Issue 2. Oxford: Update Software.

Primus G, Pummer K. (1990) Oxybutynin hydrochloride in the management of detrusor instability. *Int Urol Nephrol* 22: 243–248.

Puri VN. (1980) Urinary levels of antidiuretic hormone in nocturnal enuresis. *Ind Pediatr J Ind Acad Pediatr* 17: 675–676.

Puri P. (2003) Intestinal neuronal dysplasia. *Semin Pediatr Surg* 12: 259–264.

Rabey JM, Moriel EZ, Farkas A, Firstater M, Vardi I, Streifler M. (1979) Detrusor hyperreflexia in multiple sclerosis. Alleviation by a combination of imipramine and propantheline, a clinico-laboratory study. *Eur Neurol* 18: 33–37.

Raes A, Hoebeke P, Segaert I, Van Laecke E, Dehoorne J, Vande Walle J. (2004) Retrospective analysis of efficacy and tolerability of tolterodine in children with overactive bladder. *Eur Urol* 45: 240–244.

Rapoport JL, Mikkelsen EJ, Zavaldil A, Nee L, Gruenau C, Mendelson W, Gillin JC. (1980) Childhood enuresis II. Psychopathology, tricyclic concentration in plasma, and antienuretic effect. *Arch Gen Psychiatry* 37: 1146–1152.

333

Rasmussen PV, Kirk J, Borup K, Nørgaard JP, Djurhuus JC. (1996) Enuresis nocturna can be provoked in normal healthy children by increasing the nocturnal urine output. *Scand J Urol Nephrol* 30: 57–61.

Rasquin-Weber A, Hyman PE, Cucciara S, Fleisher DR, Hyams JS, Milla PJ, Staiano A. (1999) Childhood functional gastroinstestinal disorders. *Gut* 45 Suppl II: II60–II68.

Ravens-Sieberer U, Bullinger M. (2000) KINDLR – Fragebogen zur Erfassung der gesundheitsbezogenen Lebensqualität bei Kindern und Jugendlichen. Unpublished manual.

Raz S, Zeigler M, Caine M. (1972) Isometric studies on canine urethral musculature. *Invest Urol* 9: 443–446.

Rechtschaffen A, Hauri P, Zeitlin M. (1966) Auditory awakening thresholds in REM and NREM sleep stages. *Percept Mot Skills* 22: 927.

Redsell SA, Collier J. (2000) Bedwetting, behaviour and self-esteem: a review of the literature. *Child Care Health Dev* 27: 149–162.

Rees DL, Ransley PG. (1980) Eskornade in the treatment of diurnal incontinence in children. *Br J Urol* 52: 476–479.

Reid CJ, Borzyskowski M. (1993) Lower urinary tract dysfunction in cerebral palsy. *Arch Dis Child* 68: 739–742.

Reid G, Hsiehl J, Potter P, Mighton J, Lam D, Warren D, Stephenson J. (2001) Cranberry juice consumption may reduce biofilms on uroepithelial cells: pilot study in spinal cord injured patients. *Spinal Cord* 39: 26–30.

Reinberg Y, Crocker J, Wolpert J, Vandersteen D. (2003) Therapeutic efficacy of extended release oxybutinin chloride, and immediate release and long acting release tolterodine tartrate in children with diurnal urinary incontinence. *J Urol* 69: 317–319.

Remschmidt H, Schmidt MH, Poustka F, editors. (2001) *Multiaxiales Klassifikationsschema für psychische Störungen des Kindes- und Jugendalters nach ICD-10 der WHO (4. Auflage).* Bern: Verlag Hans H uber.

Rentzhog L, Stanton SL, Cardozo L, Nelson E, Fall M, Abrams P. (1998) Efficacy and safety of tolterodine in patients with detrusor instability: a dose-ranging study. *Br J Urol* 81(1): 42–48.

Repaske DR, Phillips JAI, Kirby LT, et al. (1990) Molecular analysis of autosomal dominant neurohypophyseal diabetes insipidus. *J Clin Endocrinol Metab* 70: 752–757.

Rew DA, Rundle JSH. (1989) Assessment of the safety of regular DDAVP therapy in primary nocturnal enuresis. *Br J Urol* 63: 352–353.

Rex DK, Fitzgerald JF, Goulet RJ. (1992) Chronic constipation with encopresis persisting beyond 15 years of age. *Dis Colon Rectum* 35: 242–244.

Riccabona M, Koen M, Schindler M, Goedele B, Pycha A, Lusuardi L, Bauer SB. (2004) Botulinum-A toxin injection into the detrusor: a safe alternative in the treatment of children with myelomeningocele with detrusor hyperreflexia. *J Urol* 171: 845–848.

Riddle MA, Nelson JC, Kleinman CS, et al. (1991) Sudden death in children receiving Norpramin®: a review of three reported cases and a commentary. *J Am Acad Child Adolesc Psychiatry* 30: 104–108.

Riddle M, Geller B, Ryan N. (1993) Another sudden death in a child treated with desipramine. *J Am Acad Child Adolesc Psychiatry* 32: 792–797.

Rintala RJ, Lindahl HG, Rasanen M. (1997) Do children with repaired low anorectal malformations have normal bowel function? *J Pediatr Surg* 32: 823–826.

Rittig S, Knudsen UB, Nørgaard JP, Pedersen EB, Djurhuus JC. (1989) Abnormal diurnal rhythm of plasma vasopressin and urinary output in patients with enuresis. *Am J Physiol* 256: F664–F671.

Rittig S, Schaumburg H, Schmidt F, Hunsballe JM, Hansen AF, Kirk J, Rasmussen PV, Djurhuus JC. (1997) Long-term home studies of water balance in patients with nocturnal enuresis. *Scand J Urol Nephrol* 31 Suppl 183: 25–27.

Rittig S, Jensen AR, Jensen KT, Pedersen EB. (1998) Effect of food intake on the pharmacokinetics and antidiuretic activity of oral desmopressin (DDAVP) in hydrated normal subjects. *Clin Endocrinol* 48: 235–241.

Roberts RO, Jacobsen SJ, Reilly WT, Pemberton JH, Talley NJ. (1999) Prevalence of combined fecal and urinary incontinence: a community-based study. *J Am Geriatr Soc* 47: 837–841.

Robertson GL. (1995) Diabetes insipidus. *Endocrinol Metab Clin North Am* 24: 549–572.

Robinson AG. (1976) DDAVP in the treatment of central diabetes insipidus. *N Engl J Med* 294: 507–511.

Robinson AG, Verbalis JG. (1985) Treatment of central diabetes insipidus. *Front Horm Res* 13: 292–303.

Robinson D, Khullar V, Cardozo L. (2001) Pharmacological management of detrusor instability. *Int Urogynecol J Pelvic Floor Dysfunct* 12: 271–278.

Robson HL, Leung AK. (1994) Side effects and complications of treatment with desmopressin for enuresis. *J Natl Med Assoc* 86: 775–778.

Robson WL, Nørgaard JP, Leung AK. (1996a) Hyponatremia in patients with nocturnal enuresis treated with DDAVP. *Eur J Pediatr* 155: 959–962.

Robson WL, Leung AKC, Bloom DA. (1996b) Daytime wetting in childhood. *Clin Pediatr* February, 91–98.

Robson WL, Jackson HP, Blackhurst D, Leung AK. (1997) Enuresis in children with attention-deficit hyperactivity disorder. *South Med J* 90: 503–505.

Robson WL, Leung AKC, Van Howe R. (2005) Primary and secondary nocturnal enuresis: similarities in presentation. *Pediatrics* 115: 956–959.

Rockney RM, McQuade WH, Days AL, Linn HE, Alario AJ. (1996) Encopresis treatment outcome: long-term follow-up of 45 cases. *J Dev Behav Pediatr* 17: 380–385.

Rodgers B. (1990) Behavior and personality in childhood as predictors of adult psychiatric disorder. *J Child Psychol Psychiatry* 31: 393–414.

Roijen LE, Postema K, Limbeek VJ, Kuppevelt VH. (2001) Development of bladder control in children and adolescents with cerebral palsy. *Dev Med Child Neurol* 43: 103–107.

Rosario DJ, Leaker BR, Smith DJ, Chapple CR. (1995) A pilot study of the effects of multiple doses of the M3 muscarinic receptor antagonist darifenacin on ambulatory parameters of detrusor activity in patients with detrusor instability. *Neurourol Urodyn* 14: 464–465.

Ruffmann R. (1988) A review of flavoxate hydrochloride in the treatment of urge incontinence. *J Int Med Res* 16: 317–330.

Ruscin JM, Morgenstern NE. (1999) Tolterodine use for symptoms of overactive bladder. *Ann Pharmacother* 33: 1073–1082.

Rushton HG, Belman AB, Zaontz MR, Skoog SJ, Sihelnik S. (1996) The influence of small functional bladder capacity and other predictors on the response to desmopressin in the management of monosymptomatic nocturnal enuresis. *J Urol* 156: 651–655.

Rutter M, Yule W, Graham P. (1973) Enuresis and behavioral deviance: some epidemiological considerations. In: Kolvin I, MacKeith RC, Meadow SR, editors. *Bladder Control and Enuresis*. London: William Heinemann Medical Books, pp 137–147.

St Laurent J, Batini C, Broughton R, Gastaut H. (1963) A polygraphic study of nocturnal enuresis in the epileptic child. *Electroenceph Clin Neurophysiol* 15: 904.

Saito M, Tahara A, Sugimoto T. (1997) 1-desamino-8-D-arginine vasopressin (DDAVP) as an agonist on V1b vasopressin receptor. *Biochem Pharmacol* 53: 1711–1717.

Sakakibara R, Hattori T, Yasuda K, et al. (1996) Micturitional disturbance after acute hemispheric stroke: analysis of the lesion site by CT and MRI. *J Neurol Sci* 137(1): 47–56.

Samuel M, Boddy SA. (2004) Is spina bifida occulta associated with lower urinary tract dysfunction in children? *J Urol* 171: 2664–2666.

Saum WR, de Groat WC. (1972) Parasympathetic ganglia: activation of an adrenergic inhibitory mechanism by cholinomimetic agents. *Science* 175: 659–661.

Sawchenko PE, Swanson LW. (1982) The organization of noradrenergic pathways from the brainstem to the paraventricular and supraoptic nuclei of the rat. *Brain Res Rev* 4: 275–325.

Scherbaum WA, Czernichow P, Bottazzo GF, Doniach D. (1985) Diabetes insipidus in children. IV. A possible autoimmune type with vasopressin cell antibodies. *J Pediatr* 107: 922–925.

Schladitz-Keil G, Spahn H, Mutschler E. (1986) Determination of bioavailability of the quaternary ammonium compound trospium chloride in man from urinary excretion data. *Arz Forsch/Drug Res* 36: 984–987.

Schmidt M, Poustka F, editors. (2003) *Leitlinien zur Diagnostik und Therapie von psychischen Störungen im Säuglings-, Kindes- und Jugendalter*, 2nd edition. Köln: Deutsche Ärzteverlag.

Scholtmeijer RJ, Nijman RJ. (1994) Reflux and videourodynamic studies: results of a prospective study after three years of follow-up. *Urology* 43: 714–718.

Schönau E, Naumann EG, Längler A, Beuth J. (2005) *Pädiatrie integrativ – konventionelle und komplementäre Therapie*. München: Urban und Fischer.

Schulman SL, Colish Y, von Zuben FC, Kodman-Jones C. (2000) Effectiveness of treatments for nocturnal enuresis in a heterogeneous population. *Clin Pediatr* 39: 359–364.

Schulte-Baukloh H, Michael T, Sturzebecher B, Knispel HH. (2003) Botulinum-a toxin detrusor injection as a novel approach in the treatment of bladder spasticity in children with neurogenic bladder. *Eur Urol* 44: 139–143.

335

Schuster T, Kellnar S. (1997) Zum aktuellen Stand der Funktionsdiagnostik des Dickdarms und Anorektums in der Kinderchirurgie. *Zentralbl Kinderchir* 2.

Schwab M, Wenzel D, Ruder H. (1996) Hyponatremia and cerebral convulsion due to short term DDAVP therapy for control of enuresis nocturna. *Eur J Pediatr* 155: 46–48.

Schwartz RD, Stephens FD, Cussen LJ. (1981) The pathogenesis of renal dysplasia. II. The significance of lateral and medial ectopy of the ureteric orifice. *Invest Urol* 19: 97–100.

Scott RJ, McIlhaney JS. (1959) The voiding rates in normal male children. *J Urol* 82: 224–230.

Scott R, Morrison LM. (1980) Diuretic treatment of enuresis. *J R Coll Surg Edinb* 25: 470–472.

Sener F, Hasanoglu E, Soylemezoglu O. (1998) Desmopressin versus indomethacin treatment in primary nocturnal enuresis and the role of prostaglandins. *Urology* 52: 878–881.

Sentovich SM, Kaufman SS, Cali RL, Falk PM, Blatchford GJ, Antonson DL, Thorson AG, Christensen MA. (1998) Pudendal nerve function in normal and encopretic children. *J Pediatr Gastroenterol Nutr* 1998: 70–72.

Serel TA, Perk H, Koyuncuoglu HR, Kosar A, Celik K, Deniz N. (2001) Acupuncture therapy in the management of persistent primary nocturnal enuresis – preliminary results. *Scand J Urol Nephrol* 35: 40–43.

Serels S, Stein M. (1998) Prospective study comparing hyoscyamine, doxazosin, and combination therapy for the treatment of urgency and frequency in women. *Neurourol Urodyn* 17: 31–36.

Shaul DB, Harrison EA. (1997) Classification of anorectal malformations – initial approach, diagnostic tests, and colostomy. *Semin Pediatr Surg* 6: 187–195.

Shelov SP, Gundy I, Weiss JC, McIntire MS, Olness K, Staub HP, Jones DJ, Haque M, Ellerstein NS, Heagarty MC, Starfield B. (1981) Enuresis: a contrast of attitudes of parents and physicians. *Pediatrics* 67: 707–710.

Shepherd AM, Tribe E, Bainton D. (1984) Maximum perineal stimulation; a controlled study. *Br J Urol* 56: 644–646.

Sher PK, Reinberg Y. (1996). Successful treatment of giggle incontinence with methylphenidate. *J Urol* 156: 656–658.

Shimura N. (1993) Urinary arginine vasopressin (AVP) measurement in children: water deprivation test incorporating urinary AVP. *Acta Paediatr Jpn* 35: 320–324.

Shin YM, Southwell BR, Stanton MP, Hutson JM. (2002) Signs and symptoms of slow-transit constipation versus functional retention. *J Pediatr Surg* 37: 1762–1765.

Shu SG, Lii YP, Chi CS. (1993) The efficacy of intranasal DDAVP therapy in children with nocturnal enuresis. *Chung Hua I Hsueh Tsa Chih* 52: 368–371.

Sibley GN. (1985) An experimental model of detrusor instability in the obstructed pig. *Br J Urol* 57: 292–298.

Siegel S, Rawitt L, Sokoloff B, Siegel B. (1976) Relationship of allergy, enuresis, and urinary infection in children 4 to 7 years of age. *Pediatrics* 57: 526–528.

Sillén U. (1999) Bladder dysfunction in children with vesico-ureteric reflux. *Acta Paediatr* 88 Suppl 431: 40–47.

Sillén U, Hellström A-L, Hermansson G, Abrahamsson K. (1999) Comparison of urodynamic and free voiding pattern in infants with dilating reflux. *J Urol* 161: 1928–1933.

Silver E. (1996) Family therapy and soiling. *J Fam Ther* 18: 415–432.

Silver E, Williams A, Worthington F, Phillips F. (1998) Family therapy and soiling: an audit of externalising and other approaches. *J Fam Ther* 20: 413–422.

Silveri M, Capitanucci MD, Capozza M, et al. (1997) Occult spinal dysraphism: neurologic voiding dysfunction and long term urologic follow up. *Pediatr Surg Int* 12: 148–150.

Simpson L. (2000) Stress incontinence in younger women: prevention and treatment. *Nurs Stand* 14: 49–54.

Sinclair DB, Wheatley M, Snyder T. (2004) Frontal lobe epilepsy in childhood. *Pediatr Neurol* 30: 169–176.

Singh B, McC Mortensen NJ, Jewell DP, George B. (2004) Perianal Crohn's disease. *Br J Surg* 91: 801–814.

Skoog SJ, Stokes A, Turner KL. (1997) Oral desmopressin: a randomized double-blind placebo controlled study of effectiveness in children with primary nocturnal enuresis. *J Urol* 158: 1035–1040.

Smedje H, Broman JE, Hetta J. (1999) Parents' reports of disturbed sleep in 5–7-year-old Swedish children. *Acta Paediatr* 88: 858–865.

Smellie JM, Tamminen-Möbius T, Olbing H, et al. (1992) The international reflux study in children. Five-year study of medical or surgical treatment in children with severe reflux: radiological renal findings. *Pediatr Nephrol* 6: 223–230.

Smellie JM, McGrigor VS, Meadow SR, Rose SJ, Douglas MF. (1996) Nocturnal enuresis: a placebo controlled trial of two antidepressant drugs. *Arch Dis Child* 75: 62–66.

336

Smith LJ. (1996) A behavioural approach to the treatment of non-retentive encopresis in adults with learning disabilities. *J Intellect Disabil Res* 40: 130–139.

Smith L, Smith P, Lee SWY. (2000) Behavioural treatment of urinary incontinence and encopresis in children with learning disabilities: transfer of stimulus control. *Dev Med Child Neurol* 42: 276–279.

Söderström U, Hoelcke M, Alenius L, Söderling AC, Hjern A. (2004) Urinary and faecal incontinence: a population-based study. *Acta Paediatr* 93: 386–389.

Song BZ, Wang XY. (1985) Short-term effect in 135 cases of enuresis treated by wrist–ankle needling. *J Tradit Chin Med* 5: 27–28.

Sonnenschein M. (2001) Kindliche und Elterliche Einschätzung der Enuresis – ein empirischer Vergleich, unter Berücksichtigung der Subtypen. Medical doctoral thesis, Universität zu Köln.

Soomro NA, Khadra MH, Robson W, Neal DE. (2001) A crossover randomized trial of transcutaneous electrical nerve stimulation and oxybutynin in patients with detrusor instability. *J Urol* 166: 146–149.

Sorensen PS, Vilhardt H, Gjerris F, Warberg J. (1984) Impermeability of the blood–cerebrospinal fluid barrier to 1-deamino-8-D-arginine-vasopressin (DDAVP) in patients with acquired, communicating hydrocephalus. *Eur J Clin Invest* 14: 435–439.

Speakman MJ, Brading AF, Gilpin CJ, Dixon JS, Gilpin SA, Gosling J. (1987) Bladder outflow obstruction – a cause of denervation supersensitivity. *J Urol* 138: 1461–1466.

Spehr C, De Geeter P. (1991) Faulty voiding and drinking habits – a contribution to the genesis of enuretic syndrome? (German). *Urologe* 30: 231–234.

Spencer T, Biederman J, Wilens T, Harding M, O'Donnell D, Griffin S. (1996) Pharmacotherapy of attention-deficit hyperactivity disorder across the life cycle. *J Am Acad Child Adolesc Psychiatry* 35: 409–432.

Stanton SL. (1973) A comparison of emepronium bromide and flavoxate hydrochloride in the treatment of urinary incontinence. *J Urol* 110: 529–532.

Starfield B. (1967) Functional bladder capacity in enuretic and nonenuretic children. *J Pediatr* 70: 777–781.

Starzl TE, Taylor CW, Magoun HW. (1951) Collateral afferent excitation of reticular formation of brain stem. *J Neurophysiol* 14: 479–496.

Stauber T, Petermann F, Bachmann H, Hampel P. (2005) Stressverarbeitung und Lebensqualität bei funktioneller Harninkontinenz im Kindesalter. *Z Gesundheitspsych* 13: 12–20.

Stauffer CM, van der Weg B, Donadini R, Ramelli GP, Marchand S, Bianchetti M. (2004) Family history and behavioral abnormalities in girls with recurrent urinary tract infections: a controlled study. *J Urol* 171: 1663–1665.

Steers WD, Kyu-Sung L. (2001) Depression and incontinence. *World J Urol* 19: 351–357.

Steffens J, Netzer M, Isenberg E, Alloussi S, Ziegler M. (1993) Vasopressin deficiency in primary nocturnal enuresis. *Eur Urol* 24: 366–370.

Stegner H, Artman HG, Leake RD, Fisher DA. (1983) Does DDAVP (1-desamino-8-D-arginine-vasopressin) cross the blood–CSF barrier? Neuroendocrinology 37: 262–265.

Steinhausen H-C, Göbel D. (1989) Enuresis in child psychiatric clinic patients. *J Am Acad Child Adolesc Psychiatry* 28: 279–281.

Steinmüller A, Steinhausen H-C. (1990) Der Verlauf der Enkopresis im Kindesalter. *Prax Kinderpsychol Kinderpsychiatr* 39: 74–79.

Stenberg A, Läckgren G. (1994) Desmopressin tablets in the treatment of severe nocturnal enuresis in adolescents. *Pediatrics* 94: 841–846.

Stenberg A, Läckgren G. (1995) A new bioinplant Deflux® system for the endoscopic treatment of vesicoureteral reflux. Experimental and clinical results. *J Urol* 154: 800–803.

Steriade M, Iosif G, Apostol A. (1969) Responsiveness of thalamic and cortical motor relays during arousal and various stages of sleep. *J Neurophysiol* 32: 251–265.

Stern HP, Stroh SE, Fiedorek SC, Kelleher K, Mellon MW, Pope SK, Rayford PL. (1995) Increased plasma levels of pancreatic polypeptide and decreased plasma levels of motilin in encopretic children. *Pediatrics* 96: 111–117.

Stoher M, Madersbacher H, Richter R, Wehnert J, Dreikorn K. (1999) Efficacy and safety of propiverine in SCI-patients suffering from detrusor hyperreflexia: a double-blind, placebo-controlled clinical trial. *Spinal Cord* 37: 196–200.

Stokland E, Andreasson S, Jacobsson B, Jodal U, Ljung B. (2003) Sedation with midazolam for voiding cystourethrography in children: a randomized double-blind study. *Pediatr Radiol* 33: 247–249.

Stores G, Wiggs L, editors. (2001) *Sleep Disturbance in Children and Adolescents with Disorders of Development: Its Significance and Management*. London: Mac Keith Press.

337

Suchoversky O, Furtado S, Rohs G. (1995) Beneficial effect of intranasal desmopressin for nocturnal polyuria in Parkinson's disease. *Mov Disord* 10: 337–340.

Sugaya K, Roppolo JR, Yoshimura N, Card JP, de Groat WC. (1997) The central neural pathways involved in micturition in the neonatal rat as revealed by the injection of pseudorabies virus into the urinary bladder. *Neurosci Lett* 223: 197–200.

Sukhai RN. (1993) Enuresis nocturna: longterm use and safety aspects of Minirin (desmopressin) spray. *Regul Pept* 10: 309–310.

Sureshkumar P, Craig JC, Roy LP, Knight JF. (2000) Daytime urinary incontinence in primary school children: a population-based survey. *J Pediatr* 137: 814–818.

Sureshkumar P, Bower W, Craig J, Knight JF. (2003) Treatment of daytime urinary incontinence in children: a systematic review of randomized controlled trials. *J Urol* 170: 196–200.

Sutphen JL, Borowitz SM, Hutchison RL, Cox DJ. (1995) Long-term follow-up of medically treated childhood constipation. *Clin Pediatr* 34: 576–580.

Sutphen J, Borowitz S, Ling W, Cox DJ, Kovatchev B. (1997) Anorectal manometric examination in encopretic-constipated children. *Dis Colon Rectum* 40: 1051–1055.

Swanson JR, Jones GR, Krasselt W, Denmark LN, Ratti F. (1997) Death of two subjects due to imipramine and desipramine metabolite accumulation during chronic therapy: a review of the literature and possible mechanisms. *J Forensic Sci* 42: 335–339.

Swithinbank LV, Brookes ST, Shepherd AM, Abrams P. (1998) The natural history of urinary symptoms during adolescence. *Br J Urol* 81 Suppl 3: 90–93.

Swithinbank LV, Donovan JL, Rogers CA, Abrams P. (2000) Nocturnal incontinence in women: a hidden problem. *J Urol* 164(3 Pt 1): 764–766.

Szabo L, Fegyvernski S. (1995) Maximum and average flow rates in normal children – the Miskolc nomograms. *Br J Urol* 76: 16–20.

Tanagho EA, Miller ER. (1970) Initiation of voiding. *Br J Urol* 42: 175–183.

Taskinen S, Valanne L, Rintala R. (2002) Effect of spinal cord abnormalities on the function of the lower urinary tract in patients with anorectal abnormalities. *J Urol* 168: 1147–1149.

Taubman B. (1997) Toilet training and toileting refusal for stool only: a prospective study. *Pediatrics* 99: 54–58.

Taubman B, Buzby M. (1997) Overflow encopresis and stool toileting refusal during toilet training: a prospective study on the effect of therapeutic efficacy. *J Pediatr* 131(5): 768–771.

Terho P. (1991) Desmopressin in nocturnal enuresis. *J Urol* 145: 818–820.

Theobald RJJ. (1995) Purinergic and cholinergic components of bladder contractility and flow. *Life Sci* 56: 445–454.

Theunis M, Van Hoecke E, Paesbrugge S, Hoebeke P, Vande Walle J. (2002) Self-image and performance in children with nocturnal enuresis. *Eur Urol* 41: 660–667.

Thrasher TN. (1989) Role of forebrain circumventricular organs in body fluid balance. *Acta Physiol Scand* 136 Suppl 583: 141–150.

Timms DJ. (1990) Rapid maxillary expansion in the treatment of nocturnal enuresis. *Angle Orthod* 60: 229–234.

Tomita R, Munakata K, Howard ER, Fujisaki S. (2004) Histological studies on Hirschsprung's disease and its allied disorders in childhood. *Hepatogastroenterology* 51: 1042–1044.

Trousseau A. (1870) Nocturnal incontinence of urine. In: Trousseau A. *Lectures on Clinical Medicine*. London: New Sydenham Society, pp 475–490.

Trsinar B, Kraij B. (1996) Maximal electrical stimulation in children with unstable bladder and nocturnal enuresis and/or daytime incontinence: a controlled study. *Neurourol Urodyn* 15: 133–142.

Turner GM, Coulthard MG. (1995) Fever can cause pyuria in children. *BMJ* 311: 924.

Turunen S, Karttunen TJ, Kokkonen J. (2004) Lymphoid nodular hyperplasia and cow's milk hypersensitivity in children with chronic constipation. *J Pediatr* 145: 606–611.

Tuvemo T. (1978) DDAVP in childhood nocturnal enuresis. *Acta Paediatr Scand* 67: 753–755.

Tuzuner F, Kecik Y, Ozdemir S, Canaku M. (1989) Electro-acupuncture in the treatment of enuresis nocturna. *Acupunct Electrother Res* 14: 211–215.

t'Veld BA, Kwee-Zuiderwijk WJ, van Puijenbroek EP, Stricker BH. (1998) Neuropsychiatrische bijwerkingen toegeschreven aan het gebruik van oxybutynine. *Ned Tijdschr Geneeskd* 142: 590–592.

Umlauf MG, Chasens ER. (2003) Sleep disordered breathing and nocturnal polyuria: nocturia and enuresis. *Sleep Med Rev* 7: 403–411.

338

Unalacak M, Aydin M, Ermis B, Ozeren A, Sogut A, Demirel F, Unluoglu I. (2004) Assessment of cardiac autonomic regulation in children with monosymptomatic nocturnal enuresis by analysis of heart rate variability. *Tohoku J Exp Med* 204: 63–69.

Usumez S, Iseri H, Orhan M, Basciftci FA. (2003) Effect of rapid maxillary expansion on nocturnal enuresis. *Angle Orthod* 73: 532–538.

Valenti G, Laera A, Gouraud S, Pace G, Aceto G, Penza R, Selvaggi FP, Svelto M. (2002) Low-calcium diet in hypercalciuric enuretic children restores AQP2 excretion and improves clinical symptoms. *Am J Renal Physiol* 28: F895–F903.

Valiquette G, Herbert J, Meade-D'Alisera P. (1996) Desmopressin in the management of nocturia in patients with multiple sclerosis. A double-blind, crossover trial. *Arch Neurol* 53: 1270–1275.

Vallotton MB. (1991) The multiple faces of the vasopressin receptors. *Mol Cell Endocrinol* 78: C73–C76.

Van Arsdalen K, Wein AJ. (1991) Physiology of micturition and continence. In: Krane RJ, Siroky M, editors. *Clinical Neuro-urology*. New York: Little Brown, pp 25–82.

Vandel S, Bertschy G, Bonin B, et al. (1992) Tricyclic antidepressant plasma levels after fluoxetine addition. *Neuropsychobiology* 25: 202–207.

Van der Plas RN, Benninga MA, Büller, HA, Bossuyt PM, Akkermanns LM, Redekop WK, Taminiau JA. (1996a) Biofeedback training in treatment of childhood constipation: a randomised controlled study. *Lancet* 348: 776–780.

Van der Plas RN, Benninga MA, Redekop WK, Taminiau JA, Büller HA. (1996b) Randomised trial of biofeedback training for encopresis. *Arch Dis Child* 75: 367–374.

Van der Plas RN, Benninga MA, Taminiau JA, Büller HA. (1997) Treatment of defecation problems in children: the role of education, demystification and toilet training. *Eur J Pediatr* 156: 689–692.

Van Ginkel R, Benninga MA, Blommart JE, Van der Plas R, Boeckstaens GE, Büller HA, Taminiau J. (2000) Lack of benefit of laxatives as an adjunctive therapy for functional nonretentive fecal soiling in children. *J Pediatr* 137: 808–813.

Van Ginkel R, Reitsma JB, Buller HA, van Wijk MP, Taminiau J, Benninga MA. (2003) Childhood constipation: longitudinal follow-up beyond puberty. *Gastroenterology* 125: 357–363.

van Gool JD. (1997) Muscular dystrophy and the pelvic floor. In: van Gool JD, editor. *Second Course on Paediatric Urodynamics*. University of Utrecht, pp 77–79.

van Gool JD, de Jonge GA. (1989) Urge syndrome and urge incontinence. *Arch Dis Child* 64: 1629–1634.

van Gool JD, Kuitjen RH, Donckerwolcke RA, Messer AP, Vijverberg MAW. (1984) Bladder-sphincter dysfunction, urinary infection and vesico-ureteral reflux with special reference to cognitive bladder training. *Contrib Nephrol* 39: 190–210.

van Gool JD, Vijverberg MAW, de Jong TPVM. (1992a) Functional daytime incontinence: clinical and urodynamic assessment. *Scand J Urol Nephrol* Suppl 141: 58–69.

van Gool JD, Vijverberg MAW, Messer AP, Elzinga-Plomp A, de Jong, TPVM. (1992b) Functional daytime incontinence: non-pharmacological treatment. *Scand J Urol Nephrol* Suppl 141: 93–105.

van Gool JD, Hjälmås K, Tamminen-Möbius T, Olbing H. (1992c) Historical clues to the complex of dysfunctional voiding, urinary tract infection and vesicoureteral reflux. The International Reflux Study in Children. *J Urol* 148: 1699–1702.

Van Hoecke E, Hoebeke P, Braet C, Vande Walle J. (2004) An assessment of internalizing problems in children with enuresis. *J Urol* 171: 2580–2583.

Van Kerrebroeck PEV. (2002) Experience with the long-term use of desmopressin for nocturnal enuresis in children and adolescents. *BJU Int* 89: 420–425.

Van Kerrebroeck P, Kreder K, Jonas U. (2001) Tolterodine once-daily: superior efficacy and tolerability in the treatment of the overactive bladder. *Urology* 57: 414–421.

van Kerrebroeck P, Abrams P, Lange R, Slack M, Wyndaele JJ, Yalcin I, Bump RC. (2004) Duloxetine versus placebo in the treatment of European and Canadian women with stress urinary incontinence. *BJOG* 111: 249–257.

Van Laecke E, Golinveaux L, Goossens L, Raes A, Hoebeke P, Vande Walle J. (2001) Voiding disorders in severely mentally and motor disabled children. *J Urol* 166: 2404–2406.

van Leerdam FJ, Blankespoor MN, van der Heijden AJ, Hirasing RA. (2004) Alarm treatment is successful in children with day- and night-time wetting. *Scand J Urol Nephrol* 38: 211–215.

van Londen A, van Londen-Barensten M, van Son M, Mulder G. (1993) Arousal training for children suffering from nocturnal enuresis: a 2½ year follow-up. *Behav Res Ther* 31: 613–615.

van Londen A, van Londen-Barensten M, van Son M, Mulder G. (1995) Relapse rate and parental reaction after successful treatement of children suffering from nocturnal enuresis: a 2½ year follow-up of bibliotherapy. *Behav Res Ther* 33: 309–311.

van Ophoven A, Pokupic S, Heinecke A, Hertle L. (2004) A prospective, randomized, placebo controlled, double-blind study of amitriptyline for the treatment of interstitial cystitis. *J Urol* 172: 533–536.

Varlam DE, Dippel J. (1995) Non-neurogenic bladder and chronic renal insufficiency in childhood. *Pediatr Nephrol* 9: 1–5.

Varley CK. (2000) Sudden death of a child treated with imipramine. Case study. *J Child Adolesc Psychopharmacol* 10: 321–325.

Varley CK, McLellan J. (1997) Case study: two additional sudden deaths with tricyclic antidepressants. *J Am Acad Child Adolesc Psychiatry* 36: 390.

Vernon S, Lundblad B, Hellström AL. (2003) Children's experience of school toilets present a risk to their physical and psychological health. *Child: Care Health Dev* 29: 47–53.

Vijverberg MAW, Elzinga-Plomp A, Messer AP, van Gool JD, de Jong TPVM. (1997) Bladder rehabilitation, the effect of a cognitive training programme on urge incontinence. *Eur Urol* 31: 68–72.

Vilhardt H. (1990) Basic pharmacology of desmopressin. A review. *Drug Invest* 2: 2–8.

Vincent SA. (1966) Postural control of urinary incontinence: the curtsey sign. *Lancet* ii: 631–632.

von Garrelts B. (1956) Micturition in the normal male. *Acta Chir Scand* 112: 326–340.

von Gontard A. (1995) Enuresis im Kindesalter – psychiatrische, somatische und molekulargenetische Zusammenhänge. Universität zu Köln: Professorial thesis.

von Gontard A. (2001) *Einnässens im Kindesalter: Erscheinungsformen – Diagnostik – Therapie*. Stuttgart: Thieme Verlag.

von Gontard A. (2002) Psychological aspects of urinary incontinence and enuresis in children. *Prog Ped Urol* 5: 135–147.

von Gontard A. (2004) *Enkopresis: Erscheinungsformen – Diagnostik – Therapie*. Stuttgart: Kohlhammer Verlag.

von Gontard A (2006a) Enuresis und funktionelle Harninkontinenz. In: Schmidt M, Poustka F, editors. *Leitlinien zur Diagnostik und Therapie von psychischen Störungen im Säuglings-, Kindes- und Jugendalter*, 3rd edition. Köln: Deutsche Ärzteverlag, in print.

von Gontard A. (2006b) Enkopresis. In: Schmidt M, Poustka F, editors. *Leitlinien zur Diagnostik und Therapie von psychischen Störungen im Säuglings-, Kindes- und Jugendalter*, 3rd edition. Köln: Deutsche Ärzteverlag, in print.

von Gontard A, Hollmann E. (2004) Comorbidity of functional urinary incontinence and encopresis: somatic and behavioral associations. *J Urol* 171: 2644–2647.

von Gontard A, Lehmkuhl G. (1996) Pharmakotherapie der Enuresis nocturna. *Z Kinder-Jugendpsychiatr* 24: 18–33.

von Gontard A, Lehmkuhl G. (2002) *Leitfaden Enuresis*. Göttingen: Hogrefe Verlag.

von Gontard A, Hollmannn E, Benden B, Eiberg H, Rittig S, Lehmkuhl G. (1997) Clinical enuresis phenotypes in familial nocturnal enuresis. *Scand J Urol Nephrol* 31 Suppl 183: 11–16.

von Gontard A, Lettgen B, Gaebel E, Heiken-Löwenau C, Schmitz I, Olbing H. (1998a) Day wetting children with urge incontinence and voiding postponement – a comparison of a pediatric and child psychiatric sample – behavioural factors. *Br J Urol* 81 Suppl 3: 100–106.

von Gontard A, Eiberg H, Hollmann E, Rittig S, Lehmkuhl G. (1998b) Molecular genetics of nocturnal enuresis: clinical and genetic heterogeneity. *Acta Paediatr* 87: 571–578.

von Gontard A, Plück J, Berner W, Lehmkuhl G. (1999a) Clinical behavioral problems in day and night wetting children, *Pediatr Nephrol* 13: 662–667.

von Gontard A, Sonnenschein M, Lehmkuhl G. (1999b) Enuretic children's subjective perceptions of wetting and body concepts. Denver: International Children's Continence Society Meeting (Abstract).

von Gontard A, Eiberg H, Schaumburg H, Rittig S. (1999c) Enuresis: associations of genotype and phenotype. *Mol Psychiatry* 4 Suppl 1, S57–S58.

von Gontard A, Eiberg H, Hollmann E, Rittig S, Lehmkuhl G. (1999d) Molecular genetics of nocturnal enuresis – linkage to a locus on chromosome no. 22. *Scand J Urol Nephrol* 33 Suppl 202: 76–80.

von Gontard A, Benden B, Mauer-Mucke K, Lehmkuhl G. (1999e) Somatic correlates of functional enuresis, *Eur Child Adolesc Psychiatry* 8: 117–125.

von Gontard A, Schaumburg H, Hollmann E, Eiberg H, Rittig S. (2001a) The genetics of enuresis – a review. *J Urol* 166: 2438–2443.

von Gontard A, Laufersweiler-Plass C, Backes M, Zerres K, Rudnik-Schöneborn S. (2001b) Enuresis and urinary incontinence in children and adolescents with spinal muscular atrophy. *BJU Int* 88: 409–413.

von Wendt L, Simila S, Niskanen P, Järvelin MR. (1990) Development of bowel and bladder control in the mentally retarded. *Dev Med Child Neurol* 32: 515–518.

Voskuijl WP, de Lorijn F, van Ginkel R, et al. (2002) Functional non-retentive fecal soiling in children: a decade of follow-up. *Gastroenterology* 122: 505.

Voskuijl WP, van Ginkel R, Taminiau J, Boeckstaens GE, Benninga MA. (2003) Loperimide suppositories in an adolescent with childhood-onset functional non-retentive fecal soiling. *J Pediatr Gastroenterol Nutr* 37: 198–200.

Voskuijl WP, Heijmans J, Heijmans HS, Taminiau J, Benninga MA. (2004a) Use of Rome II criteria in childhood defecation disorders: applicability in clinical and research practice. *J Pediatr* 145: 213–217.

Voskuijl WP, van der Zaag-Loonen HJ, Ketel IJG, Grootenhuis MA, Derkx BHF, Benninga MA. (2004b) Health related quality of life in disorders of defecation: the Defecation Disorder List. *Arch Dis Child* 89: 1124–1127.

Voskuijl WP, de Lorijn F, Verwijs W, Hogeman P, Heijmans J, Mäkle W, Taminiau J, Benninga MA. (2004c) PEG 3350 (Transipeg) versus lactulose in the treatment of childhood functional constipation: a double blind, randomised, controlled, multicentre trial. *Gut* 53: 1590–1594.

Vulliamy D. (1959) The day and night output of urine in enuresis. *Arch Dis Child* 31: 439.

Vurgun N, Yiditodlu MR, Ypcan A, Ari Z, Tarhan S, Balkan C. (1998) Hypernatriuria and kaliuresis in enuretic children and the diurnal variation. *J Urol* 159: 1333–1337.

Waites KB, Canupp KC, Armstrong S, DeVivo MJ. (2004) Effect of cranberry extract on bacteriuria and pyuria in persons with neurogenic bladder secondary to spinal cord injury. *J Spinal Cord Med* 27: 35–40.

Wald A, Hinds JP, Caruana BJ. (1989) Psychological and physiological characteristics of patients with severe idiopathic constipation. *Gastroenterology* 97: 932–937.

Watanabe H, Azuma Y. (1989) A proposal for a classification system of enuresis based on overnight simultaneous monitoring of electroencephalography and cystometry. *Sleep* 12: 257–264.

Weaver LT. (1988) Bowel habit from birth to old age. *J Pediatr Gastroenterol Nutr* 7: 637–640.

Weber J, Grise P, Roquebert M, et al. (1987) Radioopaque markers transit and anorectal manometry in 16 patients with multiple sclerosis and urinary bladder dysfunction. *Dis Colon Rectum* 30: 95–100.

Weider DJ, Sateia MJ, West RP. (1991) Nocturnal enuresis in children with upper airway obstruction. *Otolaryngol Head Neck Surg* 105: 427–432.

Weisz JR, Weiss B, Han SS, Granger DA, Morton T. (1995) Effects of psychotherapy with children and adolescents revisited: a meta-analysis of treatment outcome studies. *Psychol Bull* 117: 450–468.

Weitzman RE, Fisher DA, Di Stefano III JJ, Bennett CM. (1977) Episodic secretion of arginine vasopressin. *Am J Physiol* 233: E32–E36.

Wennerström M, Hansson S, Hedner T, Himmelmann A, Jodal U. (2000) Ambulatory blood pressure 16–26 years after the first urinary tract infection in childhood. *J Hypertens* 18: 485–491.

Wettergren B, Jodal U, Jonasson G. (1985) Epidemiology of bacteriuria during the first year of life. *Acta Paediatr Scand* 74: 925–933.

Whitten SM, Wilcox DT. (2001) Duplex systems. *Prenat Diagn* 21: 952–957.

Wiesel PH, Norton C, Roy AJ, Storrie JB, Bowers J, Kamm MA. (2000) Gut focused behavioural treatment (biofeedback) for constipation and faecal incontinence in multiple sclerosis. *J Neurol Neurosurg Psychiatry* 69: 240–243.

Wiesel PH, Norton C, Glickman S, Kamm MA. (2001) Pathophysiology and management of bowel dysfunction in multiple sclerosis. *Eur J Gastroenterol Hepatol* 13: 441–448.

Wilens TE, Faraone SV, Biederman J, Gunawardene S. (2003) Does stimulant therapy of attention-deficit/hyperactivity disorder beget later substance abuse? A meta-analytic review of the literature. *Pediatrics* 111: 179–185.

Wille S. (1986) Comparison of desmopressin and enuresis alarm for nocturnal enuresis. *Arch Dis Child* 61: 30–33.

Wille S. (1994) Nocturnal enuresis: sleep disturbance and behavioural patterns. *Acta Paediatr* 83: 772–774.

Williams TDM, Dunger DB, Lyon CC, Lewis RJ, Taylor F, Lightman SL. (1986) Antidiuretic effect and pharmacokinetics of oral 1-desamino-8-D-arginine vasopressin. 1. Studies in adults and children. *J Clin Endocrinol Metab* 63: 129–132.

Williams G, Lee A, Craig J. (2001) Antibiotics for the prevention of urinary tract infection in children: a systematic review of randomized controlled trials. *Pediatrics* 138: 868–874.

341

Wise BG, Cardozo LD, Cutner A, Benness CJ, Burton G. (1993) Prevalence and significance of urethral instability in women with detrusor instability. *Br J Urol* 72: 26–29.

Wlodek ME, Thorburn GD, Harding R. (1989) Bladder contractions and micturition in fetal sheep: their relation to behavioral states. *Am J Physiol* 257: R1526–R1532.

Wolfish NM, Pivik RT, Busby KA. (1997) Elevated sleep arousal thresholds in enuretic boys: clinical implications. *Acta Paediatr* 86: 381–384.

Wood JD. (1994) Physiology of the enteric nervous system. In: Johnson R, editor. *Physiology of the Gastrointestinal Tract*, 3rd edition. New York: Raven Press, pp 423–482.

Wood CM, Butler RJ, Penney MD, Holland PC. (1994) Pulsatile release of arginine vasopressin (AVP) and its effect on response to desmopressin in enuresis. *Scand J Urol Nephrol* Suppl 163: 93–101.

Woolf AS, Winyard PJD. (2002) Molecular mechanisms of human embryogenesis: developmental pathogenesis of renal tract malformations. *Ped Dev Pathol* 5: 108–129.

World Health Organisation. (1993) *The ICD-10 Classification of Mental and Behavioural Disorders – Diagnostic Criteria for Research*. Geneva: WHO.

Yamanishi T, Yasuda K, Murayama N, Sakakibara R, Uchiyama T, Ito H. (2000) Biofeedback training for detrusor overactivity in children. *J Urol* 164: 1686–1690.

Yang SS, Wang CC, Chen YT. (2003) Effectiveness of alpha1-adrenergic blockers in boys with low urinary flow rate and urinary incontinence. *J Formos Med Assoc* 102: 551–555.

Yaouyanc G, Jonville AP, Yaouyanc-Lapalle H, Barbier P, Dutertre JP, Autret E. (1992) Seizure with hyponatremia in a child prescribed desmopressin for nocturnal enuresis. *J Toxicol Clin Toxicol* 30: 637–641.

Yayli G, Yaman H, Demirdal T. (2003) Asymptomatic bacteriuria rates in schoolchildren: results from a rural city in Turkey. *Trop Pediatr* 49: 228–230.

Yazbeck S, Schick E, O'Regan S. (1987) Relevance of constipation to enuresis, urinary tract infection and reflux – a review. *Eur Urol* 13: 318–321.

Yerkes EB, Cain MP, King S, Brei T, Kaefer M, Casale AJ, Rink RC. (2003) The Malone antegrade continence enema procedure: quality of life and family perspective. *J Urol* 169: 320–323.

Yeung CK. (1997) Nocturnal enuresis in Hong Kong: different Chinese phenotypes. *Scand J Urol Nephrol* 31 Suppl 183: 17–21.

Yeung CK, Godley ML, Ho CKW, Duffy PG, Ransley RG, Chen CN, Li AKC. (1995) Some new insights into bladder function in infancy. *Br J Urol* 76: 235–240.

Yeung CK, Chiu HN, Sit FK. (1999) Bladder dysfunction in children with refractory monosymptomatic primary nocturnal enuresis. *J Urol* 162: 1049–1055.

Yeung CK, Sihoe JD, Sit FK, Bower WF, Sreedhar B, Lau J. (2004) Characteristics of primary nocturnal enuresis in adults: an epidemiological study. *BJU Int* 93: 341–345.

Yokoyama O, Yoshiyama M, Namiki M, et al. (1999) Glutamatergic and dopaminergic contributions to rat bladder hyperactivity after cerebral artery occlusion. *Am J Physiol* 276: R935–R942.

Yoshimura N, Sasa M, Ohna Y, Yoshida O, Takaori S. (1988) Contraction of urinary bladder by central norepinephrine originating in the locus coeruleus. *J Urol* 139: 423–427.

Young MH, Brennen LC, Baker RD, Baker SS. (1995) Functional encopresis: symptom reduction and behavioral improvement. *J Dev Behav Pediatr* 16: 226–232.

Youssef NN, Di Lorenzo C. (2001) Childhood constipation: evaluation and treatment. *J Clin Gastroenterol* 33: 199–205.

Youssef NN, Pensabene L, Barksdale EJ, Di Lorenzo C. (2004) Is there a role for surgery beyond colonic aganglionosis and anorectal malformations in children with intractable constipation? *J Pediatr Surg* 39: 73–77.

Zerbe RL, Robertson GL. (1981) A comparison of plasma vasopressin measurements with a standard indirect test in the differential diagnosis of polyuria. *N Engl J Med* 305: 1539–1546.

Zhong MQ. (1986) Percussopunctator treatment of enuresis on the basis of differential typing of the symptoms. *J Tradit Chin Med* 6: 171–174.

INDEX

treatment
    method 117–119
    resistance 119–120
desmopressin test 53–54
detrusor hyperreflexia 192
detrusor instability, type II 142–143
detrusor muscle
    cholinergic neurotransmitters 144
    contraction suppression 21
    denervation hypersensibility 144
    infantile 14
    innervation 12
    non-compliance 195
    purinergic neurotransmitters 144
    reflex contraction 12
    smooth muscle cell activity 144
detrusor overactivity 8, 141–155
    botulinum toxin 80
    cerebral palsy 212
    cystometry 9, 52
    Duchenne muscular dystrophy 212
    idiopathic 9
    myogenic causes 144–145
    neurogenic 9, 195
    neurotransmission 143–144
    nocturnal enuresis 91–92
    oxybutynin therapy 121
    peripheral efferent activity 143
    posterior urethral valves 188
    psychogenic causes 145
    structural 190
    ultrasound diagnosis 41
    urge incontinence comorbidity 132–133
    urgency 21
    UTI risk factor 132–133, *197*
    vesico-ureteric reflux 134–135
detrusor pressure
    curve 51
    intrinsic 53
detrusor underactivity 8, 74, 175–179
    aetiology 176
    assessment 177
    clinical guidelines 178–179
    clinical signs/symptoms 176–177
    course 178
    definition 6, *7*, 131, 175–176
    epidemiology 176
    ICCS definition 6, *7*
    prognosis 178
    psychological aspects 177
    treatment 177–178
detrusor–sphincter dyssynergia
    anti-adrenergic drugs 80
    pelvic floor muscle activity measurement 52
developmental disorders, voiding disorders 61–64
developmental history 283–284
developmental tests 62

diabetes insipidus 53
    catheterizable urinary diversion 85
    central 205–206
    nephrogenic 206–209
diabetes mellitus 204–205
    constipation 242
    polydipsia 22
Diagnostic and Statistical Manual of Mental
    Disorders IV (DSM-IV) 3–4, 64
    faecal incontinence 215
diarrhoea, faecal incontinence 275
diclofenac 125
diet modification
    constipation 255
    encopresis 238, 251, 255
    nocturnal enuresis 125
dimercaptoacetyltriglycine (MAG3) 46, *47,* 48, 49
dimercaptosuccinic acid (DMSA) scintigraphy *45,*
    46, 48, *49*
    vesico-ureteric reflux 135
diuretics 125
    thiazide 207
doctor–patient relationship 65–66
doxazosin 80
drinking habits 21–22, 72–73
dry bed training (DBT) 115
Duchenne muscular dystrophy 212
dyschezia, infant 240

ear, nose and throat (ENT) surgery 125
eating disorder, case study 226
ectoderm 14, 15
egocentricity 65
electroencephalogram (EEG), sleep 93
electromyography (EMG)
    biofeedback in voiding dysfunction 168–169
    detrusor underactivity 177
    voiding dysfunction 166
emotional disorder, case study 70–71
encopresis 2, 9
    ADHD 224–225
    aetiology 227–231, 258–259, 264–265
    anal manometry 54
    anxiety disorders 225
    assessment 231–238, 250, 259
    behavioural disorders 57, 247, 249–250
        comorbidity 221–223
        subclinical symptoms 222–223
    biopsy 237
    case study 226, 254, 260
    charts 30, 31, 234, 311
    chronic paediatric illness 277
    classification 214–219
    clinical guidelines 257, 261, 265–266
    clinical signs/symptoms 247, *249,* 258
    with constipation 239–247, *248,* 249–257, *271*
        case study 254